Sinusitis

From Microbiology
to Management

INFECTIOUS DISEASE AND THERAPY

Series Editor

Burke A. Cunha

Winthrop-University Hospital
Mineola, and
State University of New York School of Medicine
Stony Brook, New York

Sinusitis

From Microbiology to Management

edited by

Itzhak Brook
Georgetown University School of Medicine
Washington, D.C., U.S.A.

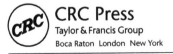

CRC Press
Taylor & Francis Group
Boca Raton London New York

CRC Press is an imprint of the
Taylor & Francis Group, an **informa** business

CRC Press
Taylor & Francis Group
6000 Broken Sound Parkway NW, Suite 300
Boca Raton, FL 33487-2742

First issued in paperback 2019

© 2010 by Taylor & Francis Group, LLC
CRC Press is an imprint of Taylor & Francis Group, an Informa business

No claim to original U.S. Government works

ISBN-13: 978-0-8247-2948-6 (hbk)
ISBN-13: 978-0-367-39215-4 (pbk)

Visit the Taylor & Francis Web site at
http://www.taylorandfrancis.com

and the CRC Press Web site at
http://www.crcpress.com

*This book is dedicated to my wife, Joyce, and my children,
Dafna, Tamar, Yoni, and Sara*

Preface

Upper respiratory tract infections and, especially, sinusitis are frequently encountered in the day-to-day practice of infectious disease specialists, allergists, pediatricians, otolaryngologists, internists, and family practitioners. The range of causative agents and available therapies and the constantly changing spectrum of antibiotic resistance can make it difficult to select the most appropriate course of treatment. Given the increasing global concerns regarding the scale of worldwide bacterial resistance, which is largely because of the misuse and overuse of antibiotics, information that can enable physicians to optimize management of infections such as sinusitis will be of great value.

This book provides state-of-the-art information on management of sinusitis tailored to the clinicians and health care providers of varied specialties. It contains a liberal number of figures and tables that clarify the underlying concepts and illustrate specific details. The authors selected to contribute to the book are the world experts and leaders in the topic(s) they address.

The book opens with a comprehensive overview of the epidemiology, clinical presentation, and diagnostic techniques of sinusitis. It then delves into the pathophysiology and the microbiology underlying the condition. The next section of the book addresses the medical management of acute and chronic sinusitis as well as the comorbid medical symptoms. We then conclude with the surgical management of these conditions and their complications. It is our hope that this book will be a useful tool and an important resource for clinicians in the management of sinusitis.

Itzhak Brook, M.D., M.Sc.

Contents

Contributors

Nafi Aygun   The Russell H. Morgan Department of Radiology and Radiological Sciences, The Johns Hopkins Medical Institution, Baltimore, Maryland, U.S.A.

Daniel G. Becker   Department of Otorhinolaryngology—Head and Neck Surgery, University of Pennsylvania, Philadelphia, Pennsylvania, U.S.A.

Luisa Bellussi   Ear, Nose, and Throat Department—University of Siena Medical School, Viale Bracci, Siena, Italy

Michael S. Benninger   Department of Otolaryngology–Head and Neck Surgery, Henry Ford Hospital, Detroit, Michigan, U.S.A.

Joel M. Bernstein   Departments of Otolaryngology and Pediatrics, School of Medicine and Biomedical Sciences, Department of Communicative Disorders and Sciences, State University of New York at Buffalo, Buffalo, New York, U.S.A.

Itzhak Brook   Departments of Pediatrics and Medicine, Georgetown University School of Medicine, Washington, D.C., U.S.A.

Nicolas Y. Busaba   Department of Otolaryngology, Harvard Medical School, VA Boston Healthcare System, Massachusetts Eye and Ear Infirmary, Boston, Massachusetts, U.S.A.

Alexander G. Chiu   Division of Rhinology, Department of Otorhinolaryngology—Head and Neck Surgery, University of Pennsylvania, Philadelphia, Pennsylvania, U.S.A.

Peter A. R. Clement Department of Otorhinolaryngology and ENT Department, University Hospital, Free University Brussels (VUB), Brussels, Belgium

Dennis A. Conrad Division of Infectious Diseases, Department of Pediatrics, University of Texas Health Science Center at San Antonio, San Antonio, Texas, U.S.A.

Valerio Damiani Ear, Nose, and Throat Department—University of Siena Medical School, Viale Bracci, Siena, Italy

Catherine F. Decker Division of Infectious Diseases, Department of Internal Medicine, National Naval Medical Center, Bethesda, Maryland, U.S.A.

Thomas M. File, Jr. Northeastern Ohio Universities College of Medicine, Rootstown, and Infectious Disease Service, Summa Health Service, Akron, Ohio, U.S.A.

Urban Forsum Division of Clinical Microbiology, Department of Molecular and Clinical Medicine, Faculty of Health Sciences, Linköping University, Linköping, Sweden

Todd D. Gleeson Division of Infectious Diseases, Department of Internal Medicine, National Naval Medical Center, Bethesda, Maryland, U.S.A.

Joshua Gottschall Department of Otolaryngology–Head and Neck Surgery, Henry Ford Hospital, Detroit, Michigan, U.S.A.

Noreen Roth Henig Adult Cystic Fibrosis Center, Advanced Lung Disease Center, California Pacific Medical Center, San Francisco, California, U.S.A.

Alexis H. Jackman Department of Otorhinolaryngology Head and Neck Surgery, University of Pennsylvania, Philadelphia, Pennsylvania, U.S.A.

Carol A. Kauffman Division of Infectious Diseases, University of Michigan Medical School, Veterans Affairs Ann Arbor Healthcare System, Ann Arbor, Michigan, U.S.A.

David W. Kennedy Department of Otorhinolaryngology Head and Neck Surgery, University of Pennsylvania, Philadelphia, Pennsylvania, U.S.A.

John H. Krouse   Department of Otolaryngology Head and Neck Surgery, Wayne State University, Detroit, Michigan, U.S.A.

David Lewis   Department of Otolaryngology, Harvard Medical School, Massachusetts Eye and Ear Infirmary, Boston, Massachusetts, U.S.A.

John Mumford   Department of Periodontics, Naval Postgraduate Dental School, Bethesda, Maryland, U.S.A.

Desiderio Passàli   Ear, Nose, and Throat Department—University of Siena Medical School, Viale Bracci, Siena, Italy

Francesco Maria Passàli   Ear, Nose, and Throat Department—University of Siena Medical School, Viale Bracci, Siena, Italy

Giulio Cesare Passàli   Ear, Nose, and Throat Department—University of Siena Medical School, Viale Bracci, Siena, Italy

Gary Schwartz   Vanderbilt University Medical Center, Nashville, Tennessee, U.S.A.

Robert J. Stachler   Department of Otolaryngology Head and Neck Surgery, Wayne State University, Detroit, Michigan, U.S.A.

Ovsev Uzunes   The Russell H. Morgan Department of Radiology and Radiological Sciences, The Johns Hopkins Medical Institution, Baltimore, Maryland, U.S.A.

Frank S. Virant   University of Washington, Seattle, Washington, U.S.A.

Ellen R. Wald   Department of Pediatrics and Otolaryngology, University of Pittsburgh School of Medicine, Allergy, Immunology, and Infectious Diseases, Pittsburgh, Pennsylvania, U.S.A.

Viveka Westergren   Division of Clinical Microbiology, Department of Molecular and Clinical Medicine, Faculty of Health Sciences, Linköping University, Linköping, Sweden

Steve White   Vanderbilt University Medical Center, Nashville, Tennessee, U.S.A.

S. James Zinreich   The Russell H. Morgan Department of Radiology and Radiological Sciences, The Johns Hopkins Medical Institution, Baltimore, Maryland, U.S.A.

SECTION I. EPIDEMIOLOGY, PRESENTATION AND DIAGNOSIS

1

Sinusitis: Epidemiology

Thomas M. File Jr.

Northeastern Ohio Universities College of Medicine, Rootstown, and Infectious Disease Service, Summa Health Service, Akron, Ohio, U.S.A.

INTRODUCTION

Respiratory tract infections are the most common type of infections managed by health care providers, and they are of great consequence (1,2). In a recent report from the Centers for Disease Control, respiratory tract infections (upper respiratory tract infections, otitis, and lower respiratory tract infections) accounted for 16% of all outpatient visits of patients to physicians (3).

Of all the respiratory infections, sinusitis is one of the most common illnesses that affect a high proportion of the population. According to the National Ambulatory Medical Care Survey data, sinusitis is the fifth most common diagnosis for which an antibiotic is prescribed (4). Sinusitis accounted for 9% and 21% of all pediatric and adult antibiotic prescriptions, respectively, written in 2002 (5). Since many cases of sinusitis are viral in etiology, these data actually suggest that antibiotics are frequently misused for the management of this illness. Such inappropriate use leads to increased resistance among respiratory tract pathogens. The inappropriate use of antibiotics is related in part to the fact that sinusitis has been a relatively poorly defined clinical syndrome which is often a self-limited illness associated with wide variations in presenting symptoms, and an incomplete understanding of the pathogenesis and clinical course of the disease. However, recent classification of the sinusitis syndrome as well as the publication of evidence-based guidelines has provided a clear approach to its management (6–8).

The appropriate classification of sinusitis as well as an awareness of its epidemiology can facilitate better management of this infection. This chapter reviews information concerning the epidemiology of acute sinusitis.

PREVALENCE AND BURDEN OF DISEASE

The true prevalence of rhinosinusitis is unclear since various types of sinusitis are often lumped into this single designation. The true prevalence rate likely varies considerably from the diagnostic rate because not all individuals seek care for rhinosinusitis, and because of the inconsistencies in definitions. Nonetheless, available statistics confirm a high overall prevalence and disease burden.

Estimates of the prevalence of acute rhinosinusitis can be extrapolated based on its association with the common cold. A reasonable estimate is that each adult has two to three colds per year, and each child has three to eight colds per year (9). Up to 80% of these upper respiratory illnesses may be associated with rhinosinusitis, equating to over one billion cases of rhinosinusitis annually in the United States (10). It has been suggested that bacterial maxillary sinusitis complicates 0.5% to 2% of all upper respiratory tract infections, which translates into approximately 20 million cases of bacterial acute rhinosinusitis annually (11). This estimate may understate the incidence of rhinosinusitis because the focus was on maxillary sinusitis. According to the 2001 National Health Interview Survey, 17.4% of the American adult population interviewed had been told by a doctor or health care professional that they had sinusitis in the past 12 months (Table 1) (12).

The prevalence of chronic rhinosinusitis may be better defined (13). According to the National Ambulatory Medical Care Survey, chronic sinusitis accounts for 12.3 million office visits to physicians, or 1.3% of total office visits annually (14). Among Canadian adults, the reported prevalence of chronic rhinosinusitis is 5% (15). Unfortunately, the term chronic sinusitis is used to characterize a wide and possibly disparate group of inflammatory disorders, and this makes any specific approach to therapy problematic.

The economic impact of rhinosinusitis is considerable. In 1996, the direct cost due to sinusitis was $5.8 billion (16). A primary diagnosis of chronic rhinosinusitis accounted for more than 50% of all expenses. To these costs, indirect costs need to be considered as well, such as days for work lost. Birnbaum et al. recently evaluated the economic burden of respiratory infection, including sinusitis, in an employed population to ascertain the impact of these infections from the perspective of the employer (17). The investigators evaluated more than 63,000 patients with at least one diagnosis for a respiratory infection in 1997 who were identified in the claims database

Table 1 Percents (With Standard Errors) of Selected Respiratory Diseases Among Persons 18 Years of Age and Over, by Selected Characteristics: United States, 2001

Selected characteristic	Selected respiratory diseases[a]: Chronic				
	Emphysema	Asthma	Hay fever	Sinusitis	Bronchitis
Total	1.5 (0.07)	10.9 (0.21)	10.0 (0.20)	17.4 (0.27)	5.5 (0.15)
Sex					
Male	1.7 (0.12)	9.4 (0.29)	8.9 (0.27)	12.8 (0.33)	3.8 (0.19)
Female	1.2 (0.09)	12.3 (0.29)	11.1 (0.28)	21.7 (0.38)	7.1 (0.23)
Age					
18–44 years	0.2 (0.03)	11.8 (0.29)	10.0 (0.27)	15.9 (0.35)	4.5 (0.19)
45–64 years	1.8 (0.14)	10.4 (0.35)	11.6 (0.38)	21.3 (0.48)	6.5 (0.28)
65–74 years	4.7 (0.40)	9.4 (0.55)	7.5 (0.54)	17.2 (0.77)	6.7 (0.48)
75 years and over	5.6 (0.51)	8.0 (0.62)	6.8 (0.54)	12.8 (0.72)	6.9 (0.63)
Race					
White	1.6 (0.08)	10.9 (0.23)	10.1 (0.22)	17.8 (0.30)	5.7 (0.40)
Black or African-American	0.7 (0.13)	11.1 (0.56)	8.8 (0.54)	17.5 (0.72)	5.3 (0.17)
American Indian or Alaska Native	1.1 (0.71)[a]	12.2 (2.62)	13.3 (2.57)	15.5 (2.72)	5.4 (1.87)[a]
Asian	0.4 (0.22)[a]	6.7 (0.98)	9.9 (1.11)	10.7 (1.20)	2.3 (0.57)
Native Hawaiian or other Pacific Islander	3.9 (2.81)[a]	16.9 (6.46)[a]	3.7 (2.74)[a]	11.1 (4.94)[a]	2.3 (2.32)[a]
Hispanic or Latino	0.6 (0.14)	8.5 (0.46)	8.4 (0.48)	11.1 (0.52)	3.1 (0.29)
Poverty status					
Poor	2.4 (0.27)	15.2 (0.71)	8.6 (0.55)	16.0 (0.71)	7.9 (0.53)
Near poor	2.9 (0.31)	11.9 (0.55)	8.7 (0.46)	16.5 (0.61)	7.1 (0.43)
Not poor	1.0 (0.08)	10.7 (0.28)	11.3 (0.29)	18.8 (0.37)	5.1 (0.20)
Region					

(Continued)

Table 1 Percents (With Standard Errors) of Selected Respiratory Diseases Among Persons 18 Years of Age and Over, by Selected Characteristics: United States, 2001 (*Continued*)

Selected characteristic	Selected respiratory diseases[a]: Chronic				
	Emphysema	Asthma	Hay fever	Sinusitis	Bronchitis
Northeast	1.3 (0.16)	11.7 (0.52)	10.8 (0.49)	16.6 (0.57)	4.8 (0.30)
Midwest	1.7 (0.16)	10.8 (0.38)	8.5 (0.37)	16.2 (0.51)	5.2 (0.31)
South	1.6 (0.13)	10.6 (0.35)	9.5 (0.34)	20.7 (0.49)	6.4 (0.27)
West	1.1 (0.12)	10.6 (0.44)	12.2 (0.45)	13.7 (0.50)	4.8 (0.29)

[a]Respondents were asked in two separate questions if they had ever been told by a doctor or other health professional that they had emphysema or asthma. Respondents were asked in three separate questions if they had been told by a doctor or other health professional in the past 12 months that they had hay fever, sinusitis, or bronchitis. A person may be represented in more than one column.

Source: From Ref. 12.

of a national Fortune 100 company. Outcome measures were compared to those of a 10% random sample of beneficiaries in the overall employed population. The authors calculated a total cost of care that included not only direct health-care costs, but also disability costs and absenteeism costs. Acute and chronic sinusitis represented the fifth and sixth most common respiratory tract infection with a total number of 9856 and 7368 patients, respectively. This compared to 10,852 treated for acute bronchitis, 5296 treated for chronic bronchitis, 4464 treated for pharyngitis, and 4036 treated for pneumonia. The total aggregate employer cost for treating acute sinusitis and chronic sinusitis was $35,126,784 and $32,824,440, respectively (compared to $46,591,584 and $6,692,439 for pneumonia and pharyngitis) (Table 2) (17).

In addition, sinusitis can adversely affect other aspects of quality of life. Matsui et al. observed an decline of cognitive function in elderly people using the Mini-Mental State Examination (18). Chronic sinusitis may affect cognitive function either by decreasing the power of concentration or affecting specific cognitive functions, which can significantly have an impact on quality of life considerations. Therefore, early medical intervention for chronic sinusitis should take into account this potentially neglected effect on cognitive function in the elderly.

EPIDEMIOLOGY AND RISK FACTORS

Individuals with allergies or asthma and those who smoke may be predisposed to rhinosinusitis (15,19). For unclear reasons, rhinosinusitis affects more females than males (12,15,20). Women patients between the ages of 25 and 64 years were seen most often (12). When results were considered by single race without regard to ethnicity, Asian adults were less likely to have been told in the preceding 12 months that they had sinusitis compared with white, black, and American Indian or native-Alaska adults (12). Adults in families that were not poor were more likely to have been told that they had sinusitis than adults in poor families. The percentage of adults with sinusitis was higher in the southern area of the United States than any other region (12).

Sokol recently reported results from a large study of sinusitis evaluated in the primary care setting, the Respiratory Surveillance Program (20). This study was undertaken over a 10-month period during the 1999–2000 respiratory infection season. Patients were evaluated from 674 community-based practices for data including patient demographics and associated risk factors (Table 3). The diagnosis of rhinosinusitis was based solely on the clinical judgment of the physician investigator. Over 16,000 patients were evaluated and similar to data presented above, females predominated (almost a two to one ratio of female to male). Underlying conditions identified in this study included smoking, diabetes, and the presence of chronic lung disease (20).

Table 2 Employer Payments in 1997 per Beneficiary by Type of Respiratory Infection, and Employer Overall Costs

	Inpatient	Outpatient	Prescription drug	Office	Other[a]	Disability costs	Absenteeism costs	Total costs	Overall costs
Symptoms of the respiratory system (n = 24,851)	3098	1822	883	602	157	776	507	7845	194,956,095
Acute upper respiratory infections of multiple or unspecified sites (n = 13,874)	613	688	455	356	81	297	301	2791	38,722,334
Acute tonsillitis and acute pharyngitis (n = 13,706)	448	628	350	315	72	156	211	2180	29,879,080
Acute bronchitis (n = 10,852)	1114	951	682	441	114	474	443	4219	45,784,588
Acute sinusitis (n = 9856)	700	889	674	449	88	335	429	3564	35,126,784
Chronic sinusitis (n = 7368)	990	1200	787	516	102	404	456	4455	32,824,440
Chronic bronchitis (n = 5296)	2054	1168	820	518	168	668	478	5874	31,108,704

Strep throat and scarlet fever, chronic pharyngitis and nasopharyngitis, chronic diseases of the tonsils and adenoids (n = 4464)	498	886	409	371	75	179	224	2642	11,793,888
Pneumonia (n = 4036)	6316	1902	973	604	242	1016	491	11,544	46,591,584
Acute nasopharyngitis (acute cold) and acute laryngitis (n = 2041)	940	787	455	449	95	252	301	3279	6,692,439
Influenza (n = 1514)	1315	1038	680	437	112	621	525	4728	7,158,192
Unique individuals in respiratory infections sample (n = 63,890)	1459	1047	598	413	97	437	346	4397	280,924,330

Aggregate employer costs is calculated by multiplying total costs by the number of beneficiaries with a specific condition.
[a]Includes care at patient's home, nursing/extended care facility, psychiatric day-care facility, substance abuse treatment facility, and independent clinical laboratories.
Source: From Ref. 17.

Table 3 Demographic Data for Sinusitis (From the Respiratory Surveillance Program)

Demographic	Overall (n = 16,135)
Age (yr), mean (range)	44 (1–97)
Sex (460 none specified) % female/% male	62/35
Ethnicity (% total)	
White	13,603 (86%)
African American	1018 (6.3%)
Hispanic	557 (3.5%)
Asian	227 (1.4%)
Other	76 (0.5%)
Unknown	654 (4.1%)
Smoker (%)	3813 (24%)
Diabetes (%)	674 (4.2%)
COPD (%)	688 (4.3%)

460 no sex specified.
Abbreviation: COPD, chronic obstructive pulmonary disease.
Source: From Ref. 20.

Predisposing Conditions of Rhinosinusitis

In addition to smoking, there are many other conditions associated with rhinosinusitis. These include allergic rhinitis, asthma, nasal polyps, aspirin hypersensitivity, cystic fibrosis, and immune deficiency [particularly immunodeficiency virus (HIV) infection] (Tables 4 and 5).

The occurrence of secondary bacterial sinusitis is highly associated with prior viral respiratory illnesses (10,11). An important area of disease leading to secondary bacterial sinusitis is obstruction at the ostiomeatal complex. A variety of factors may lead to obstruction of the ostium. The most common predisposing factor is viral infection, which causes edema and inflammation of the nasal mucosa. In addition to viral rhinosinusitis-related cases, acute bacterial sinusitis occurs related to allergy and nasal obstruction due to polyps, foreign bodies, and tumors. Less common risk factors associated with a predisposition for bacterial sinusitis are immune deficiencies such as agammaglobulinemia and human HIV infection; abnormalities of polymorphonuclear cell function; structural defects, such as cleft palate; and disorders of mucociliary clearance, including cilial dysfunction and cystic fibrosis (21).

Rhinosinusitis and the Common Cold

The relationship between rhinosinusitis and the common cold has been well established. In a sentinel prospective study of 110 adults, Gwaltney et al. evaluated the findings on CT examination of patients with rhinosinusitis (10).

Table 4 Extrinsic and Intrinsic Potential Causes of Chronic Rhinosinusitis

Extrinsic causes of CRS can broadly be broken down into:
 1. Infectious (viral, bacterial, fungal, parasitic)
 2. Noninfectious/inflammation
    a. Allergic–IgE-mediated
    b. Non–IgE-mediated hypersensitivities
    c. Pharmacologic
    d. Irritants
 3. Disruption of normal ventilation or mucociliary drainage
    a. Surgery
    b. Infection
    c. Trauma
Intrinsic causes contributing to CRS:
 1. Genetic
    a. Mucociliary abnormality
       i. Cystic fibrosis
       ii. Primary ciliary dysmotility
    b. Structural
    c. Immunodeficiency
 2. Acquired
    a. Aspirin-hypersensitivity associated with asthma and nasal polyps
    b. Autonomic dysregulation
    c. Hormonal
       i. Rhinitis of pregnancy
       ii. Hypothyroidism
    d. Structural
       i. Neoplasms
       ii. Osteoneogenesis and outflow obstruction
       iii. Retention cysts and antral choanal polyps
    e. Autoimmune or idiopathic
       i. Granulomatous disorders
          1. Sarcoid
          2. Wegener's granulomatosis
       ii. Vasculitis
          1. Systemic lupus erythematosus
          2. Churg-Straus syndrome
       iii. Pemphigoid
    f. Immunodeficiency

Source: From Ref. 13.

Among 31 patients who had CT scans performed within 24 to 48 hours of assessment, 24 (77%) had occlusion of the ethmoid sinus, 27 (87%), had abnormalities of one or both maxillary sinuses, 20 (65%) had abnormalities of the ethmoid sinuses, 10 (32%) had abnormalities of the frontal sinuses, and 12 (39%) had abnormalities of the sphenoid sinuses. Rhinovirus was

Table 5 Factors Associated with Chronic Rhinosinusitis

Systemic host factors	Local host	Environmental
Allergic	Anatomic	Microorganisms
Immunodeficiency	Neoplastic viral, bacterial, fungal	
Genetic/congenital	Acquired-mucociliary dysfunction	Noxious chemicals, pollutant, smoke
Mucociliary dysfunction	Medications	
Endocrine	Trauma	
Neuromechanism	Surgery	

Source: From Ref. 13.

detected in the secretions of 7 of 17 (41%) of these patients. The patients received no medical treatment for their infections; 14 patients with sinus abnormality as seen on the initial CT scan had repeat scans, and one of these reported resolution of symptoms. Of significance, 11 of these 14 (79%) showed clearing or marked improvement in sinus abnormalities. It is evident from this study that the common cold is associated with frequent involvement of the paranasal sinuses.

Rhinosinusitis and Allergy

Several studies suggest an association between rhinosinusitis and allergic sinusitis (22,23). Allergic rhinitis predisposes the patient to sinusitis since it can be associated with inflammation and obstruction of the ostia. Thus, allergic rhinitis and acute bacterial sinusitis can overlap.

Rhinosinusitis and Asthma

Sinusitis is often seen in patients with asthma and often exacerbates the severity of the episode (24). Although the pathophysiology of the association between asthma and sinusitis is not very clear, it may be related to damage induced by the eosinophil, a prominent component of the inflammatory process that is characteristic of both diseases. A reflex phenomenon linking inflammation in the sinuses to subsequent inflammation in the lower airways has been proposed.

PATHOGENS OF BACTERIAL SINUSITIS

Epidemiology of *Streptococcus pneumoniae* and *Haemophilus influenzae*

When sinus puncture aspirates are used to obtain secretions for culture from patients with acute sinusitis, results consistently show that *Streptococcus pneumoniae* and *Haemophilus influenzae* are the most important bacterial pathogens. Other organisms occasionally found include *Moraxella catarrhalis*, other streptococcal species (e.g., *Streptococcus pyogenes*), *Staphylococcus aureus*, and anaerobes (e.g., *Prevotella* spp., *Peptostreptococcus* spp., *Fusobacterium* spp.).

Of all the above pathogens, *S. pneumoniae* is considered the most significant from the standpoint of virulence and clinical impact. *S. pneumoniae* can be transmitted directly or through fomites; transmission is facilitated by crowding, such as in daycare centers or extended care facilities. Children are often heavily colonized with *S. pneumoniae*, and adults not exposed to children generally have a lower prevalence of *S. pneumoniae* infection. Risk factors for *S. pneumoniae* infection in adults include active or passive smoke exposure and presence of chronic diseases. *S. pneumoniae* infections occur most commonly during the winter months, in part due to the secondary relationship to viral infections.

H. influenzae is indigenous to humans and readily colonize the nasopharynx. Spread from one individual to another occurs by airborne droplets or by direct contact with secretions. The majority of sinus infections are due to nonencapsulated strains.

SINUSITIS AND HIV

In the pre-highly active anti-retroviral therapy (HAART) era, up to 70% of patients with HIV experienced at least one bout of acute sinusitis during the course of their disease, and 58% experienced recurrent infections (25). As patients are now living longer with the availability of HAART, the prevalence of acute and chronic sinusitis in HIV-infected patents has increased. In a study of 7513 HIV-infected patients enrolled from November 1990 to November 1999, the incidence of one or more diagnoses of sinusitis was 14.5% (26). The mean CD4 count at the time of sinusitis was 391. Although the authors felt the incidence of sinusitis in individuals infected with HIV is frequent, there was no association between sinusitics and an increased hazard of death after adjusting results for the level of immunodeficiency age, gender, and race.

The organisms associated with acute sinusitis in HIV patients are similar to the pathogens in other patients, with *S. pneumoniae* and *H. influenzae* being predominant. However, there is a higher occurrence of *S. aureus* and *Pseudomonas aeruginosa* in the HIV-infected patient than in the non-infected patient (Table 6) (27). The common occurrence of *P. aeruginosa* in HIV-infected patients probably reflects an impaired mucociliary transport often associated with HIV infection. In addition, more unusual organisms are also commonly found, particularly if immunodeficiency progresses. As the CD4 counts of patients dip below 200, these patients become susceptible to more opportunistic infections. Opportunistic and atypical infections include cytomegalovirus, *Aspergillus* spp., and *Mycobacterium* spp. (27).

Table 6 Sinus Pathogens in HIV

Streptococcus pneumoniae	19%
Streptococcus viridans	19%
Pseudomonas aeruginosa	17%
Haemophilus influenzae	13%
Coagulase-negative *Staphylococci*	13%
Staphylococcus aureus	9%
Candida albicans	4%
Klebsiella pneumoniae	2%
Listeria monocytogenes	2%
Torulopsis glabrata	2%

In antral washings from 41 HIV patients with acute sinusitis, four had multiple pathogens.
Source: From Ref. 27.

NOSOCOMIAL SINUSITIS

Sinusitis is a relatively common infection in patients treated in an intensive care unit (ICU). An epidemiologic study in an ICU orally-intubated population found the incidence of sinusitis, as diagnosed by cultures of maxillary sinus secretion, was 10% (28). In another study of 300 patients, the incidence of infectious sinusitis was estimated at 20% after eight days of mechanical ventilation in patients that were orotracheally or nasotracheally intubated (29). However, in a study designed to search for nosocomial sinusitis in patients who were intubated in an ICU, Holzapfel et al. found 80 patients among 199 study patients to have infectious nosocomial maxillary sinusitis (30). In this study, all patients who were nasotracheally intubated were evaluated by a sinus CT scan if body temperature was $\geq 38°C$. When CT scan showed an air-fluid level and/or an opacification within a maxillary sinus, a transnasal puncture was performed. Critieria for nosocomial sinusitis were sinus CT scan findings consistent with sinusitis, mechanical ventilation, macroscopic purulent sinus aspiration, and quantitative culture of the aspirated material with $\geq 10^3$ cfu/mL. Among the 80 patients, infection was due to polymicrobial flora in 44 patients and 138 organisms were isolated. The most common organisms were *Eshcerichia coli* (12), *P. aeruginosa* (12), *Proteus* spp. (10), *Hemophilus* spp. (7), *Klebsiella* spp. (6), *Enterobacter* spp. (6), *S. aureus* (10), *Streptococcus* spp. (30), anaerobes (15), and *Candida albicans* (10).

Multiple factors can promote nosocomial sinusitis in critically ill patients. Placement of endotracheal or gastric tubes through the nose can irritate the nasopharyngeal mucosa, causing edema in the region of the ostial meatal complex. Nasal tubes can also directly obstruct sinus drainage by acting as foreign bodies. Placing tubes via the mouth does not entirely eliminate the risk of nosocomial sinusitis, but studies suggest the risk is lessened. In one study, the incidence of sinusitis was higher in patients intubated nasotracheally as compared to those by the oropharyngeal route (31). Additional factors which may play a role in ICU patients include the supine position and limitation of head movements (which may prevent natural sinus drainage normally caused by gravity), positive-pressure ventilation, impaired ability to cough or sneeze, and the absence of airflow through the nares in ventilated patients.

REFERENCES

1. File TM Jr. The epidemiology of respiratory tract infections. Semin Respir Infect 2000; 15(3):184–194.
2. File TM Jr, Hadley JA. Rational use of antibiotics to treat respiratory tract infections. Am J Manag Care 2002; 8:713–727.
3. Armstrong GL, Pinner RW. Outpatient visits for infectious diseases in the United States, 1980 through 1996. Arch Intern Med 1999; 159:2531–2536.
4. McCaig LF, Hughs JM. Trends in antimicrobial drug prescribing among office-based physicians in the United States. JAMA 1995; 273:214–219.
5. Scott Levin Prescription Audit from Verispan, L.L.C., January–December, 2002.
6. Lanza DC, Kennedy DW. Adult rhinusitis defined. Otolaryngol Head Neck Surg 1997; 117(3 Pt 2):S1–S7.
7. Anon JB, Jacobs MR, Poole MD, Ambrose PG, Benninger MS, Hadley JA, Craig WA, and The Sinus and Allergy Health Partnership. Antimicrobial treatment guidelines for acute bacterial rhinosinusitis 2004. Otolaryngol Head Neck Surg 2004; 130(suppl 1):1–45.
8. Brook I, Gooch WM III, Jenkins SG, Pichichero ME, et al. Medical management of acute bacterial sinusitis. Recommendations of a Clinical Advisory Committee on Pediatric and Adult Sinusitis. St Louis: Annals Publishing, 2000.
9. Dingle JH, Badger GF, Jordan WS Jr. Illness in the home: a study of 25,000 illnesses in a group of Cleveland families. Cleveland: The Press of Western Reserve University, 1964.
10. Gwaltney JM Jr, Phillips CD, Miller RD, et al. Computed tomographic study of the common cold. N Engl J Med 1994; 330:25–30.
11. Gwaltney JM Jr, Wiesinger BA, Patrie JT. Acute community-acquired bacterial sinusitis: the value of antimicrobial treatment and the natural history. Clin Infect Dis 2004; 38:227–233.
12. Lucas JW, Schiller JS, Benson V. Summary health statistics for U.S. adults: National Health Interview Survey, 2001. National Center for Health Statistics. Vital Health Stat 2001; 10:218.
13. Benninger MS, et al. Adult chronic rhinosinusitis: definitions, diagnosis, epidemiology, and pathophysiology. Otolaryngol Head Neck Surg 2003; 129S(suppl 3): S1–S32.
14. Cherry DK, Burt CW, Woodwell DA. National Ambulatory Medical Care Survey: 2001 Summary. Advance Data form Vital and Health Statistics; no. 337. Hyattsville, MD: National Center for Health Statistics, 2003.

15. Chen Y, Dales R, Lin M. The epidemiology of chronic rhinosinusitis in Canadians. Laryngoscope 2003; 113:1199–1205.
16. Durr DG, Desrosiers MY, Dassa C. Impact of rhinosinusitis in health care delivery: the Quebec experience. J Otolaryngol 2001; 30:93.
17. Birnbaum HG, Morley M, Greenberg MS, Colice GL. Economic burden of respiratory infections in an employed population. Chest 2002; 122:603–611.
18. Matusi T, Arai H, Nakajo M, Mauyama M, Ebihara S, et al. Role of chronic sinusitis in cognitive functioning in the elderly. J Am Geriatr Soc 2003; 51: 1818–1819.
19. Lieu JE, Feinstein AR. Confirmations and surprises in the association of tobacco use with sinusitis. Arch Otolarynygol Head Neck Surg 2000; 126: 940–946.
20. Sokol W. Epidemiology of sinusitis in the primary care setting: results from the 1999–2000 respiratory surveillance program. Am J Med 2001; 111(9A): 19S–24S.
21. Casiano RR. Sinusitis: a complex and challenging disease. Mediguide Infect Dis 2001; 21(1):1–5.
22. Alho OP, Karttunen TJ, Karttunen R, Tuokko H, Koskela M, Suramo I, Ukhari M. Subjects with allergic rhinitis show signs of more severely impaired paranasal sinuus function during viral colds than non allergic subjects. Allergy 2003; 58:767–771.
23. Mucha SM, Baroody FM. Relationships between atopy and bacterial infections. Curr Allergy Asthma Rep 2003; 3:232–237.
24. Osur SL. Viral respiratory infections in association with asthma and sinusitis: a review. Ann Allergy Asthma Immunol 2002; 89:553–560.
25. Godofsky EW, Zinreich J, Armstrong M, et al. Sinusitis in HIV-infected patients: a clinical and radiographic review. Am J Med 1992; 93:163–170.
26. Belafsky PC, Amedee R, Moore B, Kissinger PJ. The association between sinusitis and survival among individuals infected with the human immunodeficiency virus. Am J Rhinol 2001 Sept–Oct; 15(5):343–345.
27. Milgrim LM, Rubin JS, Rosenstreich DL, et al. Sinusitis in human immunodeficiency virus infection: typical and atypical organisms. J Otolaryngol 1994; 23:450–453.
28. George DL, Falk PS, Nunally K. Nosocomial sinusitis in medical intensive care unit patients: a prospective epidemiologic study. Infect Control Hosp Epidemiol 1992; 21:497.
29. Holzapfel L, Chevret S, Madinier G, Onen F, Demingeon G, Coupry A, Chaudet M. Incidence of long term oro- or nastotracheal intubation on Nosocomial maxillary sinusitis and pneumonia: results of a randomized clinical trial. Crit Care Med 1993; 21:1132–1138.
30. Holzapfel L, Chastang C, Deningeon G, Bohe J, Piralla N, Coupry A. Randomized study assessing the systematic search for maxillary sinusitis in Nasotracheally Mechanically Ventilated Patients. Am J Respir Crit Care Med 1999; 159:695–701.
31. Rouby JJ, Laurent P, Gosnach M, et al. Risk factors and clinical relevance of nosocomial maxillary sinusitis in the critically ill. Am J Respir Crit Care Med 1996; 150:776–783.

2

Classification of Rhinosinusitis

Peter A. R. Clement

*Department of Otorhinolaryngology and ENT Department, University Hospital,
Free University Brussels (VUB), Brussels, Belgium*

INTRODUCTION

In 1972, Douek wrote that "classification has an important place in medicine, as it forms the framework upon which diagnosis is made possible, etiology recalled and separated, and treatment decided. It remains, however, an intellectual system imposed onto a nature that has rarely rigid boundaries" (1). Now, more than 30 years later, this statement is still valid.

This chapter reviews the different classifications of rhinosinusitis, and attempts to explain why in the course of time these classifications were changed. By acquiring new information about the natural history of rhinosinusitis based on novel imaging techniques such as MRI, CT scanning, and nasal endoscopy, new insights on the pathophysiology of the disease were gained. Because of better culture techniques; and recent advances in histocytochemistry of inflammation; it became obvious that the classification of this disease needed to be adapted and redefined step-by-step.

Rhinosinusitis Versus Sinusitis

There exists a general agreement that rhinosinusitis can be defined as any inflammation of the paranasal sinus mucosa (2). Johnson and Ferguson stated that because the lining of the mucosa and the paranasal sinuses is continuous, an inflammation of the nasal cavity is usually associated with inflammation of the sinus lining (3). The faculty of the staging and therapy group shared the same opinion and stated that the term rhinosinusitis is perhaps more precise than the term sinusitis. The reasons are that sinusitis does not typically develop without prior rhinitis, isolated sinus disease without rhinitis is rare, the mucous membrane lining of the nose and the paranasal sinus is continuous, and two of the prominent features of sinusitis—nasal obstruction and drainage—are associated with rhinitis symptoms (4). The Task Force on Rhinosinusitis (TFR) preferred the term rhinosinusitis as well (5). On occurrences in children, the members of the Consensus Panel on Pediatric Rhinosinusitis preferred to speak of rhinosinusitis since rhinitis and sinusitis are often a continuum of the disease (6).

Radiological Changes as Signs of Sinusitis

Havas et al. (7) found abnormal appearances of the paranasal sinuses on CT scan in 42.5% of asymptomatic adults and Bolger et al. (8) found a similar proportion of 41.7% in patients scanned for nonsinus reasons. As a possible explanation, Bolger et al (8). suggested that these abnormalities could be induced by normal variations of the sinus mucosa, asymptomatic chronic sinus disease, and mild to moderately symptomatic undiagnosed chronic sinusitis. In a CT scan study of children undergoing nonsinusitis evaluation, Diament et al. (9) detected maxillary and ethmoidal thickening in ∼50% of the patients. Similar figures were found by Gordts et al. (10,11) who demonstrated in an MRI study of a non-ENT population of adults (without any complaints and a blank surgical history) that there existed on 40% abnormalities of the mucosa, and in 45% of the cases in a non-ENT population of children.

All these imaging studies show us that imaging signs of sinusitis, in particular pathological mucosal swelling, can occur in completely asymptomatic adults and children. The meaning of these findings is unclear, and therefore, many clinicians claim that one has to treat patients and not CT or MRI scans. The problem, however, remains that subclinical, silent, or asymptomatic sinusitis exists. Whether it needs to be diagnosed or treated in order to prevent manifest sinusitis is another question that has not been investigated yet.

The aim of this chapter is to discuss the classification of symptomatic rhinosinusitis. Rhinosinusitis can be defined as any inflammation of the nasal and paranasal sinus mucosa, resulting in signs and symptoms.

Parameters Used for Classification

According to Pinheiro et al. (12), classification of rhinosinusitis should be done along five axes:

  i. Clinical presentation (duration: acute, subacute, and chronic)
 ii. Anatomical site of involvement (ethmoid, maxillary, frontal, and sphenoid)
iii. Responsible microorganism (viral, bacterial, and fungal)

iv. Presence of extra sinus involvement (complicated and uncompli-
     cated)
v.   Modifying or aggravating factors (e.g., atopy, immunosuppres-
     sion, ostiomeatal obstruction, etc.)

According to these authors, a complete classification of sinusitis
according to these five axes is essential to tailor the treatment for the particular situation. As an example of this axes system, a possibility would be
chronic (i), frontal (ii), bacterial (iii) sinusitis complicated by frontal bone
osteomyelitis (iv) and aggravated by immunosuppression due to diabetes
mellitus (v).

CLASSIFICATIONS OF SINUSITIS

Most classification systems of rhinosinusitis, however, are based on the
duration of symptoms and/or the specific sinus involved (13). In 1984, Kern
stated that a classification of sinusitis based on pathology is useful in patient
management (14). In addition to naming the involved sinuses, the classification should contain some concepts as to the duration of the sinus infection.
Kern defined *acute suppurative sinusitis*, on an arbitrary basis, as any infectious process in a paranasal sinus lasting from one day to three weeks, and
subacute sinusitis as a sinus infection that lingers from three weeks to three
months, during which period epithelial damage in the sinuses may still be
reversible (14). Irreversible changes usually occur after three months of subacute sinusitis, leading into the next phase of *chronic sinusitis* that is any
infection lasting longer than three months and requiring surgery for sinus
ventilation and drainage. From this definition, it is obvious that at that time
sinusitis was considered to be a mainly infectious process, and that after
three months the mucosal changes were considered to be irreversible. This
concept that after three months irreversible mucosal changes had occurred
corresponds with the philosophy of the Caldwell–Luc operation that insis-
ted on meticulously removing the mucus lining of the maxillary sinus in toto
(15). On the contrary Wigand showed that restoration of ventilation and
drainage after removal of cysts and polyps initiates the recovery of diseased
mucosa (16,17). At this time, a very new and important concept was introduced to preserve as much mucosa as possible because most of the mucosal
disease seemed to be reversible after adequate drainage and ventilation.

In the eighties, the basic pathological concept of sinusitis consisted of
bacterial infection due to sinus ostium obstruction, followed by hypoxia and
a series of events leading to the production of thick retained secretions creating a perfect situation for bacterial multiplication (14), i.e., the sinusitis cycle
(18). It was demonstrated, however, from standard x-ray examination of the
paranasal sinuses in 144 consecutive adult patients with perennial rhinitis,
that 20% showed major changes (total opacity of the maxillary sinus) and

another 20% showed minor changes (19). Based on a CT scan study in atopic patients, Iwens et al. concluded that signs of sinusitis exist in about 60% of the children and adults (20). Young children (three–nine years of age) showed more severe sinusitis (50% to total opacity of the involved sinuses) on the CT scans in 30% to 40% of the cases, while older children and adults more often had signs of mild sinusitis (mucosal swelling of more than 4 mm and an opacity of less than 50%).

In 1992 Shapiro et al. concluded that there existed a general agreement that sinusitis can be defined as an inflammation (not infection) of the paranasal mucosa (2). The authors proposed the following definition of sinusitis (Table 1) (2):

- *Acute sinusitis* can be defined by certain major and minor criteria that exist for longer than the typical viral upper respiratory tract infection (URTI), more than seven days. The presence of two or more minor criteria for more than seven days is highly likely to signify acute sinus disease, which is usually bacterial. If the signs and symptoms fulfill these criteria, the presence of one positive major diagnostic test result is confirmatory, whereas the minor tests may be considered supportive. Another symptom, acute onset of fever with purulent rhinorrhea, is also considered highly likely to indicate acute bacterial sinusitis.

Table 1 Clinical Diagnosis of Sinusitis

Signs and symptoms	Diagnostic tests
Major criteria	Major criteria
Purulent nasal discharge opacification	Water's radiograph or fluid level: thickening filling ≥50% of antrum
Purulent pharyngeal drainage/ mucosa	Coronal CT scan: thickening of or opacification of sinus mucosa
Purulent postnasal drip	
Cough	
Minor criteria	Minor criteria
Periorbital oedema	Nasal cytology study (smear) with neutrophils and bacterimiae
Headache	Ultrasound studies
Facial pain	
Tooth pain	
Earache	
Sore throat	Probable sinusitis
Foul breath	Signs and symptoms: 2 major, 1 minor and ≥2 minor criteria
Increased wheeze	Diagnostic tests: 1 major = confirmatory, 1 minor = supportive
Fever	

Source: Adapted from Ref. 2.

- *Chronic sinusitis* was referred as a disease that lasted more than three months that is manifested by the presence of long-term symptoms without an ongoing need for antibiotic therapy. Thus, chronic sinusitis might occur on a non-infectious basis.
- *Subacute sinusitis* was used for the gray zone between disease lasting less than a month (acute) and lasting more than three months (chronic).

Since these guidelines were published, it became more appropriate to refer to inflammation rather than infection when the term sinusitisis was used. Inflammation covers infectious as well as noninfectious mechanisms.

Using CT scans, Gwaltney et al. showed that during a common cold of two- to four-day duration, more than 80% of the cases showed abnormalities of the sinuses mucosa (21). These abnormalities of the infindibula and sinuses cleared or markedly improved within two weeks.

In a prospective study using MRI, Leopold et al. studied the evolution of acute maxillary sinusitis (manifested by facial pain, fever, and purulent rhinorrhea) in 13 previously healthy subjects (22). The MRI analysis of the volume percentage of air in the involved sinuses showed that only half of the opacification had resolved by 10 days and the sinuses were only about 80% aerated by 56 days. This study showed that although antibiotic treatment of acute maxillary sinusitis generally results in clinical resolution of symptoms within one week, mucosal changes, however, could persist for eight weeks or more.

All these new insights showed that the classification of rhinosinusi tis had to be redefined and these led in 1993 to an international conference on sinus disease, chaired by Kennedy (23) in Princeton, New Jersey. The following definitions were proposed in the Princeton meeting classification.

1. *Acute sinusitis* is defined as a symptomatic sinus infection in which symptoms persist no longer than six to eight weeks or there are fewer than four episodes per year of acute symptoms of 10 days duration. Sinusitis is acute when episodes of infection resolve with medical therapy leaving no significant mucosal damage.
2. *Chronic sinusitis* is a persistent sinusitis that cannot be alleviated by medical therapy alone, and involves radiographic evidence of mucosal hyperplasia. In adults, it is defined as eight weeks of persistent symptoms or signs, or four or more episodes per year of recurrent acute sinusitis, each lasting at least 10 days, in association with persistent changes on CT scan four weeks after medical therapy without intervening acute infection (URTI).

3. *Recurrent acute sinusitis* is defined as repeated acute episodes that resolve with medical therapy, leaving no significant mucosal damage.

The faculty of the staging and therapy group published the symptoms and signs needed for establishing the diagnosis of chronic sinusitis and divided them in major and minor ones (Table 2) (4).

In 1997, the International Rhinosinusitis Advisory Board (IRAB) published the clinical classification of rhinosinusitis in adults (24). They defined *acute rhinosinusitis* as a sinusitis with an acute onset of symptoms and a duration of symptoms less than 12 weeks and symptoms that resolve completely. *Recurrent acute rhinosinusitis* was defined as being more than one and less than four episodes of acute rhinosinusitis per year, a complete recovery between the attacks, and a symptom-free period of more than or equal to eight weeks between the acute attacks in absence of medical treatment.

The diagnosis of *acute community-acquired bacterial rhinosinusitis* (ACABRS) is judged probable if two major criteria (symptoms), or one major and two or more minor criteria, are present. The authors, however, recognize that none of these criteria are sensitive and specific for the diagnosis of ACABRS, so that an additional standard was necessary to prove the diagnostic accuracy.

Sinus puncture studies had shown that the symptoms that persist longer than 10 days without improvement are suggestive of bacterial rather than viral rhinosinusitis (25). Hence, if a patient with a cold or influenza illness does not improve or is worse after 10 days, the authors recommended treatment with antibiotics. Some symptoms such as fever, facial erythema, and maxillary toothache have high specificity but low sensitivity, and when present, the diagnosis of ACABRS is warranted.

They recognized that ACABRS needs to be differentiated from acute nosocomial or hospital-acquired bacterial rhinosinusitis (AHABRS). Nosocomial sinusitis is most often polymicrobial and is usually caused by those organisms that are most prevalent in that particular institution (12). AHABRS is often seen in critically ill or immunosuppressed patients.

Table 2 Chronic Sinusitis

Major	Minor
Nasal congestion or obstruction	Fever
Nasal discharge	Halitosis
Headache	
Facial pain or pressure	
Olfactory disturbance	

Source: Adapted from Ref. 4.

Chronic rhinosinusitis was defined as a sinusitis with a duration of symptoms more than 12 weeks, which shows persistent inflammatory changes on imaging and lasts for more than or equal to four weeks after starting appropriate medical therapy (with no intervening acute episodes). The authors also defined the acute exacerbation of chronic rhinosinusitis as a worsening of existing symptoms or appearance of new symptoms and a complete resolution of acute (but not chronic) symptoms between episodes. The authors presented their definitions and classification of infectious rhinosinusitis with a summary of current views on etiology and management. They admitted that the definitions based on the severity and duration of symptoms were imperfect, the duration of the acute episodes chosen in the various definitions was arbitrary, and the clinical significance of abnormal findings on imaging investigation was debatable. For the duration in the definition of chronic sinusitis, they followed the FDA recommendation to consider the condition if symptoms persist for more than 12 weeks (24).

From a clinical perception, the authors admitted that the definition of chronic rhinosinusitis (CRS) is often subjective and is based on symptoms that are vague, nonlocalized, and nonspecific. The relationship between the findings on endoscopic examination, the radiographic appearance and specific symptoms, and the severity is poorly defined.

The authors also realize that there appears to be an ill-defined group between the acute and the chronic conditions, and they suggest that this problem can be overcome by the use of the term "subacute" which spans the interval, but in other respects defies the definition, and it does not represent a histopathologic entity.

The IRAB also proposed another classification based on microbiological etiology, i.e., probable *viral rhinosinusitis* (nasal congestion, obstruction, nasal discharge, facial pressures/pain without fever, toothache, facial tenderness, erythema, and swelling), *acute bacterial rhinosinusitis* (same symptoms as viral rhinosinusitis) but with fever-fever is an exclusion criteria for viral rhinosinusitis or persisting without improvement for more than eight days), *recurrent acute rhinosinusitis* (incidence of more than four episodes a year), *chronic sinusitis* (with symptoms lasting longer than 12 weeks), and acute exacerbation of chronic rhinosinusitis (acute worsening of chronic sinusitis symptoms) (24). Although the IRAB recognizes the occurrence of sinusitis in allergic patients, it still considers every sinusitis to be of infectious origin. Their definition requires the inclusion of the parameter of duration in the classification based on the microbiological etiology. What was not taken into consideration by IRAB is the report by Gwaltney et al. that in maxillary sinus aspirates of patients with acute community acquired sinusitis (ACAS: the most typical example of bacterial sinusitis), viruses and fungi are found in addition to bacteria (Table 3) (26).

The same working definitions that took into account the duration of the diseases were developed by TFR, sponsored by the American Academy of Otolaryngology/Head and Neck Surgery (AAO-HNS) (5). This report

Table 3 Clinical Criteria for the Diagnosis of Acute Community-Acquired Bacterial Rhinosinusitis (ACABRS) IRAB Guidelines

Major	Minor
Purulent anterior and posterior discharge	Cough
Nasal congestion	Headache
Facial pressure or pain	Halitosis
Fever	Earache

Diagnosis of ACABRS: two major criteria, or one major criterion and two or more minor criteria. *Source*: Adapted from Ref. 24.

details the major and minor symptoms (Table 4) and defines sinusitis as the condition manifested by an inflammatory response of the nasal cavity and sinuses, and not an infection of these structures. It prefers the term rhinosinusitis to sinusitis as the mucous blanket of the sinuses is in continuity with that of the nasal cavity. They recognized that the multifactorial nature and multiple causes of rhinosinusitis make it difficult to define its cause in a given patient. They therefore concluded that it is currently impractical to define rhinosinusitis on the basis of its cause. An important differentiation between acute and chronic was made on the basis of histopathology, where

Table 4 Factors Associated with the Diagnosis of Chronic Sinusitis

Major factors	Minor factors
Facial pain, pressure (alone does not constitute a suggestive history for rhinosinusitis in absence of another major symptom)	Headache
	Fever (all nonacute)
	Halitosis
Facial congestion, fullness	
Nasal obstruction/blockage	Fatigue
Nasal discharge/purulence/discolored nasal drainage	Dental pain
	Cough
Hyposmia/anosmia	Ear pain/pressure/ fullness
Purulence in nasal cavity on examination	
Fever (acute rhinosinusitis only) in acute sinusitis alone does not constitute a strongly supportive history for acute in the absence of another major nasal symptom or sign	

Source: Adapted from Ref. 5.

acute rhinosinusitis is predominantly viewed as an exudative process associated with necrosis, hemorrhage, and/or ulceration, in which neutrophils predominate, whereas CRS is predominantly a proliferative process associated with fibrosis of the lamina propria, in which lymphocytes, plasma cells, and eosinophils predominate along with perhaps changes in bone.

Another important statement by the TRF is that a pathological review may also reveal a variety of findings that include, but are limited to, varying degrees of eosinophils in tissues and secretions, as well as the polyp formation and the presence of granulomas, bacteria, or fungi. This statement is important as it highlights the importance of inflammation (eosinophilic infiltration) rather than the infection, the presence of fungi, or the formation of nasal polyps in CRS.

The TFR also recognizes the concept of *subacute rhinosinusitis* for several reasons (5):

1. When polled, the physicians serving on the TFR indicated that they would treat rhinosinusitis lasting less than two to three weeks differently than they would treat a rhinosinusitis lasting 6 to 12 weeks.
2. Similar issues concerning otitis media had been heatedly debated until the otitis media literature arbitrarily defined acute otitis media as those lasting three weeks, subacute as lasting 3 to 12 weeks, and chronic otitis media as those lasting more than 12 weeks (27).
3. The FDA had no formal definition to describe the condition that lasts 4 to 12 weeks (less than four weeks is acute, more than four weeks is chronic).

The TFR defines five different classifications of adult rhinosinusitis (5):

1. *Acute rhinosinusitis* is a sinusitis with a sudden onset and lasting up to four weeks. The symptoms resolve completely, and once the disease has been treated, antibiotics are no longer required. A strong history consistent with acute rhinosinusitis includes two or more major factors (Table 4) or one major and two minor factors. However, the finding of nasal purulence is a strong indicator of an accurate diagnosis. A suggestive history for which acute rhinosinusitis should be included in the differential diagnosis includes one major factor, or two or more minor factors. In absence of other nasal factors, fever or pain alone does not constitute a strong history. Severe, prolonged, or worsening infections may be associated with a nonviral element. Factors suggesting *acute bacterial sinusitis* are the worsening of the symptoms after five days, the persistence of symptoms for more than 10 days, or the presence of symptoms out of proportion to those typically associated with viral URTI.

2. *Subacute rhinosinusitis* represents a continuum of the natural progression of acute rhinosinusitis that has not resolved. This condition is diagnosed after a four-week duration of acute rhinosinusitis, and it lasts up to 12 weeks. Patients with subacute rhinosinusitis may or may not have been treated for the acute phase, and the symptoms are less severe than those found in acute rhinosinusitis. Thus, unlike in acute rhinosinusitis, fever would not be considered as a major factor. The clinical factors required for the diagnosis of subacute adult rhinosinusitis are the same as for those CRS. Subacute rhinosinusitis usually resolves completely after an effective medical regimen.

3. *Recurrent acute rhinosinusitis* is defined by symptoms and physical findings consistent with acute rhinosinusitis, with these symptoms and findings worsening after five days or when persisting more than 10 days. However, each episode lasts 7 to 10 days or more, and may last up to four weeks. Furthermore, four or more than four episodes occur in one year. Between episodes, symptoms are absent without concurrent medical therapy. The diagnostic criteria for recurrent acute rhinosinusitis are otherwise identical to those of acute rhinosinusitis.

4. *Chronic rhinosinusitis* is rhinosinusitis lasting more than 12 weeks. The diagnosis is confirmed by the major and minor clinical factor complex (Table 4) with or without findings on the physical examination. A strong history consistent with chronic rhinosinusitis includes the presence of two or more major factors, or one major and two minor factors. A history suggesting that CRS should be considered in the differential diagnosis includes two or more minor factors or one major factor. Facial pain does not contribute a strong history in the absence of other nasal factors.

5. *Acute exacerbation of chronic rhinosinusitis* represents sudden worsening of the baseline CRS with either worsening or new symptoms. Typically the acute (non-chronic) symptoms resolve completely between occurrences.

The advantage of the TFR classification (5) over the Princeton meeting classification (23) is that no CT scan is needed, and the diagnosis is made on clinical grounds only (i.e., major and minor factors and duration). Williams et al. demonstrated that the overall clinical impression that takes into account 16 historical items is more accurate than a single physical examination in predicting the presence of rhinosinusitis (28). Another advantage of the TFR guidelines is that they do not include nasal endoscopy or radiological imaging, and so they are not only applicable to the specialist but also to the primary care physician. Kenny et al. (29) and Duncavage (30), in a prospective study at the Vanderbilt Asthma Sinus and Allergy Program evaluating the AAO-HNS guidelines, found that the severity of sinus pain/pressures and sinus headache did not correlate with CT scan findings. On the other hand, the severity of five other symptoms (fatigue, sleep disturbance, nasal discharge, nasal blockage, and decreased sense of smell), either alone or in combination, correlated with the severity of the CT scan findings of sinusitis.

In another study, Orlandi et al. presented their experience with the TFR guidelines in diagnosing chronic rhinosinusitis and reevaluated these guidelines three years after publication (31). They found that these criteria provide a relatively sensitive (88%) working definition of chronic sinusitis in a patient population scheduled for surgery. Nasal obstruction/blockage and facial congestion/fullness were the most common symptoms. Their "gold standard" for the definition of chronic sinusitis is a patient who has symptoms for more than 12 weeks, evidence of rhinosinusitis that was discovered on CT, and an inflammation that was found on the analysis of pathology specimens.

Hwang et al. (32) found a poor agreement between the rhinosinusitis TFR set forth positivity of symptoms—based on diagnostic guidelines for CRS—and the CT scan positivity. The sensitivity of the TFR criteria for detecting a positive scan was 89%, but the specificity was poor at only 2%. Finally, Stankiewicz et al. compared 78 patients that met the TFR criteria of subjective diagnosis with CT scan findings and endoscopy (Table 5) (33). They found that in 78 patients with a positive subjective diagnosis based on the TFR criteria, 53% had a negative CT scan and 45% had a negative endoscopy and a negative CT scan. When they looked at the number of patients with negative endoscopy and negative CT scans, and negative endoscopy and minimal disease on the CT scan, then endoscopy was correlated with CT scanning in about 80% of the patients. However, the sensitivity and specificity of endoscopy versus CT scan were 74% and 84%, respectively. On a cost-analysis basis, they conclude that endoscopy performed by a specialist should be used to corroborate the diagnosis. According to these authors, an evidence-based and reliable subjective symptom score correlating better with endoscopy and CT scan is needed (33).

Table 5 Total Patients in the Study Fulfilling the TFR Criteria for the Subjective Diagnosis of Chronic Rhinosinusitis $n = 78$ (100%)

CT scan positive for rhinosinusitis	47%
CT scan negative for rhinosinusitis	53%
Endoscopy positive, CT positive	22%
Endoscopy positive, CT negative	8%
Endoscopy negative, CT positive	26%
Endoscopy negative, CT negative	45%
Negative endoscopy correlated with CT	65%

Source: Adapted from Ref. 33.

Bhattacharyya (34) stated that the scientific basis for grouping major and minor symptoms in the TFR guidelines was not clear. According to the author, criteria justifying the classification of a symptom as "major" could include a higher prevalence in patients with CRS, a higher severity level, or an increased specificity of the symptom for the diagnosis of CRS. In a prospective study of 120 patients with CRS, the major symptoms of CRS were both more prevalent and manifest to a more severe degree than in patients without CRS. Fatigue, considered by the guidelines to be a minor symptom, was a more common and severe symptom manifestation of CRS in the patient population. When looking at the anatomical symptom domains [nasal (nasal obstruction, rhinorrhea, and sense of smell), facial (facial pain/pressure, facial congestion/fullness, and headache), oropharyngeal (halitosis, dental pain, and cuff and ear symptoms), and systemic], they found that the nasal and paranasal symptoms were the most likely manifestations to be found in patients with CRS.

Finally, in 1998 (13), part of the Joint Task Force on Practice Parameters representing the American Academy of Allergy, Asthma and Immunology, The American College of Allergy, Asthma and Immunology, and the Joint Council of Allergy, Asthma and Immunology, defined sinusitis as an inflammation of one or more of the paranasal sinuses, but they immediately add that the most common cause of sinusitis is infection. In their definition, the borderline between acute and chronic depends on the clinician and extends from three weeks to eight weeks.

It is obvious from all these classifications and definitions that there still exists a controversy between the duration of acute and chronic sinusitis and the use of the term subacute sinusitis. If the term subacute sinusitis is not used, the duration of chronic sinusitis in the adult population is defined to be more than eight weeks (23); if the term subacute is used, the duration is more than 12 weeks (TFR guidelines) (5). One of the reasons the TFR guidelines reintroduced the concept of subacute sinusitis is that a duration of 8 to 12 weeks for the term acute sinusitis was considered to be too long, whereas a duration of no more than four weeks seemed to be more appropriate.

The TFR of the AAO-HNS states that their definitions were based on an amended list of the major and minor clinical symptoms and signs believed to be most significant for the accurate clinical diagnosis of all forms of adult rhinosinusitis (5). Anterior rhinoscopy performed in the decongested nose revealed hyperemia, edema, crusting, polyps, and/or, most significantly, purulence in the nasal cavity. This statement is of importance because it included the presence of nasal polyps or nasal polyposis in the definition of CRS. Hadley et al., also a members of the TFR, stated when discussing clinical evolution of rhinosinusitis, that CRS may predispose patients to nasal polyposis, which aggravates hyposmia and may lead to anosmia. This statement supports the opinion of several authors (35) who view nasal polyposis as a subgroup of CRS. However, the lack of a good definition of nasal polyps or nasal polyposis makes utilization of this definition difficult.

According to Stedman's Medical Dictionary, a polyp is a general descriptive term with reference to any mass of tissue that bulges or projects outwards or upwards from the normal surface level, thereby macroscopically visible as a hemispheroidal, spheroidal, or irregular mound-like structure, growing from a relatively broad base or a slender stalk (36). Dorland defines a polyp as a morbid excrescence or protruding growth from mucous membrane, classically applied to a growth on the mucous membrane of the nose (37). This means that any spheroidal outgrowth of the nasal mucosa in the nose or the paranasal sinuses is to be considered a nasal polyp. Some authors, however, consider chronic sinusitis and nasal polyposis as different diseases of the respiratory mucosa of the paranasal sinuses (38). They define every polyp that can be seen by endoscopy as nasal polyposis and any polyp in the sinuses as hyperplasia. Ponikau stated that, in the Mayo Clinic, they consider nasal polyposis the end stage of the chronic inflammation process of chronic rhinosinusitis rather than two different diseases (39). According to these authors, CRS is an inflammatory disease of the nasal and paranasal sinuses that is present for more than three months, and is associated with inflammatory changes ranging from polypoid mucosa thickening to gross nasal polyps. Orlandi et al. were not able to see a significant difference between the number of major and minor factors of patients with or without nasal polyps (31). They only found that nasal dryness/crusting (not a TFR factor) was more prevalent in patients with nasal polyposis. Also, the Sinus and Allergy Health Partnership Taskforce (SAHP) described that one of the signs of inflammation must be present and identified in association with ongoing symptoms [TFR guidelines (Table 4) (5)], consistent with CRS (40). The presence of discolored nasal drainage arising from the nasal passages, nasal polyps, or polypoid swelling as identified on a physical examination with anterior rhinoscopy or nasal endoscopy. Finally, in a position paper on rhinosinusitis and nasal polyps, the European Academy of Allergy and Clinical Immunology (EAACI) stated that chronic sinusitis is the primary disease and nasal polyposis is its subpopulation (41).

According to Hamilos, (42) inflammation plays a key role in CRS. This author describes two types of inflammation that occur in sinusitis, contributing variably to the clinical expression of disease; those are the infectious inflammation that is most clearly associated with acute sinusitis, resulting from either bacterial or viral infection, and the noninfectious inflammation that is so named due to the predominance of the eosinophils and the mixed mononuclear cells, and relative paucity of neutrophils commonly seen in CRS. Mucosal thickening, sinus opacification, and nasal polyposis are seen at both ends of the spectrum (43). In some, cases intensive treatment with antibiotics and a short course of prednisone caused near-complete resolution of mucosal thickening and sustained improvement of symptoms. Such cases represent the infectious end of the spectrum. In other cases, similar treatment causes minimal regression in mucosal thickening or nasal polyposis, and minimal improvement in symptoms. Such cases can be considered as at the inflammatory end of the spectrum. Nasal polyps are most characteristic of noninfectious sinusitis but cannot be strictly categorized as infectious and noninfectious. Therefore, Hamilos (43) prefers the descriptive term "chronic hyperplastic sinusitis with nasal polyposis" or CHS/NP because it avoids implication of disease pathogenesis. CHS/NP has the following features:

1. Presence of chronic sinusitis
2. Extensive bilateral mucosal thickening
3. Nasal polyposis (usually bilateral)
4. Without obvious underlying disease, such as hypogammaglobuli-nemia, cystic fibrosis, or immotile cilia syndrome

In Hamilo's experience (43), asthma and aspirin-sensitivity are associated with CHS/NP in 62% and 49%, respectively, of their patients. According to Hamilos (43), a distinguishing feature of mucosal pathology of CHS/NP is tissue eosinophilia that is accompanied by an infiltrate of mononuclear cells, T cells, and plasma cells, neutrophilia being uncommon, occurring in only 25% of nasal polyps (44).

THE CLASSIFICATION OF FUNGAL SINUSITIS

Ponikau et al. (45,46) confirmed the presence of sinus eosinophilia in the majority (96%) of their patients with CRS by means of histological analysis of 101 consecutive patients. In the same study, they also found fungal organisms, as examined on the basis of culture (96% of patients) and histology (81%), in the sinus mucus of patients with CRS, suggesting that these organisms might be involved in the disease process of CRS. However, to their surprise, fungal organisms were also detected in the nasal mucosa of the majority of healthy control subjects. They concluded that the combination of eosinophilia and the presence of fungi explain the chronic inflammation in 96% of the patients with CRS.

As further proof of their theory, Ponikau et al. (39,45) highlighted their observation that in 51 randomly selected patients given the diagnosis of CRS and treated with intranasal amphotericin B lavage, 75% experienced a significant improvement of nasal symptoms, especially nasal discharge and nasal obstruction and 36% had a polyp-free nasal endoscopy. In those where a control CT scan was performed, they observed an improvement of the sinus opacification. The authors admit that the potential weakness of their pilot study is the fact that they did not include a placebo group. The statement of the Ponikau group from the Mayo Clinic that the majority of the CRS cases are caused by an abnormal eosinophilic response of the patient to fungi initiated an intense controversy about the validity of the fungal hypothesis (see the following sections).

In 1976, Safirstein (47) described a 24-year-old woman with allergic bronchopulmonary aspergillosis (ABPA) associated with nasal obstruction, nasal polyps, and nasal cast formation. Millar et al. (48) and Katzenstein et al. (49) mentioned the histological similarity between sinus mucoid material and mucoid impaction of the bronchi in patients with ABPA, and they named it "allergic aspergillus of the maxillary sinus" and "allergic aspergillus sinusitis," respectively. The latter (49) described the typical mucin-containing numerous eosinophils, sloughed respiratory cells, cellular debris, Charcot-Leyden crystals, and scattered fungal hyphae resembling *Aspergillus* species.

Waxman et al. (50) described the clinical features of a young adult patient with allergic aspergillus sinusitis, showing a history of asthma and recurrent polyposis, radiographic evidence of pansinusitis, and the typical mucinous material as described by Katzenstein et al. (49). The majority of their patients had positive skin tests for *Aspergillus* (60%), 85% had IgE serum levels, and 85% had precipitins to *Aspergillus*. Robson et al. (51) introduced the term "allergic fungal sinusitis" (AFS) after they described a case of an expansive tumor of the paranasal sinus caused by the rare fungal pathogen *Bipolaris hawiiensis*.

Corey et al. (52) stressed the importance of the host's immunological status, local tissue condition, and histopathological examination to differentiate among different forms of fungal disease. They differentiate between:

1. *Allergic fungal sinusitis* as the sinus counterpart of ABPA; patients showing chronic sinusitis can be atopic and show elevated IgE levels and eospinophilic counts in the peripheral blood.
2. *Fungal ball or aspergilloma* due to massive fungal exposure or local tissue anoxia. Patients are not immunocompromised.
3. *Invasive or fulminent fungal sinusitis* occurring in immunocompromised patients.

Other authors (53) also define AFS (previously allergic aspergillus sinusitis) as a chronic sinusitis with nasal polyposis in young immunocompetent patients, showing diffuse expansive sinus disease on CT scan, with the typical allergic mucine described earlier. All their patients had positive IgE RAST to fungal antigens.

Taking into account the immune status of the patient, Bent et al. (54) categorize fungal sinusitis into five subgroups: the role of the fungi, the presence of tissue invasion, the cause, and the affected sinus. A similar classification for fungal sinusitis was already published earlier by Ence et al. (55).

1. *Invasive fungal sinusitis* is an acute fungal sinusitis affecting one sinus in an immunocompromised patient, showing tissue invasion.

2. *Indolent fungal sinusitis* is a subacute sinus infection with variable tissue invasion of one or more sinuses in a nonatopic immunocompetent patient.
3. *Mycetoma or fungal ball* is a chronic saprophytic sinusitis of one sinus without tissue invasion in a non-atopic immunocompetent patient.
4. *AFS* is a chronic fungal sinusitis in an immunocompetent atopic patient, where the fungus acts as an allergen involving multiple sinuses with a unilateral predominance without tissue invasion. The patient must demonstrate the characteristic allergic mucine and have evidence of fungal etiology, either by direct observation in the surgical specimen, or by recovery of the organism in cultures of the sinus content.
5. *AFS like syndrome*: these patients have the same features as AFS patients, however, without the presence of fungi. Cody et al. (56) found that 40% of these patients with allergic mucin have AFS-like syndrome. Ferguson (57) named this AFS-like syndrome "Eosinophilic Mucin Rhinosinusitis" (EMR) stating that the driving force is not a fungus but a systemic dysregulation associated with upper and lower eosinophilia.

In 1995, deShazo et al. (58) described the criteria for the diagnosis of AFS in his study as follows:

1. Sinusitis of one or more paranasal sinuses on x-ray film
2. Identification of allergic mucin by rhinoscopy or at the time of the sinus surgery or subsequently on histopathological evaluation of material from the sinus
3. Documentation of fungal elements in nasal discharge or in material obtained at the time of surgery by stain or culture
4. Absence of diabetes, previous or subsequent immunodeficiency disease, and treatment with immunosuppressive drugs
5. Absence of invasive fungal disease at the time of diagnosis or subsequently

From the criteria for the diagnosis of AFS listed by deShazo and Swain (58), for these authors absence of atopy, asthma, nasal polyps, elevated IgE levels, and serum fungal precipitins do not exclude the diagnosis of AFS. Furthermore, bilateral involvement of the sinus on x-ray examination does not exclude the diagnosis either.

On the basis of immunopathological findings in ABPA and AFS, Corey et al. (59) concluded that both represent Gell and Coombs type I and type III response. In AFS, IgG antibodies, in addition to elevated IgE antibodies, to the specific fungus in the serum can be demonstrated. Therefore, they suggest the following immunological workup: total eosinophil count, total serum IgE, fungal antigen-specific IgE in vitro testing and/or skin test, fungal antigen-specific IgG (if available), and precipitating antibodies (if available).

In 1998, Manning et al. (60) showed that AFS is an antigen, IgE-and IgG-mediated, hypersensitivity response with a late-phase eosinophilic inflammatory reaction. On the basis of immunohistocytochemistry studying major basic protein (MBP) eosinophil-derived neurotoxin (EDN) and a neutrophils mediator (neutrophils elastase) in tissue samples of CRS, they also showed that in all cases there was evidence that MBP and EDN mediator-release predominated over neutrophils elastase, proving that AFS is a predominantly eosinophilic-driven disease.

In a controversial publication, Ponikau et al. (46) reevaluated the recurrent criteria for diagnosing AFS in CRS. By using a novel method of mucous collection and fungal-culturing technique, the authors demonstrated allergic mucin in 96% of 101 consecutive surgical cases of CRS. In the majority of their patients, they were not able to find an IgE-mediated hypersensitivity to fungal antigens. Since the presence of eosinophils in allergic mucin, and not a type I hypersensitivity, was likely the common denominator in the pathophysiology of AFS, they proposed a change of terminology from AFS to "eosinophilic fungal rhinosinusitis (EFR)." Similar results were found by Braun et al. (61). Other authors had their doubts about the validity of the Mayo Clinic hypothesis (46). Marple (62) questioned whether fungi are indeed ubiquitous and are present within 100% of normal noses, and wondered what separates those patients who develop AFS from the normal population. He also questioned if the fungal screening methods used in the study were so sensitive that normal fungal colonization was mistaken for AFS, or if CRS merely represents an early form of clinically recognized AFS.

Although it is generally accepted that eosinophils play an important role in the development of both AFS and some forms of CRS, the factors that ultimately trigger eosinophilic inflammation remain in question. Riechelmann et al. (63) disagree with the EFR theory. They were able to show the presence of fungi only in 50% of the patients with nasal polyposis when using the most sensitive detection techniques. Ragab et al. (64), using the same culture technique used by Ponikau et al. (46), were able to show positive fungal cultures in 44% of the middle meatal lavage and in 36% of the nasal cavity lavage of patients with CRS. It seems, therefore, that the rate of positive lavages is dependent of the site of collection of the sample.

The question whether fungi are present in the upper airways inducing an eventual eosinophilic response may not be relevant because the presence of these fungi can be a mere epiphenomenon of an unknown cause that initially induced the CRS. The fungi may have not been adequately removed by the mucociliary clearance and ultimately resulted in an eosinophilic response.

Novey et al. (65) showed that a normal person inhales about 50 million spores a day. With normal mucociliary clearance, these fungal spores are removed adequately and do not have the time to germinate and release their toxins. Once the fungi are not cleared because of an unknown cause, fungi start to colonize the sinuses and may contribute to the maintenance or amplification of the disease. The therapeutical results with antifungal agents such as amphotericin B lavage (39,45) or nasal spray (66) do not strongly support the role of fungi in CRS, as only in 35% to 43%, respectively, of the nasal cavities become disease-free.

Bernstein et al. (67), who are recently studying the molecular biology and immunology of nasal polyps, were unable to demonstrate that fungi play a principal role in CRS. Their data (67) support the hypothesis that *Stapylococcus aureus* releases a variety of enterotoxins (superantigens) in the nasal mucus that induce an interaction of antigen-presenting cells and lymphocytes, resulting in an up-regulation of inflammatory cells (lymphocytes and eosinophils) following an up-regulation of cytokines (TFN, IL-1β, IL-4, and IL-5). Bachert et al. (68) described IgE antibodies to *S. aureus* enterotoxins in polyp tissue, linked to a polyclonal IgE production and aggravation of eosinophilic inflammation. A similar mechanism was described by Perez-Novo et al. (69) in aspirin-sensitive nasal polyposis patients. If this hypothesis proves to be true, then the classification of fungal sinusitis needs to be reconsidered and the definitions redefined. It also illustrates that the constancy of the classifications based on the hypothetical causes is not very reliable.

Finally, Ferguson (57) described a visible growth of fungus (in AFS or EFR the fungus is not visible to the naked eye) within the nasal cavity of an asymptomatic individual and uses the term "saprophytic fungal infestation" for this condition.

THE CLASSIFICATION OF PEDIATRIC RHINOSINUSITIS

During the last decade, three manuscripts have been published that classified pediatric rhinosinusitis (6,70,71). The Lusk et al. guidelines (70) were an extension of the TFR guidelines of the AAO-HNS (5) using the same classifications. The Clement report (6) consisted of an International Consensus Meeting (ICM), primarily of otorhinolaryngologists, and the Wald et al. (71) clinical practice guideline was a consensus of the Subcommittee on Management of Sinusitis and Committee on Quality Improvement of the American Academy of Pediatricians (SMS/CQI-AAP). The three classifications of pediatric rhinosinusitis are similar, and therefore, their definitions and classification can be discussed together:

1. *Acute rhinosinusitis* in children is defined as an infection of the sinuses mostly introduced by a viral infection, where complete

Table 6 Symptoms of Severe and Non-severe Pediatric Rhinosinusitis

Non-severe	Severe
Rhinorrhea of any quality	Purulent rhinorrhea (thick, opaque, colored)
Nasal congestion	Nasal congestion
Cough	Peri-orbital edema
Headache, facial pain, and irritability (variable)	Facial pain and headache
Low grade or no fever	High fever ($\geq$39 °C)

Source: From Ref. (6).

resolution of symptoms (judged on a clinical basis only) without intermittent URTI may take up to 12 weeks (ICM) (6). Acute sinusitis can be further subdivided into severe and nonsevere (Table 6).

The SMS/CQI-AAP guideline (71) introduces the concept of *acute bacterial rhinosinusitis* (ABRS) complicating an *acute viral rhinosinusitis*. ABRS is an infection of the paranasal sinuses, lasting less than 30 days, in which symptoms resolve completely. According to Mucha et al. (72) the diagnosis of ABRS should be considered after a viral URI, when symptoms worsen after five days, are present for longer than 10 days, or are out of proportion to those seen with most viral infections.

To cover the duration gap between acute and chronic, the SMS/CQI-AAP guideline (71) also introduced the concept of "subacute bacterial sinusitis" in children as an infection of the paranasal sinuses lasting between 30 and 90 days in which symptoms resolve completely. The term subacute sinusitis was not recommended by the ICM (6) in Brussels, as the difference between acute and subacute is very arbitrary and it does not imply a different therapeutic approach in children.

2. *Recurrent acute rhinosinusitis* in children are episodes of the bacterial infection of the paranasal sinuses separated by intervals during which the patient is asymptomatic. According to the SMS/CQI-AAP guideline (71), these episodes last less than 30 days and are separated by intervals of at least 10 days.

3. *Chronic rhinosinusitis* in children is defined as a nonsevere sinus infection with low-grade symptoms that presents longer than 12 weeks.

4. Finally, *recurrent acute rhinosinusitis* in children has to be differentiated from *chronic rhinosinusitis* with frequent exacerbations (ICM) (6) or acute bacterial sinusitis superimposed on chronic

sinusitis (SMS/CQI-AAP) (71). These are patients with residual respiratory symptoms who develop new respiratory symptoms. When treated with antimicrobials, these new symptoms resolve, but the underlying residual symptoms do not.

The members of the ICM noted that medical treatment such as antibiotics and nasal steroids may modify symptoms and signs of acute and CRS, and it is sometimes difficult to differentiate infectious rhinosinusitis from allergic rhinosinusitis in a child on clinical grounds alone. According to the SMS/CQI-AAP, a viral infection in children induces a diffuse mucositis and predisposes to a bacterial infection of the sinuses in 80% of cases whereas in 20% of the cases an allergic inflammation is responsible for the bacterial superinfection.

In conclusion, an internationally well-accepted classification of rhinosinusitis in adults as well as in children that is based on duration of signs and symptoms exists. However, there still exists much controversy concerning the classification of fungal sinusitis. This classification is controversial because it is based on the eventual cause of CRS, which is still not well understood.

REFERENCES

1. Douek E. Acute sinusitis. In: Ballentyne J, Groves J, eds. Scott-Brown's Diseases of the Ear, Nose and Throat, 3rd ed. The Nose. London: Butterworths, 1972:183–213.
2. Shapiro GG, Rachelefsky GS. Introduction and definition of sinusitis. J Allergy Clin Immunol 1992; 90:417–418.
3. Johnson JT, Ferguson BJ. Infection. In: Cummings CW, Fredrickson JM, Harker LA, Krause CJ, Richardson MA, Schuller DE, eds. Otolaryngology Head and Neck Surgery. Vol. 2. 3rd ed. St Louis: Mosby, 1998:1107–1108.
4. Lund VJ, Kennedy DW, Draf W, Friedman WH, Gwaltney JM, Hoffman SR, Huizing EA, Jones JK, Lusk RP, MacKay IS, Moriyana H, Nacleirio RM, Stankiewicz JA, van Cauwenberge P, Vining EM. Quantification for staging sinusitis. Ann Otol Rhinol Laryngol 1995; 104(suppl 167):17–22.
5. Lanza D, Kennedy DW. Adult rhinosinusitis defined. Otolaryngol Head Neck Surg 1997; 117:S1–S7.
6. Clement PAR, Bluestone CD, Gordts F, Lusk RP, Otten FWA, Goossens H, Scadding GK, Takahashi H, van Buchem L, van Cauwenberge P, Wald ER. Management of rhinosinusitis in children. Arch Otolaryngol Head Neck Surg 1998; 124:31–34.
7. Havas TE, Motbey JA, Gullane PJ. Prevalence of incidental abnormalities on computed tomographic scans of the paranasal sinuses. Arch Otolaryngol Head Neck Surg 1988; 114:856–859.
8. Bolger WE, Butzin CA, Parsons DS. Paranasal sinus bony anatomic variations and mucosal abnormalities CT analysis for endoscopic sinus surgery. Laryngoscope 1991; 101:56–64.

9. Diament MJ, Senac MO, Gilsanz V, Baker S, Gillespie T, Larsson S. Prevalence of incidental paranasal sinuses opacification in pediatric patients: a CT study. J Comput Assist Tomogr 1987; 3:426–436.

10. Gordts F, Clement PAR, Buisseret Th. Prevalence of sinusitis signs in a non-ENT population. ORL 1996; 58:315–319.

11. Gordts F, Clement PAR, Destryker A, Desprechin B, Kaufman L. Prevalence of sinusitis signs on MRI in a non-ENT pediatric population. Rhinology 1997; 35:154–157.

12. Pinheiro AD, Facer GW, Kern EB. Sinusitis: current concepts and management. In: Bailey BJ, Calhoun KH, eds. Head and Neck Surgery–Otolaryngology. Vol. 1. 2nd ed. Philadelphia, New York: Lippincott-Raven, 1998:441–445.

13. Spector SL, Bernstein IL, Li JT, Berger WE, Kaliner MA, Schuller DE, Blessing-Moore J, Dykewicz MS, Fineman SF, Lee RE, Nicklas RA. Complete guidelines and references. Parameters for the Management of Sinusitis. Supplement to J Allergy Clin Immunol 1998; 102:S117–S124.

14. Kern EB. Sinusitis. J Allergy Clin Immunol 1984; 73:25–31.

15. McNab J. The Caldwell-Luc and allied operations. In: Dudley H, Carter D, Nose and Throat Consultant editor Ballantyne JC, Harrison DFN, eds. Rob and Smith's Operative Surgery. 4th ed. London: Butterworths, 1986:116–120.

16. Wigand ME. Transnasale, endoskopische Chirurgie der Nasennebenhöhlen bei Chronische Sinusitis. I. Ein bio-mechanisches Konzept der Schleimhautchirurgie. HNO 1981; 29:215–221.

17. Wigand ME. Transnasale, endoskopische Chirurgie der Nasennebenhöhlen bei Chronische Sinusitis. II. Die endonasale Kieferhöhlen Operation. HNO 1981; 29:263–269.

18. Reilly JS. The sinusitis cycle. Otolaryngol Head Neck Surg 1990; 103:856–862.

19. Mygind M. Perennial rhinitis. In: Mygind M, ed. Nasal Allergy. Oxford: Blackwell Scientific Publications, 1987:224–232.

20. Iwens P, Clement PAR. Sinusitis in allergic patients. Rhinology 1994; 32:65–67.

21. Gwaltney JM, Philips CD, Miller RD, Riker DK. Computed tomographic study of the common cold. N Eng J Med 1994; 330:25–30.

22. Leopold DA, Stafforrd CT, Sod EW, Szeverenyi NM, Allison JD, Phipps RJ, Juhlin KD, Welch MB, Saunders C. Clinical course of acute maxillary sinusitis documented by sequential MRI scanning. Am J Rhinol 1994; 8:19–28.

23. Kennedy DW. Sinus disease. Guide to first-line management. In: Kennedy DW, ed., Health Communications. Intermedia Partners, 1994:1–44.

24. Lund VJ, Gwaltney J Jr, Baquero F, Echols R, Kennedy D, Klossek J-M, MacKay I, Mann W, Ohnishi T, Stammberger H, Vinig E, Wald E, Burridge SM. Infectious rhinosinusitis in adults: classification, etiology and management. ENT J 1997;12(suppl 76):1–22.

25. Evans FO Jr, Sydnor JB, Moore WE, Moore GR, Manwaring JL, Brill AH, Jackson RT, Hanna S, Skaar JS, Holdeman LV, Fitz-Hugh S, Sande MA, Gwaltney JM Jr. Sinusitis of the maxillary antrum. N Engl J Med 1975; 293:735–739.

26. Gwaltney JM Jr, Scheld M, Sande MA, Sydnor A. The microbial etiology and antimicrobial therapy of adults with acute community-acquired sinusitis: a

fifteen-year experience at the University of Virginia and review of other selected studies. J Allergy Clin Immunol 1992:457–462.

27. Senturia BH, Bluestone CD, Lim DJ. Report of the Committee on definitions and classifications of otitis media and otitis media with effusion. Am Otol Rhinol Laryngol 1980; (suppl 68):89.

28. Williams JW Jr, Simel DL, Roberts L, Samsa GP. Clinical evaluation of sinusitis. Making the diagnosis by history and physical examination. Ann Intern Med 1992; 117:705–710.

29. Kenny TJ, Duncavage J, Bracikowski J, Yildirim A, Murray JJ, Tanner SB. Prospective analysis of sinus symptoms and correlation with paranasal computed tomographic scan. Otolaryngol Head Neck Surg 2001; 125:40–43.

30. Duncavage JA. Rhinosinusitis, Editorial Commentary. Curr Opin Otorlaryngol Head Neck Surg 2001; 9:1–2.

31. Orlandi RR, Terrell JE. Analysis of the adult chronic rhinosinusitis working definition. Am J Rhinol 2002; 16:7–10.

32. Hwang PH, Irwin SB, Griest SE, Caro JE, Nesbit G. Radiologic correlates of symptom-based diagnostic criteria for chronic rhinosinusitis. Otolaryngol Head Neck Surg 2003; 128:489–196.

33. Stankiewicz JA, Chow JM. Cost analysis in the diagnosis of chronic sinusitis. Am J Rhinol 2003; 17:139–142.

34. Bhattacharyya N. The economic burden and symptoms manifestations of chronic rhinosinusitis. Am J Rhinol 2003; 17:27–32.

35. Hadley JA, Schaefer SD. Clinical evaluation of rhinosinusitis: history and physical examination. Otolaryngol Head Neck Surg 1997; (suppl 117):S9–S11.

36. Stedman's Medical Dictionary. 26th ed. Baltimore: Williams and Wilkins, 1995:1405.

37. Dorland's Illustrated Medical Dictionary. 25th ed. Philadelphia: Saunders WB, 1965:1235.

38. Watelet J-P, Gevaert P, Bachert C, Holtappels G, van Cauwenberge P. Secretion of TGF-B1, TGF-B2, EGF and PDGF into nasal fluid after sinus surgery. Eur Arch Otorhinolaryngol 2002; 259:234–238.

39. Ponikau JU. Antifungal nasal washes for chronic rhinosinusitis: what's therapeutic—the wash or the antifungal? J Allergy Clin Immunol 2003; 111: 1137–1139.

40. Benninger MS, Ferguson BJ, Hadley JA, Hamilos DL, Jacobs M, Kennedy DW, Lanza DC, Marple BF, Osguthorpe JS, Stankiewicz JA, Anon J, Denneny J, Emanuel I, Levine H. Adult chronic sinusitis: definitions, diagnosis, epidemiology and pathophysiology. Otolaryngol Head Neck Surg 2003; 129:S1–S32.

41. Fokkens W, Lund V, Bachert C, Clement P, Hellings P, Holmstrom M, Jones N, Kalogjera L, Kennedy D, Kowalski M, Malburborg H, Mullel J, Passali D, Stammberger H, Stierna P. EAACI Position paper on rhinosinusitis and nasal polyps. Allergy 2005; 60:583–601.

42. Hamilos DL. Chronic sinusitis. J Allergy Clin Immunol 2000; 106:213–227.

43. Hamilos DL. Non infectious sinusitis. Allergy Clin Immunol Int 2001; 13: 27–32.

44. Hamilos DL, Leung DYM, Wood R, Meyers A, Stephens JK, Barkans J, Meng Q, Cunningham L, Bean DK, Kay AB, Hamid Q. Chronic hyperplastic sinusi-

tis: association of tissue eosinophilia with mRNA expression of granulocyte-macrophage colony-stimulating factor and interleukine-3. J Allergy Clin Immunol 1993; 92:39–40.

45. Ponikau JU, Sherris DA, Kita H, Kern EB. Intranasal antifungal treatment in 51 patients with chronic rhinosinusitis. J Allergy Clin Immunol 2002; 110:862–866.
46. Ponikau JU, Sherris DA, Kern EB, Homburger HA, Frigas E, Gaffey TA, Roberts GD. The diagnosis and incidence of allergic fungal sinusitis. Mayo Clin Proc 1999; 74:877–884.
47. Safirstein BH. Allergic bronchopulmonary aspergillosus with obstruction of the upper respiratory tract. Chest 1976; 70:788–790.
48. Miller JW, Johnston A, Lamb D. Allergic aspergillosus of the maxillary sinus. Prod Scott Thor Soc 1981; 36:710.
49. Katzenstein AL, Sale Sr, Greenberger PA. Pathologic findings in allergic aspergillus sinusitis. A newly recognized form of sinusitis. Am J Surg Pathol 1983; 7:439–443.
50. Waxman JE, Spector JG, Sale SR, Katzenstein A-LA. Allergic aspergillus sinusitis: concepts in diagnosis and treatment of a new clinical entity. Laryngoscope 1987; 97:261–266.
51. Robson JM, Hogan PG, Benn RA, Gatenby PA. Allergic fungal sinusitis presenting as a paranasal sinus tumour. Aust NZJ Med 1989; 19:351–353.
52. Corey JP, Delsupehe KG, Ferguson BJ. Allergic fungal sinusitis: allergic, infectious or both. Otolaryngol Head Neck Surg 1995; 113:110–119.
53. Manning SC, Mabry RL, Schaefer SD, Close LG. Evidence of IgE-mediated hypersensitivity in allergic fungal sinusitis. Laryngoscope 1993; 103:717–721.
54. Bent JP, Kuhn FA. Diagnosis of allergic fungal sinusitis. Otolaryngol Head Neck Surg 1994; 111:580–588.
55. Ence BK, Gourley DS, Jorgensen NL, Shagets FW, Parsons DS. Allergic fungal sinusitis. Am J Rhinol 1990:169–178.
56. Cody DT, Neel BN, Fereiro JA, Roberts GD. Allergic fungal sinusitis: The Mayo Clinic experience. Laryngoscope 1994; 104:1074–1079.
57. Ferguson BJ. Eosinophilic mucin rhinosinusitis: a distinct clinicopathologic entity. Laryngoscope 2000; 110:799–813.
58. deShazo RD, Swain RE. Diagnostic criteria for allergic fungal sinusitis. J Allergy Clin Immunol 1995; 96:24–35.
59. Corey JP, Romberger CF, Shaw G. Fungal disease of the sinuses. Otolaryngology 1990; 103:1012–1015.
60. Manning SC, Holman M. Further evidence for allergic pathophysiology in allergic fungal sinusitis. Laryngoscope 1998; 108:1485–1496.
61. Braun H, Buzina W, Freudenschuss K, Beham A, Stammberger H. Eosinophilic fungal rhinosinusitis: a common disorder in Europe? Laryngoscope 2003; 113:264–269.
62. Marple BF. Allergic fungal rhinosinusitis: current theories and management strategies. Laryngoscope 2001:1006–1019.
63. Riechelmann H. Pilze aund Polypen—Fakten und mythen. Laryngol Rhinol Otol 2003; 82:766–768.
64. Ragab A, Clement P, Vincken W, Simones F, Nolard N. Fungal cultures of different parts of upper and lower airways in chronic rhinosinusitis 2004. In press.

65. Novey HS. Epidemiology of allergic bronchopulmonary aspergillosis. Immunol Allergol N Am 1998; 18:641–653.
66. Lacroix J-S. Effects of antifungal local treatment on nasal polyposis.In: Mladina R, ed. Nasal Polyposis. Zagreb, Croatia: Croation Medical Association, 2002:42–44.
67. Bernstein JM, Ballow M, Schlievert PM, Rich G, Allen C, Dryja D. A superantigen hypothesis for the pathogenesis of chronic hyperplastic sinusitis with massive polyposis. Am J Rhinol 2003; 17:321–326.
68. Bachert C, van Zele T, Gevaert P, De Schrijver L, van Cauwenberge P. Superantigens and nasal polyposis. Curr Allergy Asthma Rep 2003; 3:523–531.
69. Perez-Novo CA, Kowalski ML, Kuna P, Ptasinska A, Johansson S, Bachert C. Asperin sensitivity and IgE antibodies to *Staphylococcus aureus* enterotoxins in nasal polyposis: studies on the relationship. Int Arch Allergy Immunol 2004; 133:257–260.
70. Lusk RP, Stankiewicz JS. Pediatric sinusitis. Otolaryngol Head Neck Surg 1997; 117:S53–S57.
71. Wald ER, Bordley WC, Darrow DH, Grimm KT, Gwaltney JM Jr, Marcy SM, Senac MO, Williams PV. Clinical practice guideline: management of sinusitis. Am Ac of Pediatrics, Subcommittee on management of sinusitis. Pediatrics 2001; 108:798–808.
72. Mucha SM, Baroody FM. Sinusitis update 2003. Curr Opin Allergy Clin Immunol 3:33–38.

3

Rhinosinusitis: Clinical Presentation and Diagnosis

Michael S. Benninger and Joshua Gottschall

Department of Otolaryngology–Head and Neck Surgery, Henry Ford Hospital, Detroit, Michigan, U.S.A.

INTRODUCTION

It is a widely held assertion that the diagnosis of bacterial rhinosinusitis is made too often (1). This is due to the inherent difficulty in making an accurate diagnosis. Many diagnostic challenges exist when evaluating patients with presumed rhinosinusitis. Since the sinuses cannot be observed directly, the diagnosis is dependent upon the history of present illness and is often aided by nonspecific symptoms and physical examination. Primary care physicians are at a particular disadvantage as they do not have ready access to nasal endoscopy or antral puncture with fluid analysis, which at times are helpful for establishing a diagnosis. Particularly challenging is differentiating between a self-limiting upper respiratory tract infection (URTI) or "common cold" and allergy from an acute bacterial rhinosinusitis (ABRS). The most common symptoms of rhinosinusitis include nasal congestion, purulent rhinorrhea, facial pressure or pain, and anosmia or hyposmia. These symptoms are not unique to rhinosinusitis and may be features of other inflammatory processes of the sinonasal tract. Frequently, a recent viral infection or underlying allergy precedes the development of ABRS, and thus makes the diagnosis of rhinosinusitis all the more difficult.

The current health care environment also poses inherent challenges for physicians. Reduced time per office visit, direct advertising by pharmaceutical corporations, and expectations of patients or caregivers may result in a hasty diagnosis of rhinosinusitis and the inappropriate administration of antibiotics. Clearly, prescribing antibiotics for viral or nonbacterial illness is inappropriate. However, more serious consequences of this action include the promotion of bacterial resistance, mild-to-serious drug reactions, and increased health care costs. These inherent challenges, along with the difficulty of establishing an accurate diagnosis of rhinosinusitis, have contributed to the estimated US $5.8 billion in overall health care expenditures attributed to rhinosinusitis each year (2). Thus, the accurate diagnosis of rhinosinusitis in both the adult and pediatric populations cannot be overemphasized.

DEFINITIONS

Sinusitis refers to an inflammatory process localized within one or more of the paranasal sinuses, whereas *rhinitis* is an inflammatory process within the nasal cavity. Since it is unusual for sinusitis to be present without a concurrent rhinitis, *rhinosinusitis* may be a more appropriate descriptor for this clinical disease process. Rhinosinusitis has recently been defined as "a group of disorders characterized by inflammation of the mucosa of the nose and paranasal sinuses" (3). This definition has two important features: the understanding that rhinosinusitis is a group of disorders with a number of different potential etiologies, and that the hallmark is inflammation, whether that inflammation is caused by an infection or some other inflammatory process. In this chapter, ABRS will specifically refer to a bacterial infection of the sinonasal tract unless stated otherwise. Chronic rhinosinusitis (CRS) may be associated with a number of different disorders or pathogenic mechanisms.

In order to facilitate the management of rhinosinusitis and to improve communication amongst health care professionals, definitions of rhinosinusitis for both the adult and pediatric age groups have been adopted. These definitions have been temporally related from the onset of symptoms and include ABRS, subacute bacterial rhinosinusitis, and CRS (Table 1). ABRS is defined as a bacterial infection of the paranasal sinuses lasting less than

Table 1 Rhinosinusitis: Definitions

	Duration of symptoms
Acute bacterial rhinosinusitis (ABRS)	<30 days
Subacute bacterial rhinosinusitis	>30 and <90 days
Chronic rhinosinusitis (CRS)	>90 days

Source: Adapted from Ref. 12.

30 days. In general, the symptoms resolve completely. Symptoms persisting longer than 10 days or worsening after five days more likely due to ABRS. *Subacute bacterial rhinosinusitis* is a bacterial infection of the paranasal sinuses lasting between 30 and 90 days with a similar presentation as seen in acute rhinosinusitis. CRS has recently been redefined as "a group of disorders characterized by inflammation of the mucosa of the nose and paranasal sinuses of at least 12 consecutive weeks' duration" (3). Patients often have persistent residual respiratory symptoms such as rhinorrhea or nasal obstruction. Two additional categories of rhinosinusitis further describe patients based upon frequency of infection. *Recurrent acute bacterial rhinosinusitis* is defined as multiple episodes of bacterial infection of the paranasal sinuses, each lasting for at least 7 to 10 days but less than 30 days, and separated by intervals of at least 10 days during which the patient is asymptomatic. Patients with recurrent acute bacterial sinusitis typically have four or more such infections per year. *Acute exacerbation of chronic rhinosinusitis* occurs when individuals with CRS develop new acute respiratory symptoms. When treated with antimicrobials, these new symptoms resolve, but the underlying chronic symptoms do not. True recurrent acute bacterial rhinosinusitis tends to be relatively infrequent. Patients that fit this profile are more likely to have recurrent viral URTIs or acute exacerbations of CRS rather than true recurrent acute rhinosinusitis.

To facilitate the diagnosis of rhinosinusitis, it may be useful to consider whether the sinonasal infection is a result of primary or secondary factors. Rarely is any one factor the sole cause of rhinosinusitis. More commonly, multiple medical conditions or underlying disorders can be found, which often complicates treatment. Rhinosinusitis due to primary factors is typically found in otherwise healthy individuals. The pathology is limited to the sinonasal tract. Medical treatment of the acute infection or the surgical correction of mucous outflow obstruction generally results in resolution of symptoms and overall improvement. Rhinosinusitis due to secondary factors is less common. Rhinosinusitis in these individuals is a consequence of an underlying systemic disease process or condition, predisposing patients to the development of rhinosinusitis as well as other infections. Examples of secondary factors include aspirin intolerance (Sampter's triad), immunodeficiency, primary ciliary dyskinesia, and cystic fibrosis. Treatment of the systemic disorder, in general, results in reduction in severity or resolution of the rhinosinusitis. A list of causative factors associated with the development of rhinosinusitis is seen in Table 2.

PATHOPHYSIOLOGY

The pathophysiology of rhinosinusitis is multifactorial. However, regardless of etiology, the common basis for the development of sinus disease is often associated with mucous stasis due to osteomeatal obstruction and/or

Table 2 Factors Predisposing to Bacterial Rhinosinusitis

Primary (local) factors	Secondary (systemic) factors
Viral URI	Diabetes mellitus
Allergic/nonallergic rhinitis	Inhalant/food allergies
Anatomic obstruction	Immune deficiency
Deviated septum	HIV
Concha bullosa	Hypogammaglobulinemia
Paradoxic middle turbinate	Iatrogenic
Maxillary dental disease	Asthma
Medication effects	ASA intolerance (sampter's)
Rhinitis medicamentosa	Mucociliary disorders
Cocaine	Primary ciliary dyskinesia
Air pollution/irritants	Cystic fibrosis
Gastroesphageal reflux disease	Pregnancy
Nasal polyposis	Hypothyroidism
Neoplasm	Autoimmune
	Sarcoidosis
	Wegener's granulomatosis

mucociliary dysfunction. Persistent obstruction results in decreased oxygen tension, reduced sinus pH, ciliary dysfunction, and negative pressure within the sinus cavity. Sneezing or nose blowing may cause a transient opening of the sinus drainage pathways. This, in addition to negative pressure within the sinus cavity, may result in the inoculation of pathogenic bacteria from the nasal cavity or nasopharynx into an otherwise sterile sinus cavity (4). An optimal environment for overgrowth is thereby achieved, resulting in rhinosinusitis. There has been a great interest in identifying pathways for the development of CRS. The inflammatory roles of bacteria and fungi, and the subsequent response by inflammatory cells and production of mediators of inflammation, have generated new thinking regarding the pathophysiology (3). A noninfectious inflammatory response as a result of bacterial or fungal colonization resembling "allergic or asthmatic" inflammation has been described. The resultant host inflammatory response with production of inflammatory cytokines may be the underlying cause of CRS. Of particular interest in this area are the roles of bacterial and fungal allergy, eosinophilic inflammation, biofilms, and superantigens (3).

RHINOSINUSITIS OR UPPER RESPIRATORY TRACT INFECTION?

Rhinosinusitis is most often a sequela of an acute URTI (5). Viruses responsible for URTIs include rhinovirus, parainfluenza virus, influenza virus type A and B, coronavirus, respiratory syncytial virus, and adenovirus.

Rhinovirus is implicated in approximately 50% of common colds (1). In addition to osteomeatal obstruction due to inflammation and edema, respiratory viruses may have a direct cytotoxic effect on the nasal cilia that may result in impaired mucociliary clearance long after resolution of the acute viral infection. Rhinovirus has also been shown to increase the adherence of pathogenic bacteria, such as *Streptococcus pneumoniae* and *Hemophilus influenzae* in the nasopharynx, increasing the likelihood of bacterial colonization and infection (6).

In the United States, the incidence of acute respiratory illness due to the common cold is two–three/year in the adult with 0.5% to 2% progressing into an ABRS (7). Children on average have six to eight upper respiratory infections per year, with 5% to 10% progressing into ABRS (8). Due to this reason, children may be particularly susceptible to rhinosinusitis.

The time from onset of symptoms was found to play an important role in differentiating URTI from rhinosinusitis. Most viral URTI will begin to improve within seven days and completely resolve by 10 days. Symptoms worsening after seven days or persisting for 10 days or more are highly suggestive of bacterial rhinosinusitis (1,9).

DIAGNOSIS OF RHINOSINUSITIS

Clinical investigations regarding the diagnosis of rhinosinusitis have been difficult until recently, due to a lack of consensus for the definition of rhinosinusitis. In 1996, the Rhinosinusitis Task Force of the American Academy of Otolaryngology–Head and Neck Surgery published general criteria for the diagnosis of rhinosinusitis (10). Diagnosis is based upon the time from onset of symptoms, as well as the number and type of symptoms present. Thus, the diagnosis of rhinosinusitis is dependent upon establishing a time frame for the disease and then applying clinical criteria to assure the diagnosis.

History

Individuals with rhinosinusitis may present with symptoms of nasal congestion, nasal discharge, facial pressure or pain, hyposmia, or anosmia. The pain of acute rhinosinusitis is typically a stabbing pain or ache, localized over the involved sinus. Thus, pain may provide a clue as to which sinus is involved (Table 3). Maxillary sinus pain may elicit infraorbital tenderness extending to the maxillary teeth and occasionally to the ear. Ethmoid pain is typically reported between the eyes and over the nasal dorsum. Frontal pain may present as headaches extending to the temple or occiput. Isolated sphenoid sinus pain may present with headache, particularly at the vertex of the skull. Headaches and facial pain are rarely associated with rhinosinusitis, unless a concomitant nasal symptom is present.

Table 3 Pain and Associated Sinus Involvement

Sinus	Associated pain
Maxillary	Infraorbital, maxillary teeth, referred otalgia
Ethmoid	Medial canthus, nasal dorsum
Frontal	Supraorbital, bitemporal, occipital
Sphenoid	Vertex of skull

Children with rhinosinusitis may have a different presentation compared to their adult counterparts. Since young children are unable to verbalize their complaints, they may present with irritability as their only symptom. Sinus pain is not a prominent feature; however, children may have nasal obstruction and purulent rhinorrhea. Cough is a feature that may be seen in children with rhinosinusitis, which is typically not seen with adults. It may occur during the day or night; however, the cough is particularly worse at night. Rhinosinusitis is the second most common cause of chronic cough in children (11). Other symptoms include foul breath, bronchial hyperresponsiveness, and periorbital edema. The periorbital edema is usually non-tender and is usually seen on the dependent side and is worse upon awakening.

The symptoms of nasal congestion/obstruction, facial pressure/pain, nasal purulence or rhinorrhea, and anosmia/hyposmia are considered major symptoms. The presence of two major symptoms is sufficient for the diagnosis of rhinosinusitis (12). Cough is a minor symptom in adults, but a major symptom when seen in children. Minor symptoms include headache, irritability, fever, halitosis, fatigue, dental pain, and ear pain. The presence of one major symptom and two minor symptoms is also sufficient for the diagnosis of rhinosinusitis (Table 4) (12). Although symptoms and time-based criteria may be appropriate in making the diagnosis in ABRS, they have been insufficient in CRS (3). A diagnosis of CRS is best made through a combination of symptoms and time-based criteria as in ABRS, but supported by nasal endoscopy or radiologic testing.

A thorough history of present illness is required for all patients, particularly to identify the secondary causes of rhinosinusitis. Features of the history important when evaluating an individual for rhinosinusitis include presenting symptoms, onset and duration of symptoms, and associated comorbid disorders. A history of asthma, aspirin intolerance, nasal polyposis, and rhinosinusitis is consistent with the ASA intolerance syndrome (Sampter's triad). This entity is difficult to treat, with persistent bronchial hyperreactivity, despite treatment of rhinosinusitis. Immune deficiencies including HIV, common variable immune deficiency, and IgG and IgA hypogammaglobulinemia are associated with recurrent rhinosinusitis. Patients with a history of recurrent pneumonia, otitis media, sterility,

Table 4 Factors Associated with the Diagnosis of Chronic Sinusitis

Major factor	Minor factors
Facial pain, pressure (alone does not constitute a suggestive history for rhinosinusitis in absence of another major symptom)	Headache
Facial congestion, fullness	Fever (all non-acute)
Nasal obstruction/blockage	Halitosis
Nasal discharge/purulence/discolored nasal drainage	Fatigue
Hyposmia/anosmia	Dental pain
Purulence in nasal cavity on examination	Cough
Fever (acute rhinosinusitis only) in acute sinusitis alone does not constitute a strongly supportive history for acute in the absence of another major nasal symptom or sign	Ear pain/pressure/fullness

Source: Adapted From Ref. 12.

and rhinosinusitis should be evaluated for primary ciliary dyskinesia. Patients with Kartagener's syndrome present with primary ciliary dyskinesia, rhinosinusitis, situs inversus, and bronchiectasis.

Perennial or seasonal allergies may present with symptoms such as nasal congestion, cough, and behavioral changes, which are seen in both allergic rhinitis and rhinosinusitis. It may be the underlying etiology in failed antimicrobial therapy directed at presumed rhinosinusitis. Symptoms and signs consistent with allergies include sneezing, clear nasal secretions, and itchy mucous membranes of the upper aerodigestive tract. Allergies can play a significant role in recurrent acute and chronic rhinosinusitis. All patients should be evaluated for allergies when the history is elicited, with a focus on both food and inhalant allergies, such as dust mite, mold, dander, and pollen (13). There may be a history of rhinosinusitis coinciding with the allergy season. The tendency to have allergy is genetically determined and therefore is reflected in the family history. If one parent has a history of allergy problems, any child in that family has a 20% to 40% chance of having an allergic disease. If both parents have allergy problems, any child has a 50% to 70% chance of having allergic manifestations at some time in his/her life (14). In 13% of children with a negative allergy history, skin testing is nevertheless positive. This has prompted some to advocate formal allergy testing in all cases of CRS who failed medical treatment, and prior to proceeding with surgery (15). Appropriate allergy skin testing or in vitro tests (RAST, ELISA, and IgE) may be performed. In vitro tests for allergy are useful in young children who may not tolerate skin testing.

Gastroesphageal reflux disease, or GERD, has been implicated as an underlying etiology of CRS, especially in children. Double lumen pH probe analysis of children with CRS has demonstrated esophageal reflux in 63% of patients and nasopharyngeal reflux in 32% (16). Seventy-nine percent of patients had improvement in CRS symptoms after medical treatment of GERD. In a separate study, 89% of patients initially deemed as candidates for sinus surgery avoided an operation after reflux treatment (17).

Patients with a history of maxillofacial trauma may present with recurrent rhinosinusitis or CRS due to disruption or obstruction of the osteomeatal drainage pathways. Complete resolution of recurrent symptoms may require surgical correction of the anatomic obstruction. Occasionally mucosa may be trapped within the fracture line, resulting in the development of a mucocele or a mucopyocele and CRS.

Nasal neoplasm, both benign and malignant, may be a cause of unilateral nasal symptoms and rhinosinusitis due to obstruction of the nasal cavity and sinus drainage pathways. Unilateral nasal polyposis unresponsive to corticosteroid therapy should raise the index of suspicion for a nasal neoplasm. Care must be taken to rule out CNS tissue prior to biopsy.

Inflammatory nasal polyposis is seen in bilateral nasal cavities and responds well to systemic and topical corticosteroid therapy. They may result from chronic nasal inflammation, often associated with nasal allergies. Inflammatory polyposis often has the classic "water bag" appearance. Any child with nasal polyposis should be evaluated for cystic fibrosis.

Physical Examination

Intranasal examination may provide clues for the diagnosis of rhinosinusitis. However, this is often nonspecific and thus greater emphasis is placed upon the aforementioned symptoms-driven diagnostic criteria. Intranasal examination is facilitated through the use of a nasal speculum, handheld otoscope, or nasal endoscopes, including fiber-optic and rigid types (Fig. 1). The examination of the mucosal linings of the symptomatic nose may demonstrate generalized rhinitis with erythema and edema. The inferior turbinates, often engorged, may limit visualization beyond the anterior aspect of the inferior turbinate. Topical decongestion with alpha-adrenergic agonist, such as oxymetazoline, permits an improved visualization of the middle turbinate and middle meatus. Nasal purulence may be seen along the floor of the nasal cavity. The color of the mucous is not a dependable sign to differentiate a bacterial infection from a viral URTI. Distinguishing between purulent-appearing nasal secretions from an infected sinus versus colonized stagnant secretions from the nasal cavity or chronic adenoiditis may also prove difficult. However, purulence found within the middle meatus is highly suggestive of rhinosinusitis. Nasal polyposis may be seen, and should be characterized based upon its growth beyond the anatomic limits of the middle meatus. This may be useful to document response to therapy. Occasionally, differentiating a nasal polyp from the middle

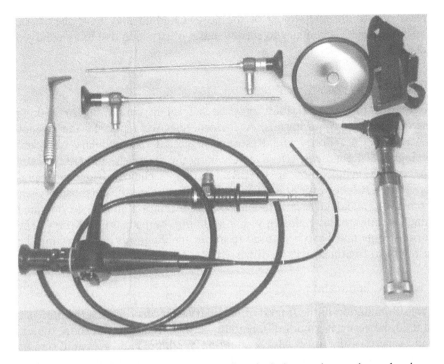

Figure 1 Tools for intranasal examination include nasal specula and mirror, otoscope, fiber-optic endoscope, and rigid telescope.

turbinate may be a source of confusion. Palpation of the structure after application of topical 2% pontocaine may reveal a firm, tender structure more consistent with that of the middle turbinate.

Significant anatomic causes of obstructed sinonasal drainage should be noted, including septal deviation or spurring, concha bullosa, and paradoxical middle turbinate. Occasionally, adequate assessment of the lateral nasal wall may be problematic. Percussion over the maxillary and frontal sinus may elicit tenderness, which is, however, largely nonspecific. Oral cavity examination may demonstrate an oro-antral fistula, poor dentition, or dental abscess. Purulent drainage from the nasopharynx may be seen in the posterior oropharynx.

In young children or adults with mental illness, a foreign body must be considered, especially in cases of unilateral purulent rhinorrhea. The drainage is usually foul-smelling. An otoscopic examination may demonstrate otitis media. Due to its communication with the nasopharynx via the eustachian tube, in children the middle ear may be considered a paranasal sinus. Children with rhinosinusitis may have an associated otitis media. If allergy is present, the patients may display allergic shiners and a supratip crease due to chronic wiping of the nose. Children may have the classic "adenoid facies" secondary to chronic nasal obstruction due to an enlarged adenoid.

Diagnostic Aids

A number of diagnostic aids may be helpful in confirming or making the diagnosis of rhinosinusitis. An evidenced-based report by the Agency for Health Care Policy and Research suggested that ancillary tests and radiographs are not cost-effective in making the diagnosis, and are typically unnecessary in uncomplicated ABRS. Rather, a clinical diagnosis is preferred. In CRS, however, it is recommended that unless the diagnosis is clear from history and physical examination, confirmation should be obtained either through nasal endoscopy, CT scanning, or plain sinus X-rays. The various tools that have been used to aid in the diagnosis and assessing the response to treatment will be discussed.

Transillumination

Transillumination of the frontal or maxillary sinus may suggest the presence of fluid; however, it cannot differentiate between fluid opacification, tumor, and agenesis of the sinus. Also, evaluation of ethmoid and sphenoid sinuses is not feasible. The utility of transillumination in the diagnosis of rhinosinusitis is questionable and would not likely facilitate the diagnosis or treatment. Transillumination may have some value in confirming the diagnosis or assessing the response to treatment, if it were positive at the onset of treatment and negative later. Since clinical response may be a better measure, transillumination has little value (18).

Rigid or Flexible Endoscopy

Rigid or flexible endoscopy gives the diagnostician unparalleled access to the nose for the evaluation of the lateral nasal wall, which may otherwise not be possible on anterior rhinoscopy (Fig. 2). The anatomy of the middle meatus can be carefully evaluated. The presence of accessory ostia may be confused for the natural os. Small polyps or purulence within the middle meatus may be seen. Evaluation of the sphenoethmoidal recess is possible by directing a fiber-optic scope along the floor of the nose and then directing the tip 90 degrees cephalad (toward the top of the head). In children, evaluation of the nasopharynx may demonstrate chronic adenoiditis.

Cultures may be taken from the middle meatus during rigid nasal endoscopy. Although culture of the sinus cavity itself is not obtained, a strong correlation between endoscopic culture of the middle meatus and antral puncture with culture has been reported. Endoscopically obtained cultures demonstrate a sensitivity of 85.7%, and a specificity of 90.6% when

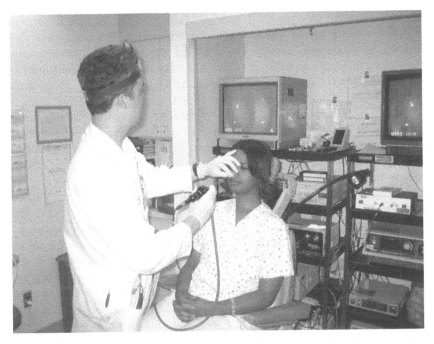

Figure 2 Intranasal examination using 0° rigid telescope with video documentation.

compared to sinus puncture (19–21). Culture of the nasal cavity in the absence of frank purulence will likely yield nasal flora, and thus would not be useful. Although culture-directed therapy is ideal, treatment of uncomplicated cases of rhinosinusitis is presumptive, and is directed at *S. pneumoniae, H. influenzae, and Moraxella catarrhalis.* However, cultures should be considered in patients who have failed previous therapy, have a history of immunodeficiency, or have poorly controlled diabetes mellitus. Although the concordance between cultures obtained from antral puncture and those endoscopically obtained from the middle meatus appear promising, not enough evidence currently exists to recommend this technique over antral puncture.

Sinus Aspiration and Culture

Although sinus aspiration and culture are considered the gold standard for the diagnosis of rhinosinusitis, they are rarely indicated in uncomplicated cases. The cost, need for specialty referral, and discomfort experienced by the patient need to be considered. Although generally safe, sinus puncture has been associated with rare but serious complications, including tissue emphysema, air embolism of venous channels, vasovagal reactions, and soft tissue or bony infection (19). Although adult patients readily tolerate the procedure in an outpatient setting, children often require a general anesthetic. As previously stated, initial treatment of ABRS is presumptive, directed at the most commonly identified organisms (*S. pneumoniae, H.Influenzae, M. catarrhalis*) (1). The majority of cases of rhinosinusitis would likely resolve even without antibiotics. Positive cultures are recovered in only 50% to 60% of patients diagnosed with rhinosinusitis (7,19,20).

The maxillary sinus is readily accessible through a canine fossa approach or via the inferior meatus. In children, an inferior meatal approach is preferred since it carries less risk to the dentition and orbit. This is performed under general anesthesia and often in conjunction with adenoidectomy.

A sublabial, canine fossa sinus puncture is well tolerated, and can be performed in the office setting with minimal morbidity. Commercial kits are readily available (Fig. 2). A specialist finds the procedure simple to perform and accurate results can be obtained as long as proper steps are taken to prevent contamination (Table 5). The aspirated fluid should be noted for its gross appearance. Aerobic and anaerobic cultures as well as gram stain should be obtained. Fungal cultures can be obtained if the index of suspicion is high.

Individuals with rhinosinusitis who have failed multiple courses of antibiotics and those with immune suppression should be considered for sinus aspiration and culture. Those individuals with infection extending to the orbit or threatened intracranial extension should be scheduled for emergency surgery. However, critically ill patients who are not operative candidates may tolerate sinus aspiration quite well. This procedure may prove to be therapeutic as well as diagnostic.

Quantitative cultures may assist in identification of the pathogenic organism from nasal flora. The recovery of bacteria in a density of at least 10^4 colony-forming units (CFU)/mL is considered representative of a true infection (8). Also, the finding of at least one organism per high power field on gram stain is significant, and correlates with the recovery of bacteria in a density of 10^5 CFU/mL (8).

Table 5   Procedure for Maxillary Sinus Puncture

Approach through the canine fossa or inferior meatus
  Prepare site with topical antiseptic (Betadine)
  Local (1% lidocaine/1:100,000 epinephrine) infiltrated with 27-gauge needle
  Trocar and catheter is inserted into maxillary sinus directed away from orbit
  Withdraw trocar and aspirate
  If no frank pus, inject 2 cc sterile saline into maxillary sinus and aspirate
  Therapeutic irrigation of maxillary sinus with 60 cc sterile saline
  Specimen sent for gram strain, aerobic, and anaerobic cultures

---

Limitations of sinus aspiration include the inability to sample the sphenoid and ethmoid sinuses. Frontal sinus sampling would engender risk to the brain and would be inadvisable. Contamination by oral or nasal flora may result in misleading results; however, quantitative cultures may prove more reliable.

Imaging

The role of imaging is discussed in detail in another chapter, and will only be briefly described here. Plain sinus radiographs have long been used to aid in the diagnosis of rhinosinusitis. Given the poor sensitivity and specificity and the likelihood of abnormal findings even with a viral URTI, plain sinus radiographs have little value in ABRS. They have not been shown to be cost-effective (18). They may be helpful in confirming the diagnosis of CRS in patients who have appropriate signs and symptoms for a sufficient duration of time, but cannot be confirmed by a nasal examination, particularly where endoscopy is not available (3). Ultrasound has also been used, particularly in Europe, but has similar if not greater limitations compared to plain sinus films (18).

CT scanning is considered the radiographic modality of choice. Although limited in differentiating ABRS from a viral URTI (22), CT scans are very useful in CRS (3) or in assessing the suspected complications of either ABRS or CRS. MRI scan is generally considered to be of limited value in the evaluation of rhinosinusitis at this time (3).

Ancillary Tests

There are a number of ancillary tests that may be helpful in assessing the severity of disease or the response to treatment. These include measures of smell (such as the University of Pennsylvania Smell Identification Test or UPSIT), measures of nasal airflow or resistance by acoustic rhinometry or rhinomanometry, the Electronic Nose, or various blood tests. As mentioned previously, allergy testing may be useful, particularly in those with a strong allergic history or family history, or who have had a poor response to directed therapy.

Outcome Evaluations

An area of great recent interest in many diseases and disorders over the last few years are the methods to evaluate quality of life (QOL) and outcomes. Rhinosinusitis has been well studied in relationship to QOL and outcomes, and a few tools or instruments have been specifically designed to evaluate this specific entity. Three commonly used instruments are the Rhinosinusitis Disability Index (RSDI) (23), the Sino–Nasal Outcomes Test (SNOT) (24), and the Chronic Sinusitis Survey (CSS) (25). The RSDI was specifically developed to assess rhinosinusitis, although it has more recently been validated for other nasal and sinus disorders, including allergic and non-allergic rhinitis. Although there are some differences between these instruments, they all serve to establish a level of function for rhinosinusitis patients and may be used to evaluate the response to treatment.

CONCLUSION

Many symptoms of rhinosinusitis are common to other nasal inflammatory diseases such as the common cold and seasonal or perennial allergy. The diagnosis of both pediatric and adult rhinosinusitis is best made based upon clinical criteria (3), with a large portion of the diagnosis being based upon the duration of symptoms into acute, subacute, and chronic subtypes. The duration of symptoms is supported by the number and type of symptoms as well as physical findings. Thus, the diagnoses are dependent upon establishing a time frame for the disease and then applying clinical criteria to assure the diagnosis. Ancillary diagnostic evaluation should be considered on a case-by-case basis. However, nasal endoscopy or CT scan should be part of the diagnostic evaluation of CRS. Culture-directed therapy is not cost-effective in cases of routine ABRS and is not recommended. The physician should rely on the understanding of the pathophysiology and natural history of rhinosinusitis to make an accurate diagnosis and institute an appropriate treatment plan.

REFERENCES

1. Sinus and Allergy Health Partnership. Antimicrobial treatment guidelines for acute bacterial rhinosinusitis. Otolaryngol Head Neck Surg 2004; 130(suppl 1): S1–S50.
2. Ray NF, Baraniuk JN, Thamer M, Rinehart CS, Gergen PJ, Kaliner M, Josephs S, Pung YH. Healthcare expenditures for sinusitis in 1996: contributions of asthma, rhinitis, and other airway disorders. J Allergy Clin Immunol 1999; 103:408–414.
3. Benninger MS, Ferguson BJ, Hadley JA, Hamilos DL, Jacobs M, Kennedy DW, Lanza DC, Marple BF, Osguthorpe JD, Stankiewicz JA, Anon J, Denneny J, Emanuel I, Levine H. Adult chronic rhinosinusitis: definitions, diagnosis, epidemiology, and pathophysiology. Otolaryngol Head Neck Surg 2003; 129(3): S1–S32.
4. Benninger MS, Anon J, Mabry RL. The medical management of rhinosinusitis. Otolaryngol Head Neck Surg 1997; 117:S41–S49.
5. Kaliner M. Medical management of sinusitis. Am J Med Sci 1998; 316(1):21–28.
6. Fainstein V, Musher DM, Cate TR. Bacterial adherence to pharyngeal cells during viral infection. J Infect Dis 1980; 141(2):172–176.
7. Gwaltney JM. Acute community-acquired sinusitis. Clin Infect Dis 1996; 23: 1209–1225.
8. Wald ER. Sinusitis. Pediatr Rev 1993; 14(9):345–351.
9. American Academy of Pediatrics. Subcommittee on Management of Sinusitis and Committee on Quality Improvement. Clinical practice guideline: management of sinusitis. Pediatrics 2001; 108(3):798–808.

10. Anon JB. Report of the rhinosinusitis task force committee meeting: alexandria, Virginia, August 17th, 1996. Otolaryngol Head Neck Surg 119;117(3 Pt 2): S1–S68.
11. Holinger LD. Chronic cough in infants and children. Laryngoscope 1986; 96: 316–322.
12. Lanza DC, Kennedy DW. Adult rhinosinusitis defined. Otolaryngol Head Neck Surg 1997; 117:S1–S7.
13. Goldsmith AJ, Rosenfeld RM. Treatment of pediatric sinusitis. Pediatr Clin North Am 2003; 50:413–426.
14. Cook PR, Nishioka GJ. Allergic rhinosinusitis in the pediatric population. Otolaryngol Clin North Am 1996; 29:29–56.
15. Parsons DS. Chronic sinusitis: a medical or surgical disease? Otolaryngol Clin North Am 1996; 29(1):1–9.
16. Phipps CD, Wood WE, Gibson WS, Cochran WJ. Gastroesophageal reflux contributing to chronic sinus disease in children. Arch Otolaryngol Head Neck Surg 2000; 126:831–836.
17. Bothwell MR, Parsons DS, Talbot A, Barbero GJ, Wilder B. Outcome of reflux therapy on pediatric chronic sinusits. Otolaryngol Head Neck Surg 1999; 121:255–262.
18. Benninger MS, Holzer S, Lau J. Diagnosis and treatment of acute bacterial rhinosinusitis: summary of the Agency on Health Care Policy and Research's Evidence Based Report. Otolaryngol Head Neck Surg 2000; 122:1–7.
19. Benninger MS, Applebaum PC, Denneny J, Osguthorpe JD, Stankiewicz J, Zucker D. Maxillary sinus puncture and culture in the diagnosis of acute bacterial rhinosinusitis: the case for pursuing other culture methods. Otolaryngol Head Neck Surg 2002; 127:7–12.
20. Talbot GH, Kennedy DW, Scheld M, Granito K. Rigid nasal endoscopy versus sinus puncture and aspiration for microbiologic documentation of acute bacterial maxillary sinusitis. Clin Infect Dis 2001; 33:1668–1675.
21. Gold S, Tami T. Role of middle meatus aspiration culture in the diagnosis of chronic sinusitis. Laryngoscope 1997; 107(12):1586–1589.
22. Gwaltney JM, Phillips CD, Miller RD, Riker DK. Computed tomographic study of the common cold. N Engl J Med 1994; 330(1):25–30.
23. Benninger MS, Senior B. The development of the rhinosinusitis disability index (RSDI). Arch Otolaryngol Head Neck Surg 1997; 123:1175–1179.
24. Piccirillo J, Merritt J, Richards M. Psychometric and clinimetric validity of the 20-item sino-nasal outcome test. Otolaryngol Head Neck Surg 2002; 126: 41–47.
25. Gliklich R, Hilinski J. Longitudinal sensitivity of generic and specific health measures in chronic rhinosinusitis. Qual Life Res 1995; 4:27–32.

4

Imaging Sinusitis

Nafi Aygun, Ovsev Uzuner, and S. James Zinreich
*The Russell H. Morgan Department of Radiology and Radiological Sciences,
The Johns Hopkins Medical Institution, Baltimore, Maryland, U.S.A.*

INTRODUCTION

Radiological imaging is complementary to the clinical and endoscopic evaluation of patients with rhinosinusitis. The diagnosis of this pathological entity is made clinically and with the help of endoscopy. Imaging is an essential part of presurgical evaluation and monitoring of difficult-to-treat, recurrent, postsurgical disease. In patients in whom there might be clinical suspicion of a noninflammatory pathology, imaging can be extremely helpful in distinguishing the various pathological entities.

AVAILABLE IMAGING MODALITIES

Plain Sinus Radiograph

Plain radiographic evaluation of the paranasal sinuses has fallen out of favor despite its wide availability and comparatively low cost. The overall sensitivity and specificity of plain radiographs for sinusitis is 40 to 50% and 80 to 90%, respectively (1). The sensitivity approaches clinically acceptable levels only for the diagnosis of maxillary sinus disease (2–4). Generally, for a comprehensive evaluation, four standard views are obtained: lateral view, Caldwell view, Waters' view, and sub-mentovertex or base view. The lateral view shows the bony perimeter of the frontal, maxillary, and sphenoid sinus (Fig. 1). The Caldwell view shows the bony perimeter of the

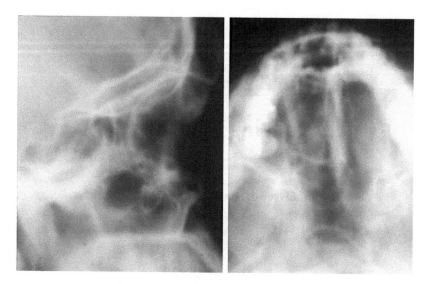

Figure 1 Lateral (*right*) and sub-mentovertical (*left*) views of the sinuses. Plain radiographs lack the sensitivity, specificity, and anatomic precision needed for the evaluation of most patients with sinusitis.

frontal sinus. The Waters' view shows the outlines of the maxillary sinuses, some of anterior ethmoid air cells, and the orbital outline. The sub-mentovertex view evaluates the sphenoid sinus and the anterior and posterior walls of the frontal sinuses (Fig. 1). Evaluation of the ostiomeatal unit (OMU) and the detail of the ethmoid morphology are precluded by this modality.

Computerized Tomography

Computerized tomography (CT) is the imaging standard for sinusitis (5). Its ability to display bone, mucosa, and air makes it a perfect tool for the imaging of the paranasal sinuses. The fine bony architecture of the nasal cavity and the paranasal sinus drainage pathways is accurately depicted with CT examination. CT is very sensitive in detection of mucosal hypertrophy and retained secretions in the paranasal sinuses.

Technique

Single channel CT (SC-CT) scanners use either incremental or helical acquisition schemes for paranasal sinus examination. Coronal images optimally display the anterior ostiomeatal unit, the relationship of the orbits and brain to the paranasal sinuses, and also correlate best with the surgical approach. The slice thickness should be 3 mm or less without interslice gap for optimal evaluation of the key structures such as OMU and frontal recess. Image acquisition in the coronal plane requires an extension of the head, which may not be possible for very young patients and patients with airway problems or neck pain. Thin axial images can be reconstructed in the coronal plane for such patients. Direct sagittal images cannot be obtained with CT.

Multichannel CT (MC-CT) (also called multidetector or multislice CT) scanners have been recently introduced. The single X-ray detector present in SC-CT has been replaced with multiple rows of detectors in MC-CT scanners that allow registration of multiple channels of data with one rotation of the X-ray tube. For example, 16-slice MC-CT equipment has a 16-fold capacity to collect image data per X-ray tube rotation compared to a SC-CT. This increased capacity affords much thinner slices from larger body parts in shorter periods of time. Thin slices permit isotropic data sets in which the voxels (the smallest elements of a data set) are cuboidal. Cuboidal voxels offer excellent reconstruction of images in essentially any plane without degradation of quality. Currently, slices as thin as 0.5 mm can easily be obtained with near-isotropic voxels. Isotropic imaging created a paradigm shift in CT imaging: we are no longer confined to the plane of acquisition. Data can be collected from a body part in any desired plane, and two-dimensional images [multiplanar reconstruction (MPR)] can be displayed in any desired plane (Fig. 2). Real-time interactive manipulation of image data and three-dimensional reconstructions are made possible by high-performance workstations equipped with special software.

Intravenous contrast administration is not necessary for assessment of uncomplicated inflammatory sinus disease. Different shades of gray inherently present in every CT image can be displayed in various "windows" to enhance visualization of certain tissues (e.g., bones and soft-tissues). A window width of 2000 Hounsfield units with a level of –200 Hounsfield units is the most advantageous for inflammatory disease of the paranasal sinuses. These "window levels" afford best display of the narrow air channels. Window settings can easily be changed to highlight certain structures and "hard-copy" films are then printed. Adjustment of window settings is not a post-processing method and does not change the raw data, whereas bone reconstruction algorithms (also called bone filters) manipulate the raw data to best demonstrate the bony detail. Images reconstructed using bone algorithm are recommended for the evaluation of the paranasal sinuses. Evaluation of the soft tissues on these images, however, is very limited, even when the window settings are adjusted for soft tissues (Fig. 3).

Radiation Exposure

The increasing number of CT examinations and desire for high-resolution images inevitably increase the radiation dose to patients. Factors inherent to the individual CT scanner and the patient greatly influence radiation dose. Among many operator adjustable scanning parameters that affect the radiation dose, tube current (milliamper-second, mAs) has the most direct and profound effect on the final radiation dose received by the

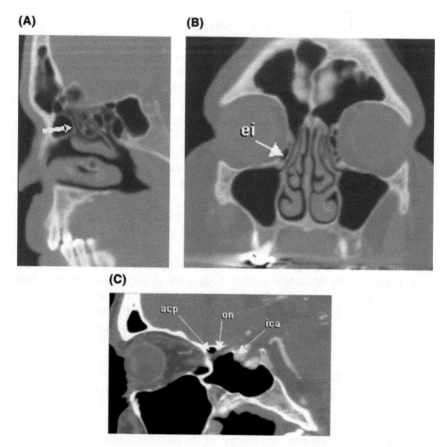

Figure 2 Paradigm shift in CT imaging: images in virtually any plane can be reconstructed from the acquired data set to better demonstrate a certain structure.
(**A**) Oblique-sagittal reconstruction along the frontal sinus outflow tract (*arrow*).
(**B**) Oblique-coronal reconstruction along the ethmoid infundibulum. (**C**) Reconstruction along the optic nerve (on) shows dehiscent nerve canal, pneumatized anterior clinoid process (acp) and protrusion of internal carotid artery (ica) to the
sphenoid sinus.

patient. A considerable reduction in radiation exposure can be achieved by
lowering mAs (6–8). Low mAs results in increased image noise and possible
loss of fine detail. A tube current of 50–80 mAs at 120 kVp tube voltage is a
reasonable compromise and diagnostic accuracy of paranasal sinus CT is
not affected at these settings compared to higher mAs values (9–13). A very
low–radiation dose CT (even lower than four view radiographs) study can
be performed with 10 mAs and noncontiguous slices for patients who
require multiple repeat studies (8). While the radiation exposure to the lens
from sinus CT examination is well below the threshold level believed to

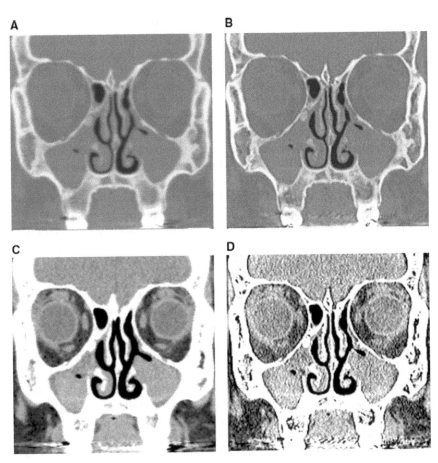

Figure 3 The effect of technical parameters on the appearance of images. (**A**) Bone window with soft-tissue algorithm, (**B**) bone window with bone algorithm, (**C**) soft-tissue window with soft-tissue algorithm and (**D**) soft-tissue window with bone algorithm. Note that the bone detail is better depicted on image (**B**) and soft-tissue is better evaluated on image (**C**). Patient has CRS and prominent osteitis. Note evidence of prior surgery.

induce cataracts, there is a theoretical risk of stochastic effects (e.g., carcinogenesis), which is not dependent on a minimum threshold of exposure. Therefore, judicious use of CT is advised. Multiple examinations with high-dose protocols should be avoided particularly in young patients.

Magnetic Resonance Imaging

Magnetic resonance imaging (MRI)'s exquisite contrast resolution makes it a perfect tool in the imaging of soft tissues. MRI is extremely sensitive to mucosal thickening. In fact, MRI's sensitivity may be too high due to the fact that small increases in volume and signal intensity of the mucosa in the ethmoid sinuses and nasal turbinates can be a reflection of physiological nasal cycle (14). Due to MRI's limited ability to display fine bone detail, its use is limited in diagnostic and presurgical evaluation of uncomplicated inflammatory sinus disease. MRI has proven most helpful in the evaluation of regional and intra-cranial complications of inflammatory sinus disease and their surgical manage-ment, in the detection of neoplastic processes, and in improved display of anatomic relationships between the intra- and extra-orbital compartments. MRI is also useful in the evaluation of mucoceles and cephaloceles.

T1- and T2-weighted MRI obtained in axial and coronal planes provide a satisfactory evaluation of the sinuses. Contrast [gadolinium–diethylenetriaminepentaacetic acid (Gd–DTPA)]-enhanced, fat-saturated T1-weighted images are recommended for a more comprehensive examination.

ANATOMY

Understanding of the anatomy of the lateral nasal wall and its relationship to adjacent structures is essential (15–17). The lateral nasal wall contains three bulbous projections: superior, middle, and inferior turbinates (con-chae). The turbinates divide the nasal cavity into three distinct air passages: the superior, middle, and inferior meati. The superior meatus drains the posterior ethmoid air cells and, more posteriorly, the sphenoid sinus (through the sphenoethmoidal recess). The middle meatus receives drainage from the frontal sinus [through the frontal sinus outflow tract (FSOT)], maxillary sinus (through the maxillary ostium and subsequently the ethmoi-dal infundibulum), and the anterior ethmoid air cells (through the ethmoid cell ostia). The inferior meatus receives drainage from the nasolacrimal duct.

The frontal aeration varies among patients. The frontal sinuses can be small and only occupy the diploic space of the medial frontal bone, or they can be large and extend through the floor of the entire anterior cranial fossa, posterior to the planum sphenoidale. In general, a central septum separates the left and the right sides. The floor of the frontal sinus slopes inferiorly toward the midline. The frontal sinus drains through an hourglass-shaped structure. Some call this entity the frontal sinus outflow tract (FSOT) (Figs. 2A and 4). The superior portion of this outflow tract is a funnel-shaped narrowing called infundibulum in the inferior and medial aspect of the frontal sinus, which leads to the frontal ostium. The frontal ostium forms the waist of the hourglass in the most medial portion of the frontal sinus. The bottom portion of the hour-glass is called the frontal recess, the narrowest portion of this outflow tract, which in turn leads to the superior portion of the middle meatus affording communication with the anterior ethmoid sinus. The frontal recess is neigh-bored by the agger nasi cell anteriorly, the ethmoid bulla posteriorly, and unci-nate process inferiorly (Fig. 4).

A

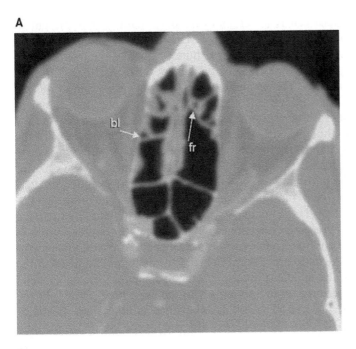

B

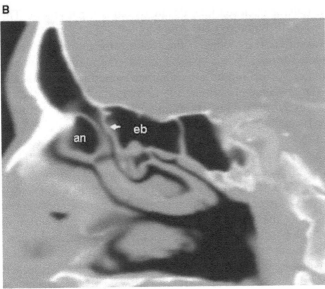

Figure 4 (**A**) Axial and (**B**) oblique sagittal images show the frontal sinus outflow tract (*arrow*) which is mildly narrowed due to circumferential mucosal thickening. *Abbreviations*: EB, ethmoid bulla; BL, basal lamella; AN, agger nasi cell.

The agger nasi cell is an ethmoturbinal remnant that is present in nearly all patients. It is aerated and represents the most anterior ethmoid air cell. It usually borders the primary ostium or floor of the frontal sinus; thus, its size may directly influence the patency of the frontal recess and the anterior middle meatus. The uncinate process is a superior extension of the lateral nasal wall (medial wall of the maxillary sinus). Anteriorly, the uncinate process fuses with the posteromedial wall of the agger nasi cell and the posteromedial wall of the nasolacrimal duct. Laterally, the free edge of the uncinate process delimits the ethmoid infundibulum, which is the air passage that connects the maxillary sinus ostium to the middle meatus. The superior attachment of the uncinate process has three major variations which determine the anatomic configuration of the frontal recess and its drainage (18). These variations are: (1) the uncinate process may extend laterally to attach to the lamina papyracea or the ethmoid bulla forming a terminal recess of the infundibulum and the frontal recess directly opens to the middle meatus (Fig. 5), (2) the uncinate process may extend medially and attaches to the lateral surface of the middle turbinate, (3) the uncinate process may extend medially and superiorly to directly attach to the skull base (Fig 5). In the latter two forms, the frontal recess drains to the infundibulum. Posterior to the uncinate is the ethmoid bulla (Fig 4b), usually the largest of the anterior ethmoid cells.

The ethmoid bulla is enclosed laterally by the lamina papyracea. The gap between the ethmoid bulla and the free edge of the uncinate process defines the hiatus semilunaris. Medially, the hiatus semilunaris communicates with the middle meatus, the air space lateral to the middle turbinate. Laterally and inferiorly, the hiatus semilunaris communicates with the infundibulum by the air channel between the uncinate process and the inferomedial border of the orbit. The infundibulum serves as the primary drainage pathway from the maxillary sinus. The structure medial to the ethmoid bulla and the uncinate process is the middle turbinate. Anteriorly, it attaches to the medial wall of the agger nasi cell and the superior edge of the uncinate process. Superiorly, the middle turbinate adheres to the cribriform plate. As it extends posteriorly, the middle turbinate emits a number of laterally coursing bony attachments. The first of these bony leaflets is the basal or ground lamella that fuses with the lamina papyracea posterior to the ethmoid bulla. The basal lamella demarcates the anterior ethmoid sinus from the posterior ethmoid sinus (Fig. 4A).

In most individuals, the posterior wall of the ethmoid bulla is intact. The air space between the basal lamella and the ethmoid bulla is the retrobullar recess or the sinus lateralis, which may extend superior to the ethmoid bulla forming the suprabullar recess (Fig. 6). The suprabullar recess opens to the frontal recess. Dehiscence or total absence of the posterior wall of the ethmoid bulla is common and may provide communication between these air spaces.

A

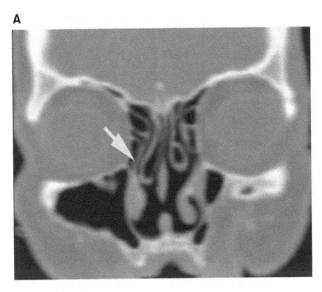

B

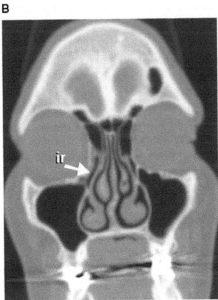

Figure 5 Coronal CT. In the most commonly seen anatomic variation, the uncinate process attaches to the lamina papyracea or the ethmoid bulla. The infundibular recess (ir) is formed between the uncinate process and the orbit. In this variation the frontal sinus outflow tract drains to the middle-meatus.

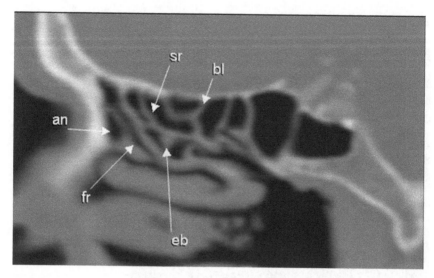

Figure 6 The anatomy of the ethmoid and frontal sinus outflow tract on sagittal CT. *Abbreviations*: AN, agger nasi cell; FR, frontal recess; EB, ethmoid bulla; SR, suprabullar recess; BL, basal lamella.

The posterior ethmoid sinus consists of air cells between the basal lamella and the sphenoid sinus. The number, shape, and size of these air cells vary significantly among persons (19–21).

The sphenoid sinus is the most posterior sinus (Fig. 7). It is usually embedded in the clivus and bordered superoposteriorly by the sella turcica. Its ostium is located medially in the anterosuperior portion of the anterior sinus wall, which in turn communicates with the sphenoethmoidal recess into the posterior aspect of the superior meatus (Fig. 8). The sphenoethmoidal recess lies just lateral to the nasal septum and can sometimes be seen on coronal images, but it is best seen in the sagittal and axial planes.

The relationship between the aerated portion of the sphenoid sinus and the posterior ethmoid sinus needs to be accurately represented so the surgeon can avoid operative complications. Usually in the paramedian sagittal plane, the sphenoid sinus is the most superior and posterior air space. More laterally, the sphenoid sinus is located more inferiorly, and the posterior ethmoid air cells become the most superior and posterior air space. This relationship is seen well on transverse and sagittal images. The number and position of the septa of the sphenoid sinus vary. Some septa can adhere to the bony wall covering the internal carotid artery, which frequently penetrates the sphenoid sinus. Note is to be made that all septations are vertically oriented within the sphenoid sinus. Horizontal bony separations within the area of the sphenoid sinus represent a bony separation between the posterior ethmoid sinus cells above and the sphenoid sinus below.

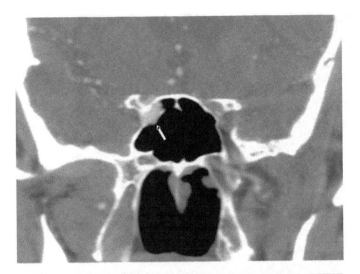

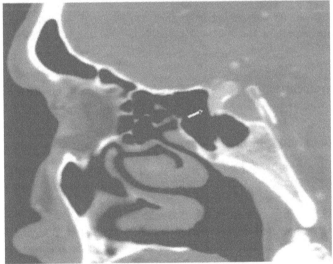

Figure 7 The sphenoid sinus and carotid artery. Contrast-enhanced (**A**) coronal and (**B**) sagittal images show protrusion of internal carotid artery (ica) into the sphenoid sinus with dehiscent carotid canal. Note that on a noncontrast CT displayed with bone windows this would be indistinguishable from a sphenoid polyp. *Arrows*: ICA.

Anatomically, the paranasal sinuses are in close proximity to the anterior cranial fossa, cribriform plate, internal carotid arteries, cavernous sinuses, the orbits and their contents, and the optic nerves as they exit the orbits (Figs. 2C and 7) (22–24). The surgeon should be cautious when

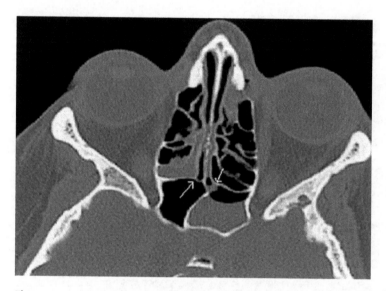

Figure 8 Axial CT image through the sphenoid sinus. The sphenoid ostium is at the medial and superior aspect of the sphenoid sinus. Note that the left ostium is obstructed by mucosal thickening.

maneuvering instruments in the posterior direction to avoid an inadvertent penetration and drainage of these structures (22,23,25,26).

Anatomic Variations and Congenital Abnormalities

The nasal anatomy is unique and similar to the uniqueness of "thumb print." Although the nasal anatomy varies significantly among patients, certain anatomic variations are common in the general population and may be seen more frequently in patients with chronic inflammatory disease (20,21,25–28). Multiple studies demonstrated an association between some anatomic variations and sinusitis, but a causal relationship has not been established. It appears that some of these variations contribute to mechanical obstruction of the ostiomeatal channels in patients with sinusitis, and need to be addressed during surgery. The significance of an anatomic variation is determined by its relationship with the ostiomeatal channels and nasal air passages. The most common variations are discussed in the following paragraphs. It is stressed that the high variability of the anatomy necessitates careful presurgical assessment on an individual basis.

Concha Bullosa

Concha bullosa is defined as an aeration of the middle turbinate (Fig. 9). Concha bullosa may be unilateral or bilateral. Less frequently, aeration of

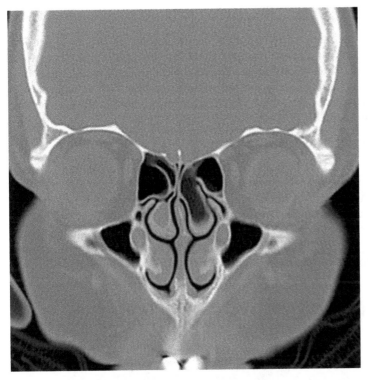

Figure 9 Concha Bullosa: coronal CT image showing bilateral concha bullosa. The right concha bullosa is opacified.

the superior turbinate may occur, whereas aeration of the inferior turbinate is infrequent. A concha bullosa in the middle turbinate may enlarge to obstruct the middle meatus or the infundibulum. The air cavity in a concha bullosa is lined with the same epithelium as the rest of the nasal cavity; thus, these cells can undergo the same inflammatory disorders experienced in the paranasal sinuses. Obstruction of the drainage of a concha can lead to mucocele formation.

Nasal Septal Deviation

Nasal septal deviation is an asymmetric bowing of the nasal septum that may compress the middle turbinate laterally, narrowing the middle meatus. Bony spurs are often associated with septal deviation. Nasal septal deviation is usually congenital but may be a post traumatic finding in some patients. Nasal septal deviation occurs with a similar frequency in asymptomatic persons with no CT evidence of sinusitis and in patients with sinusitis (29). When the angle of deviation is high, it may contribute to the mechanical obstruction of the anterior ostiomeatal complex.

Paradoxic Middle Turbinate

The middle turbinate usually curves medially towards the nasal septum. However, its major curvature can project laterally and, thus, narrow the middle meatus and infundibulum. This variant is called a paradoxic middle turbinate. The inferior edge of the middle meatus may assume various shapes with excessive curvature, which in turn may obstruct the nasal cavity, infundibulum, and middle meatus.

Variations in the Uncinate Process

The course of the free edge of the uncinate process varies. In most cases, it extends slightly obliquely toward the nasal septum with the free edge surrounding the inferior or anterior surface of the ethmoid bulla. Sometimes, the free edge of the uncinate adheres to the orbital floor or inferior/anterior aspect of the lamina papyracea. This variant is usually associated with a hypoplastic (Fig. 10), and often opacified, ipsilateral maxillary sinus resulting from closure of the infundibulum. Due to the small maxillary sinus, the

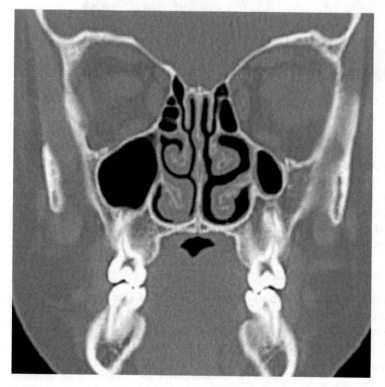

Figure 10 Hypoplastic maxillary sinus: the uncinate is attached to the floor of the orbit on this coronal CT image. Also note that the wall of the maxillary sinus is very thick.

ipsilateral orbit is more inferiorly located, giving rise to more frequent orbital complications during surgery (30,31). The posterior edge of the uncinate process may attach to the lamina papyracea, wall of the ethmoid bulla, middle turbinate, or skull base. The attachment site of the posterior edge of the uncinate process determines the drainage site of the frontal recess.

Haller Cells (Infrabullar Recess Cells)

Haller cells are ethmoid air cells that extend along the medial roof of the maxillary sinus (Fig. 11). Their appearance and size vary. They may cause narrowing of the infundibulum when they are large. Haller cells may exist as discrete cells or they may open into the maxillary sinus or infundibulum.

Onodi Cells

Onodi cells are lateral and posterior extensions of the posterior ethmoid air cells (32). They extend the paranasal sinus cavity very near the optic nerves

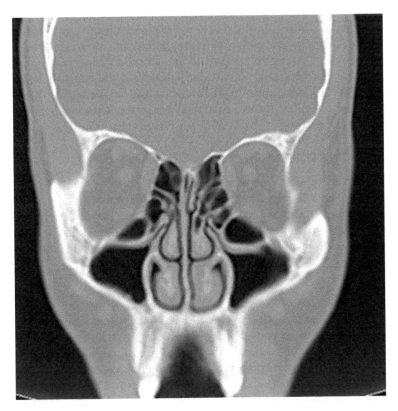

Figure 11 Haller cell: bilateral extension of ethmoid cells into the maxillary sinuses. Note the proximity of the Haller cells to the ethmoid infundibulum.

as they exit the orbits. These cells may surround the optic nerve tract and put the nerve at risk during surgery.

Giant Ethmoid Bulla

The largest of the ethmoid air cells, the ethmoid bulla may enlarge to narrow or obstruct the middle meatus and infundibulum.

Extensive Pneumatization of the Sphenoid Sinus

Pneumatization of the sphenoid sinus can extend into the anterior clinoid processes and clivus, surrounding the optic nerves. When this occurs, the risk of damage to the optic nerves is increased during surgical exploration. The carotid canal may protrude into the sphenoid sinus and there could be a bony dehiscence on the sphenoid sinus wall, increasing the risk of catastrophic carotid artery injury.

Medial Deviation or Dehiscence of the Lamina Papyracea

Medial deviation or dehiscence of the lamina papyracea may be a congenital finding or the result of prior facial trauma. Regardless, the intra-orbital contents are at risk during surgery because of the common dehiscences in the area and the ease of confusing this medial bulge with the ethmoid bulla. Excessive medial deviation and bony dehiscence tend to occur most often at the site of the insertion of the basal lamella into the lamina papyracea, thus rendering this portion of the lamina papyracea most delicate.

Aerated Crista Galli

Aeration of the crista galli, a normally bony structure, can occur (Fig. 12). When aerated, these cells may communicate with the frontal recess. Obstruction of this ostium can lead to chronic sinusitis and mucocele formation. It is important to recognize this entity preoperatively and to differentiate it from an ethmoid air cell to avoid extension of surgery into the cranial vault.

Cephalocele and Meningocele

Extracranial herniations of the brain and/or its coverings may be congenitally present or may result from previous ethmoid or sphenoid sinus surgery. Their presence needs to be considered when dealing with an isolated soft-tissue mass adjacent to the ethmoid or sphenoid roof, especially if complemented by adjacent bone erosion. The differential diagnosis includes mucocele, neoplasm, cephalocele, and less likely, a polyp associated with an adjacent bony dehiscence. Coronal CT will best display the extent of bony erosion, and sagittal and coronal MRI will be helpful in narrowing the differential diagnosis. CT cisternography is diagnostic (Fig. 13).

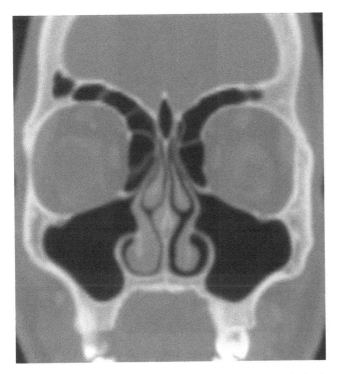

Figure 12 Supraorbital ethmoid air cells and pneumatized crista galli demonstrated on coronal CT image.

Asymmetry in Ethmoid Roof Height

It is important to note any asymmetry in the height of the ethmoid roof (Fig. 14). The incidence of intracranial penetration during functional endoscopic sinus surgery (FESS) is higher when this anatomic variation occurs. Intracranial penetration is more likely to occur on the side where the position of the roof is lower (23).

Acquired abnormalities of the sinus walls such as osteoma and fibrous dysplasia are relatively common and usually asymptomatic. They can present with sinus-related complaints when they interfere with sinus drainage.

IMAGING RHINOSINUSITIS

Acute Rhinosinusitis

Air–fluid levels and complete opacification of a sinus are the imaging hallmarks of acute rhinosinusitis (ARS) (Fig. 15). More than one sinus are usually involved, typically the maxillary and the ethmoid sinuses. CT is much more sensitive than plain radiographs. Air–fluid level is a very

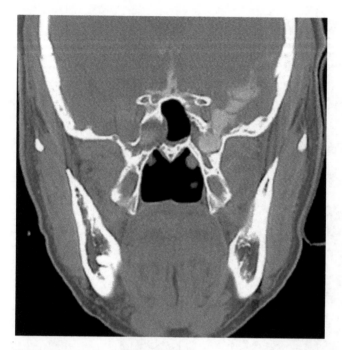

Figure 13 Cephalocele: CT-cisternogram in the coronal plane demonstrates CSF containing sacs in the pterygoid recesses of the sphenoid sinus.

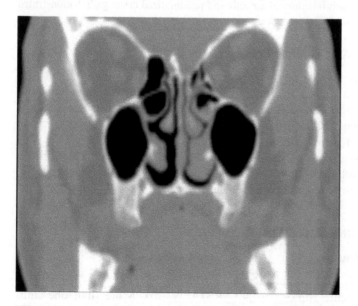

Figure 14 Low fovea ethmoidalis: the left cribriform plate is more inferiorly positioned than the right.

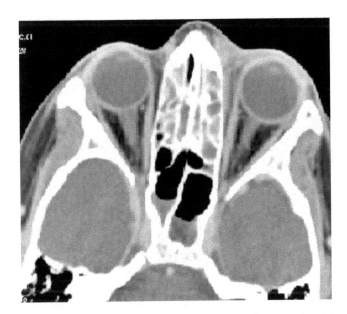

Figure 15 Characteristic CT appearance of acute sinusitis on axial contrast-enhanced image: low attenuation fluid retention in the sphenoid and ethmoid sinuses with air fluid levels. Also note that the patient has left preseptal cellulitis.

specific sign for ARS in the appropriate clinical setting. Other causes of altered air–fluid level in a sinus include trauma, prolonged supine position, and intubation (typical ICU patient), recent nasal irrigation, cerebrospinal fluid (CSF) leak, and chronic rhinosinusitis (CRS). ARS is diagnosed on the basis of history, clinical presentation, and physical examination. Imaging is not recommended for diagnosing ARS because of the cost-containment concerns and radiation exposure, unless the patient is not responding to initial treatment or there is a complicating factor (33–35). A limited sinus CT consisting of five to six axial noncontiguous images is utilized in many practices for the initial diagnosis of ARS. The charge for limited sinus CT is only slightly higher than the charge for plain radiographs and the radiation dose is reduced, while the diagnostic accuracy remains reasonably high. The cost-effectiveness of limited sinus CT exam, which changes with evolving technology and its impact on treatment plan, has not been well studied (36). When the clinical question is whether there is sinusitis or not, a limited sinus CT would be adequate. The reduced cost and radiation dose of limited sinus CT cannot be used as a justification for imaging of uncomplicated ARS. Authors believe that the diagnosis of ARS should be made clinically, and that when imaging is necessary, a "high quality" CT exam should be performed.

ARS is often a self-limited disease and symptoms subside with or even without treatment; however, in rare instances, catastrophic complications

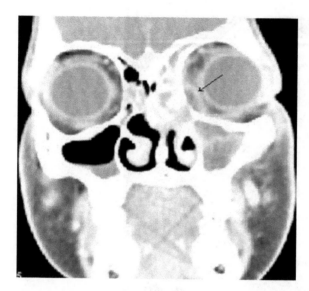

Figure 16 Sub-periosteal abscess: contrast-enhanced coronal CT shows acute sinusitis of the left maxillary and ethmoid with a peripherally enhancing fluid attenuation mass in the left extraconal orbit.

occur. Because of the close proximity of the sinuses to the brain and orbit, and the naturally present dehiscences and vascular channels in the sinus walls, infection can spread to the orbit and intracranial compartment. Sub-periosteal phlegmon and abscess result when the infection is limited by the intact periorbita (Fig. 16). Penetration of the periorbita allows infection to spread to the orbital soft tissues causing orbital cellulitis, which may lead to permanent loss of vision. Intracranial complications such as meningitis, epidural and subdural empyema, brain abscess, and cavernous sinus thrombophlebitis typically occur in the setting of frontal and sphenoid sinusitis (Fig. 17). Early identification and treatment are essential in preventing catastrophic results. Contrast-enhanced CT detects most orbital complications. MRI is the study of choice for intracranial extension.

Subacute Rhinosinusitis

Subacute rhinosinusitis is clinically defined as persistence of symptoms for more than four weeks and up to 12 weeks. There is no specific radiological sign for subacute rhinosinusitis and a typical CT study shows some opacification of one or more sinuses.

Chronic Rhinosinusitis

The term chronic rhinosinusitis (CRS) is preferred because rhinitis almost always precedes sinusitis and sinusitis occurs concurrently with inflammation

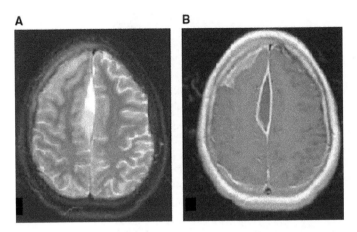

Figure 17 Subdural empyema: axial (**A**) T2-weighted and (**B**) post-contrast T1-weighted MRI show subdural collections on this patient who was diagnosed with acute frontal sinusitis one week prior to this MRI.

of the nasal passages (37,38). CRS diagnosis is symptom-based and requires persistence of patient complaints for more than 12 consecutive weeks. Since many clinical symptoms of CRS are vague, subjective, and nonspecific, objective demonstration of mucosal inflammation is necessary to confirm the clinical diagnosis (37,39–41). Anterior rhinoscopy may not always be able to confirm the presence of mucosal inflammation, and nasal endoscopy is required to visualize the middle meatus and ethmoid bulla (41). CT, as the imaging standard for evaluation of the sinuses, is an excellent tool to confirm the presence and assess the extent of inflammation in the sinonasal cavity beyond what is permitted by endoscopy (5,42). The plain radiographs lack the sensitivity, specificity, and anatomic precision needed for the management of these patients and are simply inadequate. Limited sinus CT examinations which employ selected, noncontiguous axial slices may be adequate in some clinical scenarios when the patient had a thorough evaluation of the anatomy with a high quality CT previously. One has to keep in mind, though, that the limited sinus study is limited not only in cost and radiation exposure, but in information as well.

Although CT provides excellent information about the extent and distribution of mucosal disease and status of the nasal air passages, it does not yield much information about the origin of the changes (e.g., infection, allergies, granulomatous inflammation, postsurgical scarring, etc.).

The CT signs suggestive of CRS include diffuse or focal mucosal thickening, partial or complete opacification, and bone remodeling and thickening caused by osteitis from adjacent chronic mucosal inflammation and polyposis (Fig. 18). The distribution of the inflammatory mucosal changes

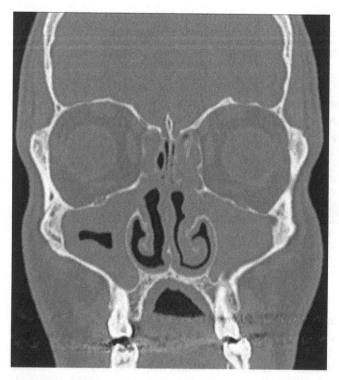

Figure 18 Diffuse nonspecific CRS: bilateral ethmoid and maxillary opacification. Note prior uncinectomy, middle turbinectomy, and ethmoidectomy.

in the nasal cavity and sinuses may provide a clue as to the level of mechanical obstruction. Babble et al. (43) defined five recurring patterns of inflammatory sinonasal disease including infundibular, OMU, sphenoethmoidal recess, sinonasal polyposis, and sporadic or unclassifiable disease. In this study, the infundibular pattern (26% of patients) referred to the focal obstruction within the maxillary sinus ostium and ethmoid infundibulum that was associated with maxillary sinus disease. The OMU pattern (25% of patients) referred to ipsilateral maxillary, frontal, and anterior ethmoid sinus disease. This pattern was caused by obstruction of the middle meatus. The frontal sinus is sometimes spared because of the variability in frontal sinus drainage pathway. The sphenoethmoidal recess pattern (6% of patients) resulted in sphenoid or posterior ethmoid sinus inflammation caused by sphenoethmoidal recess obstruction. Diffuse nasal and paranasal sinus polyps occurred in 10% of the study population (sinonasal polyposis pattern). One-fourth of the patients in this study did not show a recognizable pattern. Zinreich and others found middle-meatus opacification in 72% of patients with chronic sinusitis; 65% of these patients had mucosal thickening of the maxillary sinus (20,21,26). The patients with frontal sinus inflamma-tory disease had opacification of the frontal recess (20,21,26). Frontal sinus opacification involving the OMU without maxillary or anterior ethmoid sinus inflammatory disease was rare (20,21,26). Yousem et al. (44) found that when the middle meatus was opacified, associated inflammatory changes occurred in the ethmoid sinuses in 82% of patients and in the maxillary sinuses in 84%. Bolger et al. (45) found that when the ethmoid infundibulum was free of disease, the maxillary and frontal sinuses were clear in 77% of patients. Certain anatomic variants, as described, have been implicated as causative factors in the presence of chronic inflammatory disease. Lidov and Som (46) found that a large concha bullosa could produce signs and symptoms by narrowing the infundibulum. However, Yousem et al. (44) found that the presence of a concha bullosa did not increase the risk of sinu-sitis. This was corroborated by Bolger et al. (45) who found that concha bul-losa, paradoxic turbinates, Haller cells, and uncinate pneumatization were not significantly more common in patients with chronic sinusitis than in asymptomatic patients. Yousem et al. (44) found that nasal septal deviation and a horizontally oriented uncinate process were more common in patients with inflammatory sinusitis. Although these variants may not necessarily pre-dispose to sinusitis, the size of a given anatomic variant and its relationship to adjacent structures are important in the development of sinusitis (19).

When sinus secretions are acute and of low viscosity, they are of inter-mediate attenuation on CT (10–25 Hounsfield units). In the more chronic state, sinus secretions become thickened and concentrated, and the CT attenuation increases with density measurements of 30 to 60 Hounsfield units (Fig. 19) (47).

Sinonasal polyposis has been recognized as a distinct form of CRS, both clinically and radiographically, although polyp formation is a nonspecific response to variety of inflammatory stimuli (Fig. 20). There is an obvious association with asthma, aspirin-sensitivity, and eosinophilia. The pathogenesis of sinonasal polyposis is very complex and not clearly understood (48–50). However, high recurrence rate of sinonasal polyposis is well documented (51–54). Antrochoanal and sphenochoanal polyps appear as well-defined masses that arise from the maxillary or sphenoid sinus and extend to the choana through the middle meatus or sphenoeth-moid recess, respectively (Fig. 21). They can present as nasopharyngeal masses. It is important to recognize their origin and relation to the maxillary or sphenoid ostium in treatment planning.

Retention cysts are very common incidental findings in imaging studies and seen as very well-defined rounded masses, typically in the maxillary sinus floor (Fig. 22). Their clinical significance is not clear (55). They may become symptomatic if large enough to interfere with drainage pathways (56).

Mucoceles, a complication of CRS, result from the obstruction of the sinus drainage and subsequent expansion of the sinus (Fig. 23). Mucoceles

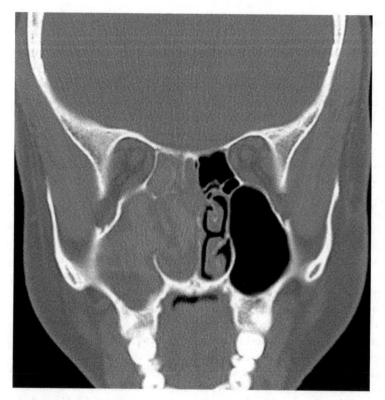

Figure 19 Right-sided ethmoid and maxillary sinusitis with obstruction of the ostio-meatal unit is demonstrated on this coronal CT image. The central high attenuation in the maxillary sinus suggests chronic secretions with high protein content.

are more commonly seen in the ethmoid and frontal sinuses and present with symptoms secondary to compression of the adjacent structures in addition to usual symptoms of CRS. Thickening and sclerosis of the bony walls of the sinuses (Fig. 24) have been traditionally attributed to the secondary reaction of the bone to a chronic mucosal inflammation. More recent work suggests that the bone may actually play an active part in the disease process and that the inflammation associated with CRS may spread through the haversian system within the bone (57,58). The combination of a surgical procedure and experimentally induced sinusitis creates an inflammatory process within bone with the classic histological features of osteomyelitis. Furthermore, bone inflammation may induce chronic inflammatory changes in the overlying mucosa at a significant distance from the site of infection. Identification of bone thickening and sclerosis on CT exam is straightforward, due to CT's exquisite ability to show the bone detail.

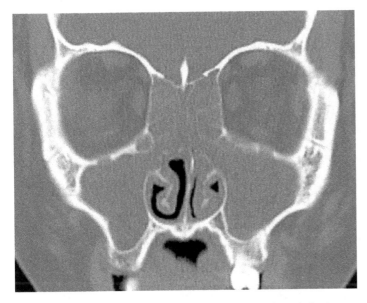

Figure 20 Typical CT appearance of sinonasal polyposis in the coronal plane.

On MRI, the appearance of CRS varies because of the changing concentrations of protein and free water protons (59). Som and Curtin (47) describe four patterns of MRI signal intensity that can be seen with chronic sinusitis: (1) hypointense on T1-weighted images and hyperintense on T2-weighted images with a protein concentration less than 9%; (2)

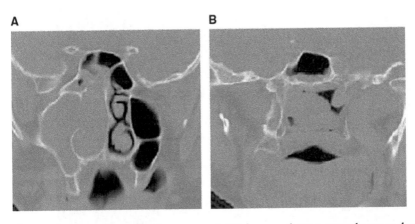

Figure 21 Antrochoanal polyp: coronal CT images show a nasopharyngeal mass that can be followed to the expanded maxillary ostium. The right maxillary sinus and nasal fossa are opacified.

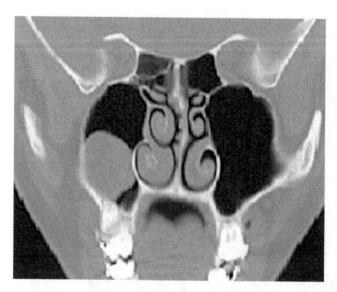

Figure 22   Typical appearance of a retention cyst.

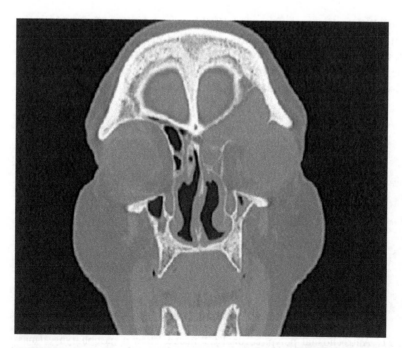

Figure 23   Frontal mucocele. Coronal CT image shows expansion of the left frontal sinus into the orbit with marked thinning of the sinus wall.

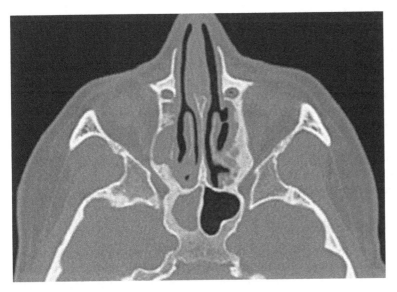

Figure 24 CRS and osteitis: marked thickening of the sinus walls.

hyperintense on T1-weighted images and hyperintense on T2-weighted images with total protein concentration increased by 20% to 25%; (3) hyperintense on T1-weighted images and hypointense on T2-weighted images with total protein concentration of 25% to 30%; and (4) hypointense on T1-weighted images and T2-weighted images with a protein concentration greater than 30% and inspissated secretions in an almost solid form. MRI of inspissated secretions (i.e., those with protein concentrations greater than 30%) may have a pitfall in that the signal voids on T1- and T2-weighted images may look identical to normally aerated sinuses.

The correlation between patient symptoms and CT findings is difficult to determine partly due to the fact that chronic mucosal inflammation may be present without the findings identified on CT examinations such as mucosal hypertrophy and retained secretions and that a modest amount of inflammation diagnosed by CT may be present in asymptomatic persons. Several studies failed to show a correlation between symptom severity and severity of CT findings (40,41,60–62). Particularly, symptoms such as headache and facial pain do not correlate with CT findings at all (63–65). A positive correlation between the severity of symptoms and CT findings may be demonstrated when certain symptoms and negative CT exams are eliminated (66,67). The nasal endoscopy findings correlate with CT findings, though the correlation is less than perfect (41,63,68). The positive predictive value of abnormal endoscopy for abnormal CT is greater than 90%, whereas the negative predictive value of normal endoscopy for normal CT is only 70% (41,63).

To better classify patients into diagnostic and prognostic categories, various symptom-, CT-, and endoscopy- scoring systems have been used. The Lund–MacKay scoring system is the most popular method applied to CT description of sinus disease because of its simplicity and reproducibility (69). A score of 0, 1, or 2 is given to each of the five sites (anterior ethmoid, posterior ethmoid, frontal, maxillary, and sphenoid) on both sides of the sinonasal cavity for normal pneumatization, partial opacification, or complete opacification, respectively (70,71). The ostiomeatal complex receives either 0 or 2. This yields a maximum score of 12 for one side.

In a small study, the impact of CT on treatment decision was evaluated (36). CT changed the treatment in one-third of the patients and provided better agreement on treatment plan among ENT surgeons (36).

Fungal Rhinosinusitis

Fungal rhinosinusitis (FRS) differs from bacterial and other types of sinusitis not only in etiology but also in demographics of the effected population, clinical approach, diagnosis, treatment, and prognosis. There are two main forms of FRS: invasive and noninvasive (72). Within these categories, five clinicopathologically distinct entities are defined (73): (i) acute invasive, (ii) chronic invasive granulomatous form, (iii) chronic invasive nongranulomatous form, (iv) fungus ball and (v) allergic fungal sinusitis. It must be emphasized that FRS is a spectrum of disease and the differences in clinical presentation are largely determined by the host defense system. Therefore, it is not uncommon to see overlapping clinical and imaging features.

Acute Invasive FRS

Acute invasive FRS is seen primarily in immunocompromised patients and is fatal if untreated. A high index of clinical suspicion and biopsy of the middle turbinate are necessary for early diagnosis, which may be life-saving (74). CT study obtained early in the disease course may be normal or show nonspecific mucosal thickening indistinguishable from the appearance of bacterial/viral disease (75) (Fig. 25). Bone destruction and swelling of the soft tissues adjacent to the paranasal sinuses occur in advanced disease.

Chronic Invasive FRS

Chronic invasive FRS has been associated primarily with immunocompromised patients; however, it does occur in the non-immunocompromised as well and has a more protracted course with relatively slow progression of disease, sometimes despite treatment, and high recurrence rate. There is no apparent difference in clinical and radiological features of the granulomatous and nongranulomatous forms. The radiological hallmark of chronic invasive FRS is bone destruction, which is better depicted with CT, whereas MRI better defines the soft-tissue extent of disease and brain involvement.

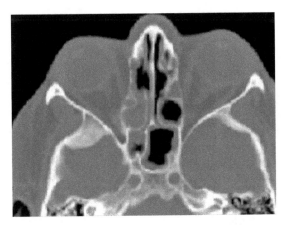

Figure 25 Acute invasive fungal sinusitis. On this patient with advanced leukemia and prior sinus surgery, axial CT shows nonspecific mucosal thickening in the ethmoid cells. Biopsy proven acute invasive sinusitis.

Foci of increased attenuation (on CT) in the sinus mucosal thickening may indicate fungal colonization as found in 74% of our patient population (76). The radiological differential diagnosis of chronic invasive FRS is broad and includes benign and malignant neoplasms, infectious and idiopathic granulomatous diseases, and allergic fungal sinusitis.

Fungus Ball

Fungus ball refers to a sinus mass that consists of packed hyphae. Patients with fungus ball are typically immunocompetent and present with varying nonspecific sinus-related complaints. Serendipitous identification of fungus balls is not uncommon. Diffuse opacification of a single sinus is the most common radiographic feature (77). Foci of hyperattenuation in the center of the sinus mass is seen in approximately 50 to 74% of the patients (75,77,78). Large calcified concretions are characteristic of the disease but uncommonly found (Fig. 26). Thickening of the sinus walls is common. Bone erosion may occasionally be seen.

Allergic FRS

Allergic FRS, an immunologically mediated hypersensitivity reaction to fungi, is the most common fungal disease of the sinuses (79). A central area of hyperattenuation on sinus CT is almost always present and corresponds to markedly decreased T2 signal on MRI. This appearance is due to the metabolized ferromagnetic elements (primarily iron) and calcium within the concretion (Fig. 27). Expansion of the involved sinuses with bone remodeling or destruction is common.

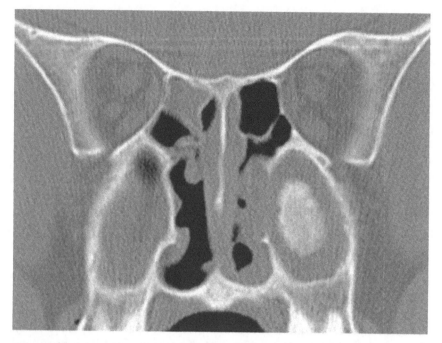

Figure 26 Fungus ball: dense calcification in the center of the completely opacified left maxillary sinus is shown on this coronal CT image.

Saprophytic Colonization

Saprophytic colonization of the sinonasal mucosa is very common, particularly in patients who had undergone sinus surgery, and mere presence of fungi on the mucosa does not necessarily constitute the disease.

PRESURGICAL IMAGING EVALUATION

Using a systematic approach is helpful when interpreting sinus CT studies. One must identify and describe the important structures of the paranasal sinuses including the frontal sinus, the FSOT, the agger nasi cell and anterior ethmoid sinus, the ethmoid roof, the ethmoid bulla, the uncinate process, the infundibulum, the maxillary sinus, the middle meatus, the nasal septum and nasal turbinates, the basal lamella, the sinus lateralis, the posterior ethmoid sinus, the sphenoid sinus, and the sphenoethmoidal recess.

The symmetry of the ethmoid roof should be noted. If not recognized, discrepant heights of the ethmoid roof may lead to inadvertent penetration of the cranial vault during surgery (23).

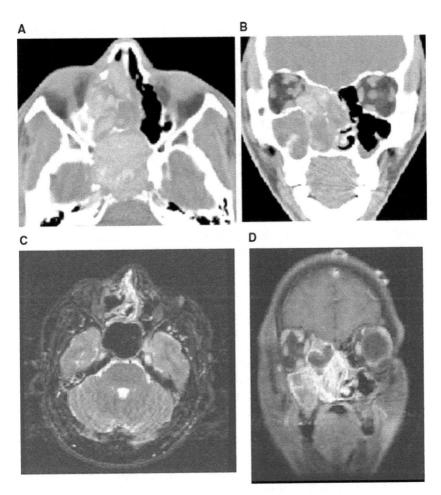

Figure 27 Allergic fungal sinusitis (AFS): axial (**A**) and coronal (**B**) CT, axial T2-weighted and post-contrast coronal T1-weighted MRI. Predominantly high attenuation, heterogeneous mass in the right-sided sinuses with erosion into the orbit, the middle, and posterior cranial fossae. Note that the mass in the sphenoid and parts of the ethmoid sinuses shows essentially no signal on T2-weighted MRI.

Careful attention should be paid to the status of the lamina papyracea, and any dehiscence or excessive medial deviation of this bone should be reported. The relationship of the sphenoid sinus and posterior ethmoid air cells with the internal carotid artery and optic nerves should be noted. In particular, extensive expansion of the sinuses around the internal carotid artery or the optic nerve and bony dehiscences adjacent to either structure should be noted. The incidence of bony dehiscence around the parasellar portions of the internal carotid artery is 12% to 22% (80). The carotid canal frequently penetrates the aerated portion of the sphenoid sinus; in many cases, the sphenoid sinus septa will adhere to the bony covering of the carotid canal. The surgeon needs to be aware of this variation to prevent fracture of the sphenoid sinus septum–carotid canal junction and avoid puncturing the carotid canal. Cephaloceles can be present in the sphenoid and ethmoid sinuses and mimic inflammatory disease. Any bony dehiscence should be evaluated with the possibility of encephalocele in mind.

The relationship between the posterior paranasal sinuses and the optic nerves is important to note to avoid operative complications (Fig. 28). Delano et al. (81) classified this relationship into four categories depending on the relationship of optic canal and sphenoid and posterior ethmoid sinuses. In this study, the optic nerve canal was dehiscent in all cases in which it traveled through the sphenoid sinus (type 3), in 82% of cases in which the nerve impressed on the sphenoid sinus wall (type 2), and in 77% of cases in which the anterior clinoid process is pneumatized. The presence of anterior clinoid process pneumatization is an important indicator of optic nerve vulnerability during FESS because of frequent associations with bony dehiscence and type 2 and 3 configurations.

Hypoplastic maxillary sinus is usually accompanied by variations in the lateral nasal wall anatomy and orbital floor, which may give rise to surgical complications, if not recognized (30,31).

The bony outline of the nasal cavity and paranasal sinuses must be examined with particular attention to absence of bone. Surgical removal of bone should be documented. Bone erosion or destruction may be secondary

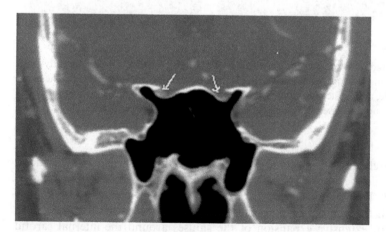

Figure 28 Contrast-enhanced coronal CT image of the sphenoid sinus: aerated anterior clinoid processes with bulging of the optic nerves into the sphenoid sinus.

to mucocele or neoplasm; the associated mAss and pattern of bone involvement are helpful clues as to the cause, and MRI may distinguish between these processes.

POSTSURGICAL IMAGING EVALUATION

The presence or absence of important structures should be identified and mentioned. The nasal cavity and paranasal sinus boundaries and important anatomical relationships should be inspected. Areas of bony thickening or dehiscence should be noted.

The following merit close scrutiny on follow-up CT scan:

The frontal recesses should be identified to determine their patency. Postoperatively, recurrence of disease is caused by persistent obstruction in this area, which is the narrowest channel within the anterior ethmoid complex and is difficult to access surgically. Therefore, the frontal recess is most likely to be affected with inflammatory disease in a patient who underwent previous surgery in the paranasal sinuses. The agger nasi cell (if it remains) should be noted because of its persistence may continue to narrow the frontal recess. In patients who had partial middle turbinate resection, one should look for lateralization of the remnant middle turbinate which may be the cause of obstruction of the frontal recess, middle meatus, and/or infundibulum.

The extent of the excision of the uncinate and removal of the ethmoid bulla should be noted. The course of the infundibulum should be examined for persistent anatomic narrowing. Careful attention should be paid to the vertical attachment of the middle turbinate to the cribriform plate and to the attachment of the basal lamella to the lamina papyracea. Traction on the vertical attachment and basal lamella of the middle turbinate during the course of middle turbinectomy can fracture the lamina papyracea or the cribriform plate.

The course of the lamina papyracea should be inspected to evaluate the integrity of this structure. Postoperative dehiscences are commonly found posterior to the nasolacrimal duct and may be caused by the uncinate resection.

Asymmetry in position of the roof of the ethmoid sinus should be noted. Intracranial penetrations are usually on the side where the position of the roof is lower.

SURGICAL COMPLICATIONS

In general, complications can be divided into minor and major (22,23,82). Minor complications include periorbital emphysema, epistaxis, postoperative nasal synechiae, and tooth pain. Although these can commonly occur, they are usually self-limited and do not require postoperative radiological evaluation.

Major complications are rare but can be severely devastating or fatal (22). A preexisting loss of integrity of the lamina papyracea can permit intraorbital fat to herniate into the ethmoid sinuses. Preexisting dehiscence of the lamina papyracea may be caused by prior trauma or erosion from chronic sinus disease. Disruption of the lamina papyracea can occur during resection of the middle turbinate if the basal lamella is resected back to its attachment to the lamina papyracea.

The medial rectus muscle, superior oblique muscle, or other orbital contents can be directly damaged if preexisting or intraoperative disruption of the lamina papyracea occurs (83). If intra-orbital and intraocular pressure builds up as a result of an expanding hematoma or air being forced into the orbit from the nasal cavity (through a dehiscent lamina papyracea), then visual impairment or blindness secondary to ischemia can result (83).

Temporary or permanent blindness caused by injury of the optic nerve can occur during posterior ethmoidectomy if the bony limit of the sinus is violated (22,23,82,83). Trauma to the vessels supplying the optic nerve also can result in visual loss.

Perforation of the cribriform plate can lead to intracranial hematoma, infection, and cerebrospinal fluid (CSF) leak.

Massive hemorrhage from direct injury to major vessels can occur. Laceration of the internal carotid artery has been reported and is often fatal (22,23). Emergent angiography and balloon occlusion of the lacerated artery have been performed. Patients who report severe postoperative headache or photophobia or who have signs that suggest subarachnoid hemorrhage should undergo noncontrast head CT. If subarachnoid blood is found, cerebral angiography is recommended to detect vascular injury. Injury to the nasolacrimal duct can result during anterior enlargement of the maxillary ostium in the middle meatus. Injury to the membranous portion of the duct may be self-limited and remit by spontaneous fistulization into the middle meatus. Stenosis or total occlusion of the nasolacrimal duct can result from more severe injury (83).

Postoperative CSF leak due to inadvertent penetration of the dura is another major complication of FESS. A CSF leak may not become clinically apparent for up to two years after surgery (23). CSF leaks will often close spontaneously with conservative measures (e.g., lumbar drain). However, if they persist, radiological workup is indicated. In many institutions, a radionuclide CSF study is the initial radiological screening examination in such patients. Three to four absorbent pledgets are placed on each side of the nasal cavity and 400 to 500 µCi of indium-111 (111-In)-labeled DTPA is instilled into the subarachnoid space through a cervical or lumbar puncture. Then, the patient undergoes imaging with a gamma camera at multiple intervals for up to 24 hours. Any position or activity known to provoke the leak is encouraged. Although images of the head and neck are obtained, evidence of the leak is unusual on these images. Rather, indirect signs of leaking are sought. Images over the abdomen are done to search for activity in the bowel, which indicates that the patient is swallowing CSF as it leaks into the nasal cavity.

At 24 hours, the nasal pledgets are removed and assayed. The results are compared with 111-In activity in a serum sample drawn at the same time. A ratio of pledget activity to serum activity is determined. It is then possible to predict the general area of the leak based on which pledgets show increased activity. If none of the pledgets have increased activity but activity over the abdomen is increased, the radionuclide test is considered positive.

When the radionuclide test is positive (directly or indirectly), a contrast CT-cisternogram, which involves intrathecal administration of 3–5 ml of water-soluble contrast media and coronal CT scanning, is done to define the anatomy and pinpoint the site of leakage.

COMPUTER-AIDED SURGERY

Computer-aided surgery (CAS) is being increasingly utilized in FESS (84). CAS offers many advantages including real-time correlation of CT images, surgical field, and position of the surgical devices. Delicate anatomic dissection, yielding more complete surgeries in difficult places and fewer complications, is afforded by CAS. Several CAS systems such as SAVANT (CBYON, Palo Alto, CA), InstaTrak (Visualization Technology, Woburn, MA), LandMarX (Medtronic Xomed, Jacksonville, FL), and VectorVision (BrainLab, Tottlingen, Germany) are in use, and they allow projection of the location of surgical instruments in the operative field on the CT image data set. The most important components of a CAS system include registration and tracking units. Registration involves mapping of certain points in the preoperative image data set to the corresponding points in the operative field. To accomplish this, certain anatomic landmarks, special headsets, or radiopaque fiducial markers placed on the patient's skull can be used. Tracking systems, using electromagnetic or optical sensors, monitor the ever-changing position of surgical instruments. The position of instruments is displayed on the image data. The navigational accuracy is dependent on the accuracy of registration, tracking, and also the quality of CT image data set. Through technological advancements, a high level of accuracy (usually within 1 mm) has been achieved (85–91). An inherent limitation of CAS is that the surgically created changes are not reflected on CT images since there is no intraoperative image acquisition.

REFERENCES

1. Engels EA, Terrin N, Barza M, Lau J. Meta-analysis of diagnostic tests for acute sinusitis. J Clin Epidemiol 2000; 53:852–862.

2. Aalokken TM, Hagtvedt T, Dalen I, Kolbenstvedt A. Conventional sinus radiography compared with CT in the diagnosis of acute sinusitis. Dentomaxillofac Radiol 2003; 32:60–62.

3. Chen LC, Huang JL, Wang CR, Yeh KW, Lin SJ. Use of standard radiography to diagnose paranasal sinus disease of asthmatic children in Taiwan: comparison with computed tomography. Asian Pac J Allergy Immunol 1999; 17:69–76.

4. Varonen H, Makela M, Savolainen S, Laara E, Hilden J. Comparison of ultrasound, radiography, and clinical examination in the diagnosis of acute maxillary sinusitis: a systematic review. J Clin Epidemiol 2000; 53:940–948.

5. Benninger MS, Ferguson BJ, Hadley JA, Hamilos DL, Jacobs M, Kennedy DW, Lanza DC, Marple BF, Osguthorpe JD, Stankiewicz JA, Anon J, Denneny J, Emanuel I, Levine H. Adult chronic rhinosinusitis: definitions, diagnosis, epidemiology, and pathophysiology. Otolaryngol Head Neck Surg 2003; 129:S1–S32.

6. Dammann F, Momino-Traserra E, Remy C, Pereira PL, Baumann I, Koitschev A, Claussen CD. Radiation exposure during spiral-CT of the paranasal sinuses. Rofo Fortschr Geb Rontgenstr Neuen Bildgeb Verfahr 2000; 172:232–237.

7. Duvoisin B, Landry M, Chapuis L, Krayenbuhl M, Schnyder P. Low-dose CT and inflammatory disease of the paranasal sinuses. Neuroradiology 1991; 33:403–406.

8. Hagtvedt T, Aalokken TM, Notthellen J, Kolbenstvedt A. A new low-dose CT examination compared with standard-dose CT in the diagnosis of acute sinusitis. Eur Radiol 2003; 13:976–980.

9. Hein E, Rogalla P, Klingebiel R, Hamm B. Low-dose CT of the paranasal sinuses with eye lens protection: effect on image quality and radiation dose. Eur Radiol 2002; 12:1693–1696.

10. Kearney SE, Jones P, Meakin K, Garvey CJ. CT scanning of the paranasal sinuses—the effect of reducing mAs. Br J Radiol 1997; 70:1071–1074.

11. Sohaib SA, Peppercorn PD, Horrocks JA, Keene MH, Kenyon GS, Reznek RH. The effect of decreasing mAs on image quality and patient dose in sinus CT. Br J Radiol 2001; 74:157–161.

12. Tack D, Widelec J, De Maertelaer V, Bailly JM, Delcour C, Gevenois PA. Comparison between low-dose and standard-dose multidetector CT in patients with suspected chronic sinusitis. Am J Roentgenol 2003; 181:939–944.

13. Zammit-Maempel I, Chadwick CL, Willis SP. Radiation dose to the lens of eye and thyroid gland in paranasal sinus multislice CT. Br J Radiol 2003; 76:418–420.

14. Zinreich SJ, Kennedy DW, Kumar AJ, Rosenbaum AE, Arrington JA, Johns ME. MR imaging of normal nasal cycle: comparison with sinus pathology. J Comput Assist Tomogr 1988; 12:1014–1019.

15. Zinreich SJBM, Oliverio PS. Sinonasal cavities: CT normal anatomy, imaging of the osteomeatal complex, and functional endoscopic surgery. In: Som PCH, ed. Head and Neck Imaging. 3rd ed. St Louis: Mosby, 1996.

16. Hosemann W. Dissection of the lateral nasal wall in eight steps. In: Wigand M, ed. Endoscopic Surgery of the Paranasal Sinuses and Anterior Skull Base. New York: Thieme, 1990.

17. Harnsberger HR. Imaging for the sinus and nose. In: Harnsberger HR, ed. Hand and Neck Imaging Handbook. St Louis: Mosby, 1990.

18. Daniels DL, Mafee MF, Smith MM, Smith TL, Naidich TP, Brown WD, Bolger WE, Mark LP, Ulmer JL, Hacein-Bey L, Strottmann JM. The frontal sinus drainage pathway and related structures. Am J Neuroradiol 2003; 24: 1618–1627.
19. Yousem DM. Imaging of sinonasal inflammatory disease. Radiology 1993; 188:303–314.
20. Zinreich SJ. Imaging of chronic sinusitis in adults: X-ray, computed tomography, and magnetic resonance imaging. J Allergy Clin Immunol 1992; 90: 445–451.
21. Zinreich SJ. Paranasal sinus imaging. Otolaryngol Head Neck Surg 1990; 103:863–868; discussion 868–869.
22. Maniglia AJ. Fatal and other major complications of endoscopic sinus surgery. Laryngoscope 1991; 101:349–354.
23. Hudgins PA, Browning DG, Gallups J, Gussack GS, Peterman SB, Davis PC, Silverstein Am, Beckett WW, Hoffman JC Jr. Endoscopic paranasal sinus surgery: radiographic evaluation of severe complications. Am J Neuroradiol 1992; 13:1161–1167.
24. Buus DR, Tse DT, Farris BK. Ophthalmic complications of sinus surgery. Ophthalmology 1990; 97:612–619.
25. Zinreich J. Imaging of inflammatory sinus disease. Otolaryngol Clin North Am 1993; 26:535–547.
26. Zinreich SJ, Kennedy DW, Rosenbaum AE, Gayler BW, Kumar AJ, Stammberger H. Paranasal sinuses: CT imaging requirements for endoscopic surgery. Radiology 1987; 163:769–775.
27. Jones NS, Strobl A, Holland I. A study of the CT findings in 100 patients with rhinosinusitis and 100 controls. Clin Otolaryngol 1997; 22:47–51.
28. Laine FJ, Smoker WR. The ostiomeatal unit and endoscopic surgery: anatomy, variations, and imaging findings in inflammatory diseases. Am J Roentgenol 1992; 159:849–857.
29. Collet S, Bertrand B, Cornu S, Eloy P, Rombaux P. Is septal deviation a risk factor for chronic sinusitis? Review of literature. Acta Otorhinolaryngol Belg 2001; 55:299–304.
30. Erdem T, Aktas D, Erdem G, Miman MC, Ozturan O. Maxillary sinus hypoplasia. Rhinology 2002; 40:150–153.
31. Salib RJ, Chaudri SA, Rockley TJ. Sinusitis in the hypoplastic maxillary antrum: the crucial role of radiology in diagnosis and management. J Laryngol Otol 2001; 115:676–678.
32. Driben JS, Bolger WE, Robles HA, Cable B, Zinreich SJ. The reliability of computerized tomographic detection of the Onodi (Sphenoethmoid) cell. Am J Rhinol 1998; 12:105–111.
33. McAlister WH, Parker BR, Kushner DC, Babcock DS, Cohen HL, Gelfand MJ, Hernandez RJ, Royal SA, Slovis TL, Smith WL, Strain JD, Strife JL, Kanda MB, Myer E, Decter RM, Moreland MS. Sinusitis in the pediatric population. American College of Radiology. ACR Appropriateness Criteria. Radiology 2000; 215(suppl):811–818.
34. Benninger MS, Sedory Holzer SE, Lau J. Diagnosis and treatment of uncomplicated acute bacterial rhinosinusitis: summary of the Agency for Health Care

Policy and Research evidence-based report. Otolaryngol Head Neck Surg 2000; 122:1–7.

35. Snow V, Mottur-Pilson C, Hickner JM. Principles of appropriate antibiotic use for acute sinusitis in adults. Ann Intern Med 2001; 134:495–497.

36. Anzai Y, Yueh B. Imaging evaluation of sinusitis: diagnostic performance and impact on health outcome. Neuroimaging Clin North Am 2003; 13:251–263, xi.

37. Hwang PH, Irwin SB, Griest SE, Caro JE, Nesbit GM. Radiologic correlates of symptom-based diagnostic criteria for chronic rhinosinusitis. Otolaryngol Head Neck Surg 2003; 128:489–496.

38. Bhattacharyya N. Chronic rhinosinusitis: is the nose really involved? Am J Rhinol 2001; 15:169–173.

39. Chester AC. Symptoms of rhinosinusitis in patients with unexplained chronic fatigue or bodily pain: a pilot study. Arch Intern Med 2003; 163:1832–1836.

40. Stankiewicz JA, Chow JM. A diagnostic dilemma for chronic rhinosinusitis: definition accuracy and validity. Am J Rhinol 2002; 16:199–202.

41. Stankiewicz JA, Chow JM. Nasal endoscopy and the definition and diagnosis of chronic rhinosinusitis. Otolaryngol Head Neck Surg 2002; 126:623–627.

42. Bhattacharyya N, Fried MP. The accuracy of computed tomography in the diagnosis of chronic rhinosinusitis. Laryngoscope 2003; 113:125–129.

43. Babbel RW, Harnsberger HR, Sonkens J, Hunt S. Recurring patterns of inflammatory sinonasal disease demonstrated on screening sinus CT. Am J Neuroradiol 1992; 13:903–912.

44. Yousem DM, Kennedy DW, Rosenberg S. Ostiomeatal complex risk factors for sinusitis: CT evaluation. J Otolaryngol 1991; 20:419–424.

45. Bolger WE, Butzin CA, Parsons DS. Paranasal sinus bony anatomic variations and mucosal abnormalities: CT analysis for endoscopic sinus surgery. Laryngoscope 1991; 101:56–64.

46. Lidov M, Som PM. Inflammatory disease involving a concha bullosa (enlarged pneumatized middle nasal turbinate): MR and CT appearance. Am J Neuroradiol 1990; 11:999–1001.

47. Som PM, Curtin HD. Chronic inflammatory sinonasal diseases including fungal infections. The role of imaging. Radiol Clin North Am 1993; 31:33–44.

48. Bachert C, Hormann K, Mosges R, Rasp G, Riechelmann H, Muller R, Luckhaupt H, Stuck BA, Rudack C. An update on the diagnosis and treatment of sinusitis and nasal polyposis. Allergy 2003; 58:176–191.

49. Bernstein JM. The molecular biology of nasal polyposis. Curr Allergy Asthma Rep 2001; 1:262–267.

50. Pawankar R. Nasal polyposis: an update: editorial review. Curr Opin Allergy Clin Immunol 2003; 3:1–6.

51. Drutman J, Harnsberger HR, Babbel RW, Sonkens JW, Braby D. Sinonasal polyposis: investigation by direct coronal CT. Neuroradiology 1994; 36:469–472.

52. Subramanian HN, Schechtman KB, Hamilos DL. A retrospective analysis of treatment outcomes and time to relapse after intensive medical treatment for chronic sinusitis. Am J Rhinol 2002; 16:303–312.

53. Scadding GK. Comparison of medical and surgical treatment of nasal polyposis. Curr Allergy Asthma Rep 2002; 2:494–499.

54. 'Rugina M, Serrano E, Klossek JM, Crampette L, Stoll D, Bebear JP, Perrahia M, Rouvier P, Peynegre R. Epidemiological and clinical aspects of nasal polyposis in France; the ORLI group experience. Rhinology 2002; 40:75–79.

55. Bhattacharyya N. Do maxillary sinus retention cysts reflect obstructive sinus phenomena? Arch Otolaryngol Head Neck Sur 2000; 126:1369–1371.

56. Hadar T, Shvero J, Nageris BI, Yaniv E. Mucus retention cyst of the maxillary sinus: the endoscopic approach. Br J Oral Maxillofac Surg 2000; 38:227–229.

57. Perloff JR, Gannon FH, Bolger WE, Montone KT, Orlandi R, Kennedy DW. Bone involvement in sinusitis: an apparent pathway for the spread of disease. Laryngoscope 2000; 110:2095–2099.

58. Khalid AN, Hunt J, Perloff JR, Kennedy DW. The role of bone in chronic rhinosinusitis. Laryngoscope 2002; 112:1951–1957.

59. Som PM, Dillon WP, Fullerton GD, Zimmerman RA, Rajagopalan B, Marom Z. Chronically obstructed sinonasal secretions: observations on T1 and T2 shortening. Radiology 1989; 172:515–520.

60. Stewart MG, Sicard MW, Piccirillo JF, Diaz-Marchan PJ. Severoty staging in chronic sinusitis: are CT scan findings related to symptoms? Am J Rhinol 1999; 13:161–167.

61. Bhattacharyya T, Piccirillo J, Wippold FJ II. Relationship between patient-based descriptions of sinusitis and paranasal sinus computed tomographic findings. Arch Otolaryngol Head Neck Surg 1997; 123:1189–1192.

62. Ashraf N, Bhattacharyya N. Determination of the "incidental" Lund score for the staging of chronic rhinosinusitis. Otolaryngol Head Neck Surg 2001; 125:483–486.

63. Rosbe KW, Jones KR. Usefulness of patient symptoms and nasal endoscopy in the diagnosis of chronic sinusitis. Am J Rhinol 1998; 12:167–171.

64. Shields G, Seikaly H, LeBoeuf M, Guinto F, LeBoeuf H, Pincus T, Calhoun K. Correlation between facial pain or headache and computed tomography in rhinosinusitis in Canadian and U.S. subjects. Laryngoscope 2003; 113:943–945.

65. Mudgil SP, Wise SW, Hopper KD, Kasales CJ, Mauger D, Fornadley JA. Correlation between presumed sinusitis-induced pain and paranasal sinus computed tomographic findings. Ann Allergy Asthma Immunol 2002; 88:223–226.

66. Kenny TJ, Duncavage J, Bracikowski J, Yildirim A, Murray JJ, Tanner SB. Prospective analysis of sinus symptoms and correlation with paranasal computed tomography scan. Otolaryngol Head Neck Surg 2001; 125:40–43.

67. Arango P, Kountakis SE. Significance of computed tomography pathology in chronic rhinosinusitis. Laryngoscope 2001; 111:1779–1782.

68. Kennedy DW, Wright ED, Goldberg AN. Objective and subjective outcomes in surgery for chronic sinusitis. Laryngoscope 2000; 110:29–31.

69. Friedman WH, Katsantonis GP. Staging systems for chronic sinus disease. Ear Nose Throat J 1994; 73:480–484.

70. Lund VJ, Mackay IS. Staging in rhinosinusitus. Rhinology 1993; 31:183–184.

71. Lund VJ, Kennedy DW. Quantification for staging sinusitis. The Staging and Therapy Group. Ann Otol Rhinol Laryngol Suppl 1995; 167:17–21.

72. deShazo RD, O'Brien M, Chapin K, Soto-Aguilar M, Gardner L, Swain R. A new classification and diagnostic criteria for invasive fungal sinusitis. Arch Otolaryngol Head Neck Surg 1997; 123:1181–1188.

73. Ferguson BJ. Definitions of fungal rhinosinusitis. Otolaryngol Clin North Am 2000; 33:227–235.

74. Gillespie MB, Huchton DM, O'Malley BW. Role of middle turbinate biopsy in the diagnosis of fulminant invasive fungal rhinosinusitis. Laryngoscope 2000; 110:1832–1836.

75. DelGaudio JM, Swain RE Jr, Kingdom TT, Muller S, Hudgins PA. Computed tomographic findings in patients with invasive fungal sinusitis. Arch Otolaryngol Head Neck Surg 2003; 129:236–240.

76. Zinreich SJ, Kennedy DW, Malat J, Curtin HD, Epstein JI, Huff LC, Kumar AJ, Johns ME, Rosenbaum AE. Fungal sinusitis: diagnosis with CT and MR imaging. Radiology 1988; 169:439–444.

77. Klossek JM, Serrano E, Peloquin L, Percodani J, Fontanel JP, Pessey JJ. Functional endoscopic sinus surgery and 109 mycetomas of paranasal sinuses. Laryngoscope 1997; 107:112–117.

78. Dhong HJ, Jung JY, Park JH. Diagnostic accuracy in sinus fungus balls: CT scan and operative findings. Am J Rhinol 2000; 14:227–231.

79. Manning SC, Holman M. Further evidence for allergic pathophysiology in allergic fungal sinusitis. Laryngoscope 1998; 108:1485–1496.

80. Johnson DM, Hopkins RJ, Hanafee WN, Fisk JD. The unprotected parasphenoidal carotid artery studied by high-resolution computed tomography. Radiology 1985; 155:137–141.

81. DeLano MC, Fun FY, Zinreich SJ. Relationship of the optic nerve to the posterior paranasal sinuses: a CT anatomic study. Am J Neuroradiol 1996; 17: 669–675.

82. Stankiewicz JA. Complications in endoscopic intranasal ethmoidectomy: an update. Laryngoscope 1989; 99:686–690.

83. Neuhaus RW. Orbital complications secondary to endoscopic sinus surgery. Ophthalmology 1990; 97:1512–1518.

84. Citardi MJ. Computer-aided frontal sinus surgery. Otolaryngol Clin North Am 2001; 34:111–122.

85. Khan M, Ecke U, Mann WJ. The application of an optical navigation system in endonasal sinus surgery. HNO 2003; 51:209–215.

86. Kherani S, Javer AR, Woodham JD, Stevens HE. Choosing a computer-assisted surgical system for sinus surgery. J Otolaryngol 2003; 32:190–197.

87. Olson G, Citardi MJ. Image-guided functional endoscopic sinus surgery. Otolaryngol Head Neck Surg 2000; 123:188–194.

88. Han D, Zhou B, Ge W. Application of an image-guidance system in endoscopic sinus surgery. Zhonghua Er Bi Yan Hou Ke Za Zhi 2001; 36:126–128.

89. Koele W, Stammberger H, Lackner A, Reittner P. Image guided surgery of paranasal sinuses and anterior skull base—five years experience with the Insta-Trak-System. Rhinology 2002; 40:1–9.

90. Zinreich SJ, Tebo SA, Long DM, Brem H, Mattox DE, Loury ME, vander Kolk CA, Koch WM, Kennedy DW, Bryan RN. Frameless stereotaxic integration of CT imaging data: accuracy and initial applications. Radiology 1993; 188:735–742.

91. Anon JB, Klimek L, Mosges R, Zinreich SJ. Computer-assisted endoscopic sinus surgery. An international review. Otolaryngol Clin North Am 1997; 30:389–401.

5

Anatomy and Physiology of the Paranasal Sinuses

John H. Krouse and Robert J. Stachler

Department of Otolaryngology Head and Neck Surgery, Wayne State University, Detroit, Michigan, U.S.A.

INTRODUCTION

A thorough understanding of the functional anatomy and physiology of the nose and paranasal sinuses is essential in approaching the diagnosis and treatment of sinonasal diseases in children and adults. By considering the sequential development of the sinuses with maturation and the intricate anatomic and physiological mechanisms that are involved in the function of the sinuses in disease and in health, clinicians will be able to apply these principles in the effective management of sinonasal pathology. The present chapter will first review the embryology of the developing nose and sinuses, and discuss their developmental anatomy throughout childhood (Table 1). It will also present the anatomy of the adult nose and sinuses in detail, with

Table 1 Developmental Anatomy of the Sinuses in Childhood

Sinus	Develops by	Radiographically present by	Completed development by
Ethmoid	In fetal life	Soon after birth	12 years of age
Maxillary	In fetal life	Soon after birth	12 years of age
Frontal	Age 1 or 2	Age 3–6	18 years of age
Sphenoid	Age 3 or 4	Age 8 or 9	Young adulthood

a focus on how these anatomical features affect the sinonasal functions. Finally, it reviews the relevant aspects of the normal physiology of the nose and sinuses, and discusses how alterations in these normal physiological mechanisms can result in acute and chronic diseases in children and adults.

EMBRYOLOGY OF THE NOSE AND PARANASAL SINUSES

The first nasal structures are seen as paired lateral nasal placodes and the midline frontonasal process by the fourth week of fetal life (1). These nasal placodes will eventually develop into the nasal cavities and their mucosal linings. The frontonasal process will become the nasal septum. The nasal placodes will invaginate to form pits that will extend back to the nasopharynx to define the nasal cavities (Fig. 1).

The initial development of the paranasal sinuses is attributable to the formation of the lateral nasal wall ridges known as ethmoturbinals (2). These ethmoturbinals develop throughout fetal life into the various processes that will form the mature ethmoid bone. In the seventh to eighth week of development, five to six ridges begin to appear. Three to four of these ridges will persist in the mature ethmoid bone. The first ethmoturbinal regresses and its ascending portion form the agger nasi. The descending portion forms the uncinate process. The second and third ethmoturbinals form the middle turbinate and the superior turbinate, respectively. The fourth and fifth ethmoturbinals form the supreme turbinate. In contrast to the ethmoid structures described above, the inferior turbinate arises from a ridge, the maxilloturbinal, which is located inferior to those structures. It is thus formed from the maxillary bone.

The nasal meati and recesses develop from primary furrows that lie between the ethmoturbinals (Fig. 1). The furrow between the first and second ethmoturbinals is called the primary furrow. Its anterior segment develops into a portion of the frontal recess. The posterior (descending) portion develops into the ethmoid infundibulum, hiatus semilunaris, and the middle meatus. The maxillary sinus primordium develops from the inferior aspect of the ethmoid infundibulum. The second and third furrows form the superior meatus and the supreme meatus, respectively. The ethmoturbinals cross the ethmoid complex to attach to the lamina papyracea of the orbit and skull base. There are numerous furrows that become invaginations or evaginations. Ultimately, these furrows will develop into the ethmoid labyrinth. The secondary concha or accessory concha of the middle meatus are the names given to the evaginations. Invaginations are called secondary furrows or accessory meati of the middle meatus. The ethmoid bulla arises from a secondary lateral nasal wall evagination. The suprabulbar and retrobulbar recesses (sinus lateralis) arise from secondary furrows forming above and behind the ethmoid bulla.

The maxillary sinus thus develops from a bud of the infundibulum. The bud continues to enlarge throughout fetal development. At birth, its

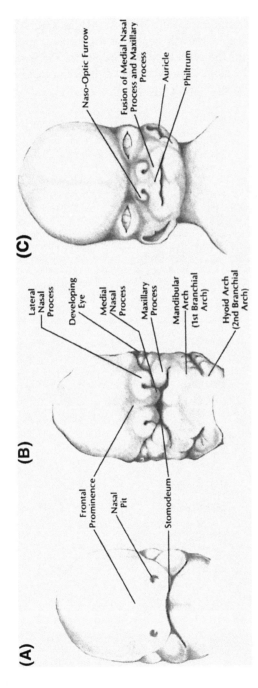

Figure 1 Development of the fetal face, frontal view, at: (**A**) four to five weeks, (**B**) five to six weeks, and (**C**) seven to eight weeks. *Source:* From Ref. 3.

size is estimated to be 6 to 8 cm^3 (Fig. 2). At four to five months after birth, the sinus can be seen radiographically as a triangular area medial to the infraorbital foramen. Rapid growth begins and continues until age three when growth slows until the seventh year. Growth of the maxillary sinus then accelerates until the sinus approximates adult size at age 12. Complete development ends in the late teens (Fig. 3) (3).

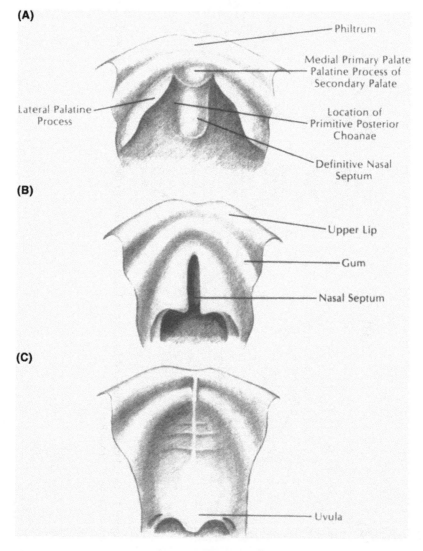

Figure 2 Nasal development, ventral view, at: (**A**) six to seven weeks, (**B**) seven to eight weeks, and (**C**) eight to nine weeks. *Source*: From Ref. 3.

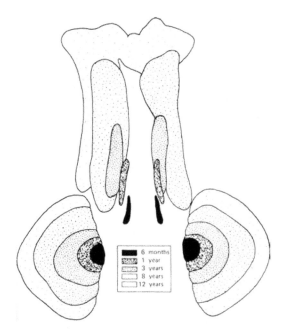

Figure 3 Development of the maxillary and frontal sinuses at various ages. *Source:* From Ref. 3.

Frontal sinus and frontal recess development is more varied. Debate still exists regarding the exact details. Three theories have been promoted. The frontal sinus may arise (1) from direct extension of the frontal recess, (2) from an anterior ethmoid cell, or (3) from the anterior superior aspect of the ethmoid infundibulum. The frontal sinus is barely perceptible at age one. Development of the frontal sinus does not characteristically begin until about the fourth year. Its adult size is attained at nearly age 12. The sinus continues to develop until the late teens.

A cartilage capsule surrounds the primordial nasal cavity and is responsible for the bony development of this region. The uncinate process begins to form by the 10th to 12th week as a bud of cartilage. By the 13th to 14th weeks, a lateral space develops that becomes the ethmoid infundibulum. At 16 weeks, the future maxillary sinus begins to form from the infundibulum. The cartilage will resorb or ossify, depending on its location.

The ethmoid sinus can be visualized radiographically at birth; however, its visualization is more difficult than the maxillary sinuses. The ethmoid and the maxillary sinuses are the only sinuses to be sufficiently developed at birth to be clinically significant in the pathogenesis of acute rhinosinusitis. The ethmoid sinuses continue to develop and are more readily seen at one year of age. By age 12, they have reached their adult size.

The sphenoid sinus is the last sinus to develop. The posterior nasal capsule is invaginated by nasal mucosa at three to four months of fetal growth. This area enlarges to become a pouch or cavity called the cartilaginous copular recess of the nasal cavity. When the walls around the cartilage ossify, it is referred to as the ossiculum Bertini. This ossification occurs in the later months of fetal development. The cavity does not definitely become the sphenoid sinus until the cartilage is resorbed as the ossiculum Bertini becomes attached to the sphenoid in the second to third year. Only in the sixth to seventh year does the sphenoid become pneumatized. Complete pneumatization does not occur until the 9th to 12th years. Further minor modifications of the sphenoid sinus occur until the late teens or into early adult life (Fig. 4).

ANATOMY OF THE NOSE AND PARANASAL SINUSES

Understanding the relationship of the bony anatomy of the face and the pneumatized cells within this bony framework is essential in appreciating the anatomy of the paranasal sinuses. The structures that make up the framework of the face include the nasal bones and cartilages, the ethmoid bones, the maxillary bones, and the frontal and sphenoid bones. The outer structure of the nose is formed by the paired nasal bones, as well as the upper lateral and lower lateral cartilages inferiorly. These structures provide prominence to the nasal pyramid, as well as allowing for an aperture to provide airflow through the nasal cavity (Fig. 5).

The midline of the nose consists of a structure known as the *nasal septum*. This structure is composed of both bone and cartilage, and divides the nasal cavity roughly into two equal halves. The anterior portion of the nasal septum is composed of the *quadrilateral cartilage*, while the more posterior portion of the septum is composed of the *perpendicular plate of*

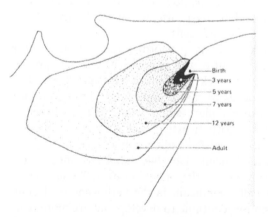

Figure 4   Development of the sphenoid sinus at various ages. *Source*: From Ref. 3.

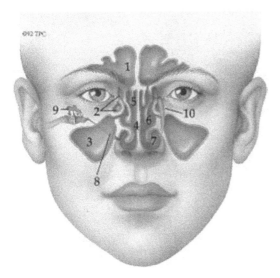

Figure 5 Coronal view of the paranasal sinuses. 1. Frontal sinuses. 2. Ethmoid sinuses. 3. Maxillary sinuses. 4. Nasal septum. 5. Superior turbinate. 6. Middle turbinate. 7. Inferior turbinate. 8. Eustachian tube. 9. Middle ear. 10. Nasolacrimal duct.

the ethmoid bone superiorly and the *vomer* inferiorly. At its posterior limit, the vomer ends at the posterior choanae of the nose.

The lateral nasal wall consists of bony prominences covered with respiratory epithelium that project into the nasal cavity. These prominences are known as the *nasal turbinates* (Fig. 6). There is a space that exists under each of these turbinates that is described as the *meatus.* There are usually three turbinates and three meati present in the lateral nasal wall bilaterally. The largest of these turbinates is the *inferior turbinate,* which arises from the maxillary bone and projects into the nasal cavity. In the underlying *inferior meatus,* the nasolacrimal duct opens into the nose at the *valve of Hassner.*

The *middle turbinate* is a projection of the ethmoid bone into the nasal cavity. The associated *middle meatus* is important in understanding paranasal sinus anatomy and physiology because it is into this meatus that the anterior sinuses communicate with the nose. More superiorly, a small *superior turbinate* is usually present in the nose, and forms the medial wall of the posterior ethmoid sinuses. In the associated *superior meatus* is an area referred to as the *sphenoethmoidal recess,* which is an important region in that the posterior ethmoid sinuses and sphenoid sinuses communicate with the nose in this location.

The superior portion of the nose is bounded by a portion of the skull base that is referred to as the *cribriform plate.* This thin bony plate extends from the sphenoid sinuses posteriorly to the frontal recess anteriorly. The perpendicular plate of the ethmoid attaches in the midportion of this structure. The cribriform plate is perforated by branches of the olfactory nerve that terminate

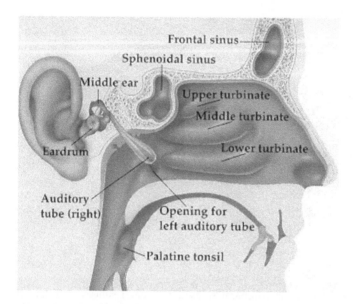

Figure 6 Sagittal view of the nose, paranasal sinuses, Eustachian tube, and middle ear.

within the nose to provide sensory input to the olfactory cortex. The cribriform plate is very thin, usually measuring only 1 to 2 mm in thickness (4).

Ethmoid Sinuses

The primary structure that forms the foundation for the bony anatomy of the face and sinuses is the ethmoid bone. The ethmoid bones are bilateral and are bound in the midline by the perpendicular plate. The superior boundary of the ethmoid bones is the cribriform plate, and the lateral boundary is the *lamina papyracea*, a thin bony plate that separates the ethmoid sinuses from the orbits laterally. Inferiorly, the ethmoid bone includes the middle turbinates and the lateral nasal wall at the area in which it fuses with the maxillary bone inferiorly.

The lamina papyracea is an important structure in that it forms the barrier between the ethmoid sinuses and the orbits. This lamina is very thin and can be compromised by a variety of processes that originate within the ethmoid sinuses. Acute infections of the ethmoid sinuses can easily cross this thin bony barrier, resulting in periorbital or orbital cellulitis or abscess formation. Inflammatory masses of the ethmoid sinuses, such as mucoceles, mucopyoceles, and neoplasms, can also compromise this barrier through erosion or expansion, resulting in orbital injury.

The anatomy of the ethmoid sinuses is complex, due to the variable pneumatization that occurs within the ethmoid bone during early development. The ethmoid sinuses can be best conceptualized as a cluster of cells that are divided into discrete anatomic regions by a series of vertical bony partitions. The cluster of cells that occurs within each ethmoid bone numbers in the range of 12 to 18 cells and is often referred to as the *ethmoid labyrinth*. The pneumatized cells of the ethmoid sinuses can be grouped into two functional units: the *anterior ethmoid cells*, which are more numerous and smaller in size and which communicate with the nose in the middle meatus, and the *posterior ethmoid cells*, which are less numerous, larger, and communicate with the nose in the sphenoethmoidal recess. The ethmoid sinuses are apparent by the third to fourth month of fetal life, and can be appreciated radiologically during the first year of life.

The anterior ethmoid cells, along with the frontal sinus and the maxillary sinus, communicate with the nose through an anatomic region that is referred to as the *ostiomeatal complex* (OMC) (Fig. 7). The OMC is important as a structural unit, in that this area is commonly conceptualized as of primary importance in the normal functioning of the anterior paranasal sinuses. When the structural integrity of the OMC is compromised and the normal ventilation and drainage of the sinuses is adversely affected, it is common for the associated sinuses to become secondarily infected.

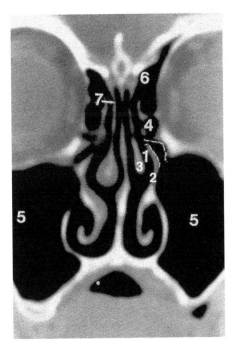

Figure 7 Coronal CT radiograph of the paranasal sinuses with ostiomeatal complex outlined. 1. Middle meatus. 2. Uncinate process. 3. Middle turbinate. 4. Ethmoid sinuses. 5. Maxillary sinuses. 6. Frontal recess. 7. Middle turbinate. Dashed lines outline the area of the infundibulum and OMC. *Abbreviation*: OMC, ostiomeatal complex.

The posterior ethmoid sinuses are composed only of several larger air cells. Posteriorly, the ethmoid sinuses are contiguous with the rostrum of the sphenoid sinus. Occasionally a single large posterior ethmoid cell will pneumatize posteriorly and laterally to the sphenoid sinus. This sphenoethmoidal or *Onodi* cell is of importance in that the optic nerve travels along its lateral aspect and can often be dehiscent.

Maxillary Sinuses

The maxillary bones are bilateral structures that form the projection of the anterior face. The maxilla consists of a main body and four processes: the frontal, orbital, alveolar, and palatal processes. It forms the midface and provides support for the maxillary teeth. The opening of the nasal cavity enters anteriorly through the maxillary bone at the nostrils bilaterally. The right and left maxillary bones are contiguous in the midline below the nose, and their palatal processes extend centrally to form the anterior portion of the hard palate. The oral cavity is separated from the nose and maxillary sinuses by this process. The alveolar processes of the maxillary bones contain the roots of the maxillary teeth.

The orbital processes of the maxillary sinuses make up the medial portion of the floor of the orbit and support the orbital contents inferiorly. The roof of the maxillary sinuses, therefore, is bilaterally contiguous with the orbital floor.

Within the maxillary bones are the *maxillary sinuses*, the largest of the four pairs of paranasal sinuses (Fig. 8). These sinuses are well developed at birth and are extensively pneumatized. They are apparent by the third to fourth month of fetal life, and can be appreciated radiologically during the first year of life. The maxillary sinuses are surrounded on all sides by bony walls. The medial wall of the maxillary sinus has an opening between the maxillary sinus and the nose, referred to as the *maxillary ostium*. This opening provides the normal communication between the maxillary sinuses and the nasal cavity, and it is through this small ostium that the maxillary sinus is both drained and ventilated. The ostium is a small opening into the ethmoid infundibulum that is located high on the medial wall of the maxillary sinus, about in the midportion of the anterior–posterior plane. This ostium is not normally visible, as it is lateral to the uncinate process of the ethmoid bone. There are also areas in the medial wall of the maxillary sinuses where there is the absence of bone and a membranous area separates the nose from the sinuses. These areas are referred to as *fontanelles*, and while more commonly found in the posterior portion of the medial wall, can also be present more anteriorly as well.

Frontal Sinuses

The superior portion of the face and anterior portion of the skull is composed of a large, flat bone referred to as the *frontal bone*. The frontal

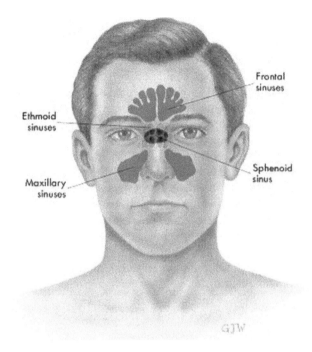

Ethmoid
sinuses

Frontal
sinuses

Sphenoid
sinus

Maxillary
sinuses

GJW

Figure 8 Coronal view of the four pairs of paranasal sinuses.

bone forms the contour of the forehead and the floor of the anterior cranial fossa. It is contiguous with the zygoma laterally and forms the roof of the orbits medially. It divides into two tables in the forehead, the anterior and posterior tables, which contain the pneumatized space referred to as the *frontal sinus*. The anterior table is palpable and visible as the forehead, while the posterior table forms the anterior wall of the anterior cranial fossa.

The frontal sinuses are of variable size and development. They are absent in up to 10% of individuals. While the average size of each frontal sinus is about 10 cc, an individual sinus can be much larger. The natural ostia of the frontal sinuses are found inferomedially, near the midline septum between the right and left sinuses. They communicate with the nose through an inverted funnel-shaped region known as the *frontal recess*. This area can be narrowed by large ethmoid cells that sometimes interfere with normal ventilation and drainage of the frontal sinuses.

The frontal bones are not pneumatized until the first or second year of life, and their definitive shape is not apparent until the third year of life. The frontal sinuses become pneumatized during this period, and are apparent as discrete structures between three and six years of age. They continue to enlarge as frontal pneumatization increases through adolescence.

Sphenoid Sinuses

Within the center of the skull is the *sphenoid bone*. This structure forms the major portion of the central skull base, as well as portions of the orbit, lateral skull, and cranial floor. Superiorly to the sphenoid bone is the sella turcica and middle cranial fossa. Within the midportion of the sphenoid bone are the *sphenoid sinuses*, small pneumatized spaces measuring 5 to 10 cc in size, that pneumatize in childhood and often do not complete their pneumatization until early adult life. These sinuses communicate with the nasal cavity in the sphenoethmoidal recesses bilaterally. The natural ostium of the sphenoid sinus is located in the anterior wall of the sphenoid bone at a location near the superior aspect of the sinus. This opening is at the inferomedial edge of the superior turbinate, in a narrow space along the sphenoid rostrum and lateral to the nasal septum.

The sphenoid sinuses are the final sinuses to pneumatize. They begin as an invagination in the nasal capsule, but are not recognizable as discrete units until age three or four. They are not radiographically apparent until age eight or nine, and continue to develop into young adulthood as the sphenoid bone completes its pneumatization.

PHYSIOLOGY OF THE NOSE AND PARANASAL SINUSES

The function of the nose is to allow inspired air to enter the upper respiratory system and to be delivered to the tracheobronchial tree. The presence of the turbinates on the lateral nasal walls allows this airflow to be turbulent, creating eddies in flow as the air moves posteriorly from the nostrils to the posterior choanae. This flow pattern directs the inspired air to come into contact with a large surface area of the nasal mucosa as it moves posteriorly, which allows three physiological functions during flow: filtration, warming, and humidification (5) (Table 2).

The mucosa of the nasal cavity is a respiratory-type pseudostratified columnar epithelium. This epithelium is contiguous with the paranasal sinuses, and it is lined with a surface layer of cilia. The ciliated surface is involved in a variety of processes, including the transport of mucus and particulate matter from the nasal cavity into the nasopharynx, where it can be swallowed. This process is known as *mucociliary clearance*, and is an essential component of the normal physiology of the nose and paranasal sinuses. As mucus is produced by goblet cells in the nasal mucosa, this mucus forms a blanket that lines the surface of the nasal epithelium. This mucous blanket is involved in filtration of particulate matter as it enters the nose. This particulate population can be composed of viral and bacterial organisms; foreign proteins such as animal dander, dust mite debris, and pollen grains; and irritants such as tobacco smoke. The filtration and transport of this particulate mass is necessary for normal sinonasal function. When mucociliary clearance mechanisms are disrupted, as from allergic or infectious rhinosinusitis, changes can occur in the underlying mucosa that can lead to chronic dysfunction and disease.

Table 2 Functions of the Nose and Sinuses

Filtration
   Removal of particulate matter
   Transport of foreign organisms, irritants, and allergens
   Prevention of large particles from reaching the lower airway
Warming
   Increasing temperature of inspired, cold air
   Delivering warm air to the lower airway
Humidification
   Increasing humidity of inspired, dry air
   Delivering moist air to the lower airway
   Mucociliary clearance
   Movement of mucus blanket through the sinuses and nose
   Transport of mucus blanket to the pharynx
Ventilation
   Increases oxygen tension in the sinuses
   Allows normal environment for respiratory epithelium

In addition to the filtration function of the nasal cavity, the nose is involved in both the warming and humidification of inspired air. The inhalation of warm, moist air into the lower respiratory tract is important in maintaining optimal function of the bronchopulmonary system. When this important function of the nose is inoperative, cold, dry air can be delivered to the lungs, which can increase the likelihood of acute bronchospasm, shortness of breath, and infection. Chronic nasal dysfunction can contribute significantly to lower respiratory diseases such as asthma and chronic bronchitis.

This mucociliary clearance mechanism is also present in the paranasal sinuses. Since the epithelium is the same throughout the upper respiratory system, the mucosa lining the sinus cavities also actively produces mucus that must be cleared into the nasopharynx and swallowed. Mucociliary clearance within the sinuses is genetically programmed in such a manner as to direct the flow of mucus from the sinuses in a predetermined, predictable pattern from the interior of each sinus to the natural opening or *ostium* of the sinus, and into the nose itself (6). Disruptions in the normal clearance of mucus from the sinus chambers results in mucous stasis within the sinuses, which leads to a sequence of events that predisposes those sinuses to both acute and chronic dysfunction and infection. Ventilation of air into the sinuses and drainage of mucus from the sinuses is central in the normal physiologic function of the sinuses, and interference with this ventilation and drainage is a key component in the pathogenesis of acute and chronic rhinosinusitis (7).

As was previously discussed, each of the sinuses communicates with the nasal cavity through a precise anatomical location. The anterior ethmoid and maxillary sinuses communicate with the nose through a common passage way, known as the OMC. Since the ethmoid infundibulum is the final space through which these sinuses communicate with the nose, disease in the ethmoid is common in most cases of acute and chronic rhinosinusitis. For this reason, the ethmoid sinuses are often considered to be the "seat of sinus disease."

The frontal sinuses also communicate with the nose anteriorly, but their pattern of ventilation and drainage is somewhat variable. In about two-thirds of individuals, the frontal sinuses communicate with the ethmoid infundibulum directly, with the frontal recess opening lateral to the bulla ethmoidalis into the hiatus semilunaris superior. In the remaining one-third of individuals, the frontal recess communicates medial to the bulla, and opens directly into the middle meatus just lateral to the attachment of the middle turbinate. In both of these cases, however, the communication with the nose is through the middle meatus inferiorly.

Both the posterior ethmoid sinuses and the sphenoid sinus communicate with the nose more posteriorly in an area known as the sphenoethmoidal recess. This area is in direct communication with the nasopharynx. While disease in the sphenoethmoidal recess is less frequent than that seen in the OMC, it is still quite common among patients with acute and chronic sinus infections.

CONCLUSION

An understanding of the embryology, developmental and adult anatomy, and physiology of the nose and paranasal sinuses is important in assisting clinicians with appropriate diagnosis and management of the patient with nasal and sinus diseases. Ongoing study of the intricate nature of sinonasal function in disease and in health can provide physicians with a better appreciation of these complex diseases, and can facilitate better outcomes in children and adults with acute and chronic rhinosinusitis.

REFERENCES

1. Hengerer AS. Embryologic development of the sinuses. Ear Nose Throat J 1984; 63:134–136.
2. Van Alyea OE. Nasal Sinuses: an Anatomic and Clinical Consideration, 2nd ed., Baltimore: Williams & Wilkins, 1951.
3. Naspitz CK, Tinkelman DG. Childhood Rhinitis and Sinusitis: Pathophysiology and Treatment. New York: Marcel Dekker, 1990.
4. Kennedy DW, Bolger WE, Zinreich SJ. Diseases of the Sinuses: Diagnosis and Management. Philadelphia, BC: Decker, 2001.
5. Abramson M, Harker LA. Physiology of the nose. Otolaryngol Clin North Am 1973; 6:623–635.
6. Stamberger H. Functional Endoscopic Sinus Surgery: the Messerklinger Technique. Philadelphia, BC: Decker, 1991.
7. Corren J, Togias A, Bousquet J. Upper and Lower Respiratory Disease. New York: Marcel Dekker, 2003.

6

Pathophysiology of Sinusitis

Alexis H. Jackman and David W. Kennedy
*Department of Otorhinolaryngology Head and Neck Surgery,
University of Pennsylvania, Philadelphia, Pennsylvania, U.S.A.*

INTRODUCTION

A complete understanding of the pathophysiology of rhinosinusitis remains elusive, but several infectious and inflammatory pathways have been identified. Microbial agents, such as viruses, bacteria, and fungus, are well-established etiologies of rhinosinusitis, especially in the acute situation, but numerous host and environmental factors have also been implicated, either individually or in combination in the chronic disease state. This chapter will discuss these various factors as well as the individual and symbiotic roles they play in the development of rhinosinusitis. Particular emphasis will be placed on current hypotheses regarding the etiology of chronic rhinosinusitis (CRS) and important new areas of research such as biofilms, superantigens (sags), and osteitis.

Local Paranasal Sinus Defense Mechanisms

The main function of the paranasal sinuses (PNS) is to eliminate foreign material and defend the body against infection. Essential local factors in maintaining normal paranasal sinus function include:

- Ostiomeatal complex (OMC) patency
- Mucociliary transport
- Normal mucus production

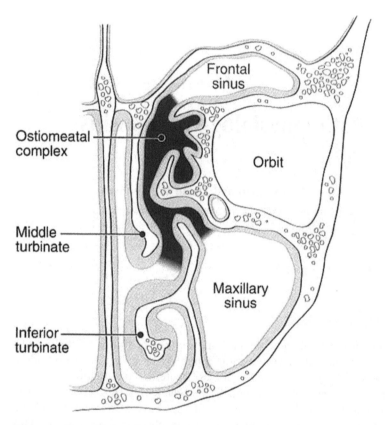

Figure 1 The ostiomeatal complex. *Source*: Kennedy DW. The concept of the ostio-meatal complex. Diseases of the Sinuses: Diagnosis and Management. Hamilton: B.C. Decker, 2001:197.

Ostiomeatal complex (OMC) is the common drainage site of the frontal, ethmoid, and maxillary sinuses. Although a myriad of variations in the size and architecture of the OMC exist, patency of this area and its respective outflow tracks is necessary for the removal of mucus and debris and mainte-nance of sufficient oxygen tensions to prevent bacterial overgrowth. (Fig. 1).

Recently, acknowledgment of an overemphasis on the role of OMC patency in CRS has been made, but nonetheless the OMC remains one of the several important factors in normal paranasal sinus function, and osteo-meatal obstruction remains a common final pathway in sinus disease becom-ing chronic. Another major factor in PNS function is mucociliary transport (MCT). MCT is dependent on both ciliary activity and the rheologic proper-ties of the mucus. Characteristics of the cilia, such as their structure and population, as well as the coordination of their movement are important in their ability to function effectively. Likewise, mucus characteristics, such as

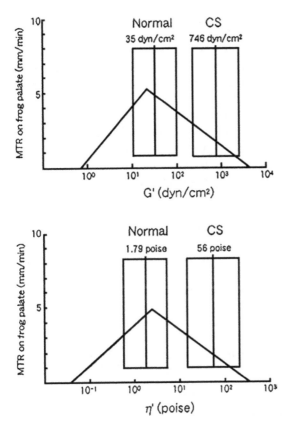

Figure 2 Effects of elasticity and viscosity on mucociliary clearance. *Source*: Adapted from Ref. 1.

the volume that is secreted and its viscoelastic properties, are known to affect overall MCT, with maximal velocities being reported for mucus with an elasticity (G') of about 20 dyn/cm^2 and a viscosity (η') of 2 poise (1) (Fig. 2).

Systemic Paranasal Sinus Defense Mechanisms

Acquired and innate immunity are systemic defense mechanisms against infection in the sinonasal tract. Humoral immunity, which is a function of B-lymphocytes, is predominately mediated by IgA antibodies. Normal mucus contains large amounts of IgA, which detects and initiates the removal of foreign material through a process termed opsinization. Additional antibodies present in nasal mucosa include IgG and IgE. Although IgE is detected in only trace amounts in normal individuals, large increases in its relative concentration are observed in atopic patients with CRS, thereby implicating IgE as a participant in allergic CRS. IgG plays a less prominent role and is present only in minimal concentrations. Cell-mediated immunity involves activated T-lymphocytes, macrophages, and cytokines. Defensins are antimicrobial cytokines that are present in the airway surface liquid of the paranasal mucosa. The cationic defensin polypeptide binds to the outer membrane of target bacterial, viral, or fungal cells, causing membrane disruption, internalization of defensin, and finally cell death (2,3). In a study comparing the level of expression of defensins in control patients versus patients with chronic sinusitis, β-defensins were detected only in patients with sinusitis. Furthermore, levels of β-defensins were significantly higher in nasal polyp (NP) tissue than in inferior turbinate tissue in these patients, supporting the role of this inflammatory mediator in the pathophysiology of CRS (4).

Interruption of the normal functions of the PNS changes the physiological milieu and creates an environment that fosters microbial proliferation and initiates an inflammatory response. A combination of local and systemic factors are involved in normal sinus function. An example of this is given by Goldman et al. (5) in their description of the mucosal surface of the airway as a "chemical shield," with the airway epithelium producing mucus-containing salt-sensitive defensins and the mucus having a low-salt (<50 mM NaCl) liquid on the surface that renders the defensins active. Interruption of any one of the many factors, involved in normal sinus functioning can impact other factors often initiating a cascade of events leading to CRS, with pathological changes in the sinuses that often begin in or are accompanied by similar changes in the nasal airway (5,6) (Fig. 3).

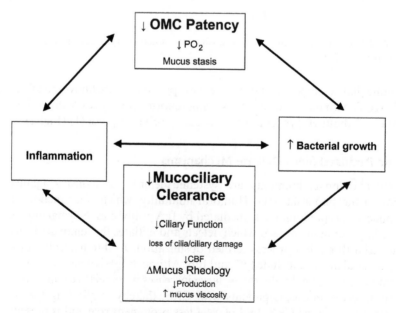

Figure 3 The pathological cycle of CRS.

DEFINITIONS OF RHINOSINUSITIS

Rhinosinusitis is an umbrella term that includes a continuum of inflammatory changes in both the nose and sinuses. Rhinosinusitis describes many different pathological processes that result in mucosal inflammation of the nose and PNS. In 1996, a multidisciplinary rhinosinusitis task force (RSTF) was formed in part to develop working definitions to describe the wide spectrum of pathological entities represented. The seminal article, "Adult Rhinosinusitis Defined," which summarized these proceedings, defined five separate categories: acute, subacute, chronic, recurrent acute, and acute exacerbation of CRS. These categories were defined according to specific major and minor signs and symptoms associated with rhinosinusitis and the time course over which they occurred without regard to their specific pathogenesis (7) (Table 1).

Acute rhinosinusitis (ARS) was defined by the presence of specific signs and symptoms for a duration of up to four weeks. Using similar clinical criteria, subacute rhinosinusitis was defined as lasting between 4 weeks and 12 weeks, and recurrent acute rhinosinusitis was defined by four or more episodes of acute sinusitis with complete symptom remission between episodes. CRS was defined by the presence of several clinical symptoms for duration of at least 12 weeks, whereas patients with sudden worsening of persistent symptoms are classified as having an acute exacerbation of CRS. These definitions put forth by the RSTF are independent of hypothesized etiologies and associated disease states, reflecting its members' view of CRS as an inflammatory disease of uncertain etiologies (7).

ACUTE RHINOSINUSITIS

ARS is most commonly associated with an infectious etiology in both children and adults. The type and species of microorganism implicated has been shown to be age-related in several studies. In children, viral agents such as adenovirus, influenza virus, parainfluenza virus, and rhinovirus predominate, although bacterial agents are also common with the major pathogens being *Streptococcus pneumoniae*, non-typeable *Haemophilus influenzae*, and *Moraxella catarrhalis* (8,9). Similarly, *S. pneumoniae, H. influenzae,* and *M. catarrhalis* were also identified as the predominant microorganisms in cases of pediatric subacute rhinosinusitis (10). Anaerobic bacteria have not been shown to play a major role in pediatric rhinosinusitis. Wald et al. reported that only one of 47 sinus aspirates was positive for anaerobic bacteria (11). In adults, *S. pneumoniae* and non-typeable *H. influenzae* account for over 75% of cases of community-acquired acute sinusitis, and two bacterial species in high density were identified in 25% of cases. Although *S. aureus* and *Streptococcus pyogenes* are uncommon causes of ARS, they have been associated with serious suppurative processes such

Table 1 Classification of Adult Rhinosinusitis[a]

Classification	Duration	Strong history	Include in differential	Special notes
Acute	≤4 weeks	≥2 major factors, 1 major factor and 2 minor factors, or nasal purulence on examination	1 major factor or ≥2 minor factors	Fever or facial pain does not constitute a suggestive history in the absence of other nasal signs or symptoms. Consider acute bacterial rhinosinusitis if symptoms worsen after 5 days, if symptoms persist for > 10 days, or in presence of symptoms out of proportion to those typically associated with viral infection
Subacute	4–12 weeks	Same as chronic	Same as chronic	Complete resolution after effective medical therapy
Recurrent acute	≥4 episodes per year, with each episode lasting ≥7 to 10 days and absence of intervening signs and symptoms of chronic rhinosinusitis	Same as acute	—	—

Chronic	≥12 weeks	≥major factors, 1 major factor and 2 minor factors, or nasal purulence on examination	1 major factor or ≥2 minor factors	Facial pain does not constitute a suggestive history in the absence of other nasal signs or symptoms
Acute exacerbations of chronic	Sudden worsening of chronic rhinosinusitis, with return to baseline after treatment	—	—	

[a]Rhinosinusitis may be clinically defined as condition manifested by an inflammatory response involving in the mucous membranes (possibly including neuroepithelium) of nasal cavity and paranasal sinuses, fluids within these cavities, and/or underlying bone. Fluids within these cavities are dynamic and are related to dynamic pathologic changes in bone and soft tissues of nasal cavity and paranasal sinuses. Symptoms associated with rhinosinusitis include nasal obstruction, nasal congestion, nasal discharge, nasal purulence, postnasal drip, facial pressure and pain, alteration in sense of smell, cough, fever, halitosis, fatigue, dental pain, pharyngitis, otologic symptoms (e.g., ear fullness and clicking), and headache.

as orbital and intracranial abscesses. Furthermore, anaerobic bacteria are also rarely implicated in ARS in adults, and when they are, they are almost always associated with a primary dental pathology (12).

The pathophysiologic reaction to infectious agents in ARS is the initiation of an inflammatory response, the intent of which is to promote the removal of foreign material, interrupt inflammatory cascade, and restore normal sinus function. On a macroscopic level, pathologic changes include mucosal edema with infiltrates of lymphocytes and plasma cells and loss of cilia from the respiratory epithelium. Luminal exudates are also found, which consist of primarily neutrophils and limited amounts of eosinophils (13–15). Several inflammatory cytokines have been demonstrated in conjunction with these histopathologic changes. Cytokines such as IL-1B, IL-6, and TNF-α are important in inducing the expression of adhesion molecules and activating endothelial cells and T-lymphocytes. Subsequently, these activated T-lymphocytes release IL-8, a neutrophil chemotaxic factor, which further enhances the inflammatory response and eventually leads to evacuation of the initiating organism (16–19). As the infection resolves, the inflammatory reaction subsides and the physiologic state is restored.

CHRONIC RHINOSINUSITIS

The specific pathogenesis of CRS remains to be determined. Although in some cases it may result from a persistent acute infection. It is thought to arise from multiple heterogeneous etiologies either independently, or more likely, in combination. The latest publications of chronic rhinosinusitis task force (CRTF) emphasize the position that it is the resulting end-stage inflammatory state that defines this disease. Furthermore, the concept of an integrated airway syndrome has been hypothesized along with rhinitis, rhinosinusitis, and asthma as a spectrum of manifestations of this single disease state (8).

In contrast to ARS, the etiology of CRS is thought to be more multifactorial with the contribution of several systemic host, local host, and environmental factors. Systemic host factors include genetic predisposition, immunosuppression, and primary ciliary dyskinesia (PCD). Local host factors include anatomical sinus obstruction or local tumors or masses obstructing the sinuses, and localized persistent inflammation, such as that in the case of bony inflammation. Environmental factors include bacteria, viruses, and fungi, as well as pollution, smoking, and allergy. Several microorganisms, such as bacteria and fungi, are associated with CRS, but additional research in this area is necessary to more clearly define their relative roles. Further understanding of these factors may provide new approaches to diagnosis and treatment of this disease.

The pathological mechanisms involved in CRS share many similarities with those of ARS, although distinct differences have been demonstrated.

The gross pathological expression of CRS is more variable, and has been divided into two major categories—CRS with nasal polyps (CRSwNP) and CRS without nasal polyps (CRSsNP). CRSwNP is characterized by extensive mucosal edema with goblet cell hyperplasia and mononuclear cell infiltration, whereas CRSsNP is often noted to have epithelial damage with very limited neural structures and goblet cell hypoplasia. Fibrosis is common in both, but occurs to a greater extent in CRSwNP (20,21). An increased number of eosinophils is the predominant difference in the cellular infiltrate between CRSwNP and CRSsNP. Also, increased local production of IgE has been reported (22). A wide variety of inflammatory mediators have been demonstrated to be increased in patients with CRSsNP and include IL-1, IL-6, IL-8, TNF-α, GM-CSF, ICAM-1, MPO (myeloperoxidase), and ECP (eosinophilic cationic protein) (23–26). Patients with nasal polyposis (NP) have also been shown to have increased amounts of these mediators, but additional inflammatory mediators in the subset of patients with NP include a subset of the IL-8 superfamily referred to as regulated on activiation- normal T expressed and secreted (RANTES) as well as IL-4 and IL-5, which have been shown to directly activate and increase the survival of eosinophils (27,28).

ETIOLOGIES OF CHRONIC RHINOSINUSITIS

A myriad of potential factors predispose an individual to the development of CRS, and several classification schemes have been developed to assist in the understanding of the relationship between these factors. One approach to the variety of proposed etiologies is to divide them into three categories: systemic factors, local host factors, and environmental factors (Table 2).

Systemic Host Factors

Genetic/Congenital Disorders

Several systemic host factors contribute to the development of CRS. Genetic abnormalities such as cystic fibrosis (CF) and primary ciliary disorders are intimately associated with CRS. Although these diseases are commonly diagnosed during childhood, adults with a lifelong history of CRS associated with bronchial infection, infertility, or situs inversus should be further evaluated (29). In patients with CRS, diagnosis of a primary ciliary disorder usually requires a tracheal biopsy because, intranasally, the acquired ciliary deformities associated with CRS can be difficult to differentiate from the congenital variant.

CF is one of the most common hereditary diseases and affects approximately 30,000 people in the United States, having a gene frequency of 1 in 20–25 (30,31). The disease was mapped to the long arm of chromosome 7 (7q31), which encodes a protein product that acts as a chloride channel. Genetic alterations of this protein allow for increased water absorption from

Table 2 Etiologic Factors in Chronic Rhinosinusitis

Systemic host factors
Genetic/congenital conditions—cystic fibrosis (CF), primary ciliary disorders (PCD)
Immunodeficiencies/immunosuppression—HIV, iatrogenic-s/p transplant,
  chemotherapy
Autoimmune—
    Granulomatosis (sarcoid, Wegener's)
    Vasculitis (SLE)
Idiopathic—Samter's syndrome
Local host factors
Anatomic abnormalities
Bony inflammation
Neuromechanisms
Mucoceles
Neoplasms (benign and malignant)
Environmental factors
Infectious—bacterial, fungal, biofilms, superantigens
Allergy—IgE-mediated, non-IgE-mediated hypersensitivities
Pollutants—pollution, smoke, dust, volatile organic compounds

the respiratory cells, resulting in increased viscosity and impaired mucociliary clearance (32). Furthermore, bacterial colonization and infection with *Pseudomonas aeruginosa, H. influenzae,* and anaerobes are frequent and thought to induce cellular changes such as goblet cell hyperplasia, loss of cilia, and squamous cell metaplasia. Gross pathological changes include nasal polyposis, which is usually noted in early childhood. In contrast to atopic patients, NP in patients with CF is not associated with a thickened basement membrane and an eosinophilic infiltrate (33). Other gross pathological changes include osteomeatal obstruction secondary to local inflammation and tenacious mucus (34). Recently, there has been significant interest in whether minor CF variations may be a factor in CRS. At this point, the evidence for this is limited. However, some patients with homozygous CF do present only with CRS, and CF should be suspected in any patient who has had an operation before the age of 18 years (35).

Another group of genetic disorders commonly associated with CRS is termed primary ciliary disorder (PCD), which include Kartagener's syndrome, immotile cilia syndrome, ciliary dysmotility, and primary ciliary orientation defects. Although it is rare with a prevalence of approxiamately 1:20,000, the effects on the sinonasal tract are significant (36). PCD is hypothesized to be a genetically heterogeneous condition as several loci on various chromosomes have been identified. Abnormalities in ciliary structure resulting in malfunction characterize this disorder and include a number of ultrastructural alterations in the ciliary architecture, which range from complete ciliary aplasia to defects in ciliary orientation (37–39).

Resulting mucus stasis leads to pathological mechanisms similar to CF in the development of CRS.

Immunodeficiency Diseases

Chronic medically refractive CRS is common in patients with congenital and acquired immunodeficiencies, as well as those who are immunosupressed. IgG deficiencies are the most common cause of immunodeficiencies associated with CRS (40). CRS frequently occurs in patients with the human immunodeficiency virus, with a reported rate of 68% of patients with this disease (41). Endoscopic surgery has been advocated as a treatment for patients who meet the surgical criteria for surgery regardless of their CD4 count (42). CRS is also commonly diagnosed in patients receiving chemotherapy and in patients being treated with long-term immunosuppressive therapies, such as in post-transplant recipients. Furthermore, specific types of immunodeficiency syndromes are associated with certain infectious pathogens. Patients with antibody deficiencies are known to have a predisposition to infections with encapsulated aerobic gram-positive organisms as well as gram-negative organisms. In contrast, CRS patients with T-cell deficiencies is associated with fungal, viral, and protozoal organisms. In patients with complement deficiencies, aerobic gram-negative organisms predominate.

Autoimmune/Idiopathic Diseases

CRS is associated with several autoimmune or idiopathic diseases and may be their presenting illness. Granulomatous disorders frequently associated with CRS include sarcoidosis and Wegener's granulomatosis (WG). Sarcoidosis, a chronic granulomatosis disease of unknown etiology, can involve the upper respiratory tract, although lower respiratory tract involvement is more common. The pathological hallmark of this disease is a chronic inflammatory response, which includes non-caseating granulomas. Local tissue changes range in severity from destruction of cilia and mucus-producing glands to local tissue destruction (43). WG is a necrotizing granulomatosis of the upper and lower respiratory tract, and is currently classified as one of the antineutrophil cytoplasmic antibodies (ANCA)-associated small vessel vasculitides. WG is characterized by autoantibodies to proteinase 3, a component of neutrophil azurophilic granules, although their detection is not required for diagnosis (44,45). Sinonasal manifestations, and therefore CRS, is common in this population and can be severe. Other vasculitides associated with CRS include systemic lupus erythematosus, Churg–Strauss vasculitis, relapsing polychondritis, and Sjogrens syndrome (46). Samter's syndrome, the triad of nasal polyps, bronchial asthma, and intolerance to aspirin, is a condition of unknown etiology, which is associated with an early onset of CRS. Typically, these patients present between the ages of 20 and 30 years with nasal congestion and polyposis that respond poorly to medical and

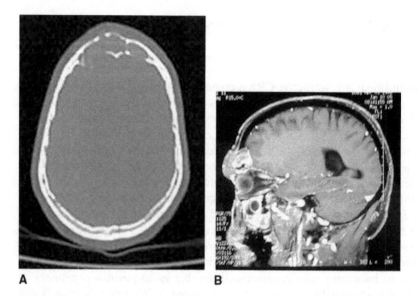

A   **B**

Figure 4   Coronal CT view of frontal sinus and sagittal MRI view of a patient with Samter's triad. *Note*: Sinus opacification and erosion of anterior and posterior table bone.

surgical management, although they may also present with asthma later in life (47). Although a genetic component of this syndrome has been suggested, few studies to date have been conducted (Fig. 4).

Local Host Factors

Anatomic Abnormalities

Local host factors can also play a role in the development of CRS. Anatomic abnormalities of the sinuses, particularly those causing obstruction or narrowing of the OMC either chronically or intermittently due to an acute inflammatory response, can be associated with CRS. Moreover, since the OMC is immediately adjacent to the site where the majority of inhaled particulate matter is deposited, it is one of the most common sites for mucosal inflammation. Obstruction in the area of the OMC will result in secondary obstruction of the dependent maxillary and frontal sinuses, and persistent inflammation of the OMC can result in persistent or recurrent infections (Fig. 5).

The relative contribution of anatomic abnormalities to the development of CRS is controversial. The rate of structural sinonasal variations on CT scans has not been shown to correlate with the rates of development of CRS (48). However, it appears reasonable that anatomical variations, such as a markedly deviated nasal septum and aerated middle turbinate (concha bullosa), both of which narrow the OMC, may predispose to muco-

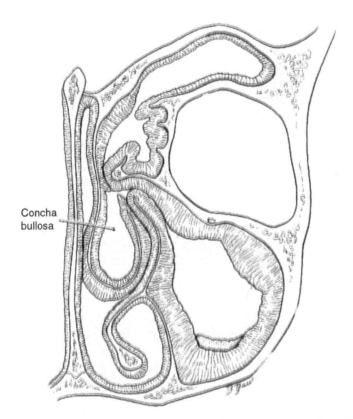

Concha
bullosa

Figure 5 Diagram of ostiomeatal complex with concha bullosa. *Source*: Cummings CW: Otolaryngology – Head and Neck Surgery, Update 1, Chapter 4: Kennedy DW, Zinreich SJ: Endoscopic Sinus Surgery, page 83, figure 4–4, CV Mosby Co. 1989.

ciliary obstruction, subsequent infection, and CRS in patients who also have other risk factors for CRS. Also, it has been demonstrated that certain anatomical abnormalities were associated with the degree and rate of ethmoid, maxillary, and sphenoid sinus opacification as determined by CT scan during an upper respiratory tract infection. These anatomical abnormalities included septal deviation, horizontal processes of the uncinate, concha bullosa, and Haller cell pneumatization (49).

Iatrogenic Anatomic Abnormalities

Previous surgery and sinonasal trauma may also predispose to sinusitis as a result of malpositioning and scarring of the sinonasal structures, particularly within the region of the OMC. In a review of the causes of failure of endoscopic sinus surgeries, Richtsmeier reported obstructed natural ostia and mucus maltransport among the ten most common reasons for persistent disease (50).

Sinonasal Cysts, Mucoceles, and Neoplasms

Local obstruction of the PNS by benign cysts, mucoceles, as well as benign and malignant neoplasms, can result in rhinosinusitis. Although mostly asymptomatic, mucous retention cysts that result from the blockage of seromucinous glands in the sinus respiratory epithelium can lead to sinus obstruction and CRS; mucoceles, expanding mucus-filled cysts that are lined by entrapped respiratory epithelium, are frequently associated with symptoms of unilateral CRS such as sinus tenderness and headache. Mucoceles commonly arise from an obstructed sinus ostium or sinus septation or from sequestered sinus epithelium a sinus fracture site. If superinfection occurs, a mucopyocele is produced. Sinus neoplasms, such as juvenile nasopharyngeal angiofibroma, inverting papilloma, and various carcinomas, typically present with unilateral nasal obstruction, but may also present with symptoms of unilateral CRS or recurrent ARS, sometimes associated with epistaxis. Accordingly, tumors need to be considered in the differential diagnosis of etiology of this disease (51,52).

Persistent Inflammation/Osteitis

Persistent inflammatory changes within the paranasal sinus bones is another local host factor associated with CRS. Investigations into the role that bony inflammatory changes play in CRS has begun recently. Histological, and radiographical changes in the bone are commonly termed "osteitic changes," and current research focuses on determining whether or not these areas are a potential source of persistent inflammation. Using histomorphometry and radioactive labeling bone studies, the rates of bony turnover in patients with CRS was found to be markedly increased and comparable to that of patients with osteomyelitis (53) (Fig. 6).

Although these findings raise the possibility that bacteria may be present in these areas, PCR studies have yet to confirm their presence. In studies of pseudomonas-induced maxillary sinusitis using a rabbit model, inflammatory changes in the bone were noted not only in the adjacent regions but also distally, apparently from spread through the Haversian canals (54). Additional studies by Khalid et al. using Pseudomonas and *S. aureus*-induced maxillary sinusitis have demonstrated similar results of increased vascularity, inflammatory infiltrates, and later fibrosis occurring in the canals of the Haversian system (55).

In summary, there is clear evidence that the bone becomes involved in the disease process in CRS and that, at least in rabbits, the inflammation in the bone may be present at a site away from the primary infection. The pathological changes seen are histologically compatible with chronic osteomyelitis, but no organisms have been identified within the bone. Although it appears very likely that this inflammation within the bone contributes significantly to the refractory nature of the disease process, this has not

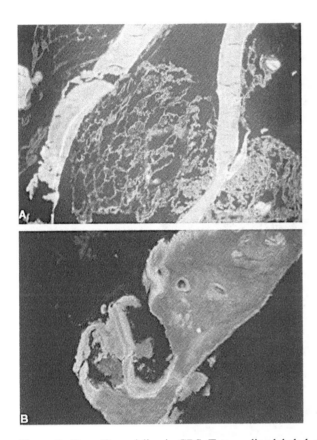

Figure 6 Bony Remodeling in CRS. Tetracycline-labeled ethmoid bone at the time of surgery in a control patient without evidence of infection (**A**) and in patients with chronic sinusitis (**B**). Two doses of tetracycline were given 14 days apart. (**A**) There is one line labeling, indicating little bone turnover. (**B**) There is marked separation of the two lines of fluorescence, indicating significant bone remodeling within the 14-day period. *Source*: Kennedy DW. Diseases of the Sinuses: Diagnosis and Management. Hamilton: B.C. Decker, 2001: 197.

yet been proven. Continuing work in this area will help to better define the pathophysiology of bony inflammation.

Environmental Factors

Microorganisms

Bacterial infections: Several prospective and retrospective studies have been conducted to assess the microbiological etiologies of CRS in both children and adults. Infectious pathogens such as *H. influenzae, S. pneumoniae* and *M. catarrhalis*, account for up to 55% of cases in pediatric CRS. The

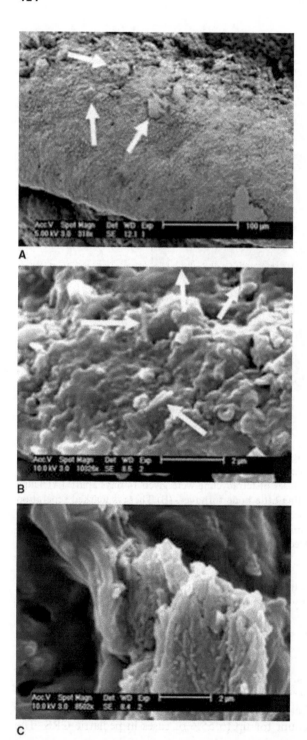

Figure 7 (*Caption on facing page*)

relative contribution of anaerobic bacteria has been debated, and the large variations in rates of isolation have been attributed to culture techniques. Brook reported that up to 50% of cases of CRS were culture-positive for anaerobic bacteria, with the predominance of *Prevotella, Fusobacterium,* and *Peptostreptococcus* spp. (56,57). In adults, infectious CRS is commonly polymicrobial, and both gram-positive and gram-negative aerobic and anaerobic bacteria are frequently isolated. A wide variety of aerobic bacteria, such as coagulase negative Staphylococcus, *S. aureus, Streptococcus viridans, P.aeruginosa, Klebsiella pneumoniae, Proteus mirabilis,* and *Enterobacter* spp. have been isolated. Also, several different anaerobic species have been demonstrated, including *Prevotella, Fusobacterium,* and *Peptostreptococcus* spp. (56–64).

Biofilms. Biofilms are sessile bacterial microcolonies that are enclosed in a highly hydrated polysaccharide matrix with interstitial voids in which nutrients and signaling molecules can be circulated. The structural and functional heterogeneity of bacterial cells within these communities protects them against the body's natural defenses and provides them with antimicrobial resistance. Through genetic alterations, bacteria in biofilms are also able to transition to the mobile planktonic form, which has been the traditional model for studying bacterial diseases (65,66). Bacterial biofilms have been demonstrated on many areas of mucosa in the human body, including the ear mucosa and tympanostomy tubes removed from patients with chronic effusions and infections (67,68). It has been hypothesized that biofilms may play an important role in cases that are refractory to antibiotic therapy, and antibiotic resistance has been demonstrated to be up to 1000-fold greater in bacteria in the biofilm form versus the planktonic form (66–70). Similarities between chronic otitis media and CRS exist. Both of these disease processes take place in the ciliated respiratory epithelium and are largely associated with an infectious etiology. The presence of bacterial biofilms in CRS patients with culture-positive Pseudomonas has been demonstrated using scanning electron microscopy (71) (Fig. 7).

Although further work in this area is required, knowledge of the presence, structural characteristics, and pathological mechanism of biofilms in CRS may help to identify new treatment modalities.

Superantigens. Another new area of interest in infectious CRS involves a group of potent mitogens termed superantigens sags. Sags are most commonly associated with bacteria, particularly *S. aureus* and *S. pyogenes* species, but can also be produced by viruses and fungi. Unlike conventional antigens whose activation requires multiple steps in only a limited number of T-lymphocytes, sags can directly stimulate a multitude of different T-lymphocytes.

Figure 7 (*Facing page*) Biofilms in Human CRS. *Source*: Cyer J, Schipor I, Perloff JR, Palmer JN. Densely coated sinonasal epithelium with tower-like structures (*white arrows*) visible near the top edge of the specimen. *Source*: From Ref. 71.

In the traditional pathway, the antigen is phagocytosized by an antigen-presenting cell (APC), degraded into numerous peptide fragments, which are then processed for cell surface display in conjunction with a major histocompatibility complex (MHC) II receptor. A compatible T-helper cell then recognizes this MHC II/peptide complex, and an inflammatory response is initiated. Sags are able to bypass these processing and presenting steps and bind directly to the outside surfaces of the HLA-DR alpha domain of MHC class II and V beta domain of the T-cell receptors (picture) (72–75). Through this mechanism, they are able to stimulate a massive expression of IL-2 at femtomolar concentrations (76). In turn, IL-2 stimulates the production of other cytokines such as TNF-α, IL-1, Il-8, and platelet activating factor (PAF), leading to an overwhelming inflammatory response. Additionally, sags also act as traditional antigens, as well as stimulate the production of anti-superantigen antibodies.

Recently, upregulation of IgE sags antibodies have been demonstrated in patients with chronic obstructive pulmonary disease (COPD) exacerbation (77). Likewise, a study by Basher et al. found increased levels of sags in patients with NP versus control patients (78). Evidence of the roles of superantigen-producing bacterial strains in the pathologic mechanism of Kawasaki disease, atopic dermitits, and rheumatoid arthritis has also been reported, and a pathophysiological mechanism in which microbial persistence and superantigen-induced T-cell inflammatory responses in CRS has also been proposed (79). Further studies in this area, as well as in other areas of CRS, may provide new diagnostic and treatment modalities.

Fungal infections: Fungal species play a variety of roles in chronic sinusitis from colonization to invasive, life-threatening disease. Invasive disease is characterized by histopathological evidence of hyphal forms within the sinus mucosa, submucosa, blood vessels, or bone, and has been associated with either fulminate or a more indolent chronic course of fungal rhinosinusitis. In addition, chronic invasive disease may or may not be associated with a giant cell response. The pathophysiology of these different disease courses has been attributed primarily to the host's immune response to the fungus, although the fungal species also appears to play some role in the disease course. Fungal species associated with fulminate forms of fungal sinusitis include *Absidia, Aspergillus, Basidobolus, Mucor,* and *Rhizopus* spp., and most often occur in immunocompromised patients (80). Species associated with chronic invasive fungal sinusitis include *Aspergillus, Mucor, Alternaria, Curvularia, Bipolaris,* and *Candida* spp., *Sporothrix schenckii,* and *Pseudallescheria boydii,* and can occur in both immunocompetent and immunocompromised patients (81,82).

Two major forms of non-invasive fungal sinusitis—allergic fungal sinusitis and sinus mycetoma—exist, with allergic fungal rhinosinusitis (AFS) forming a distinct subcategory of CRS. Diagnostic criteria for AFS

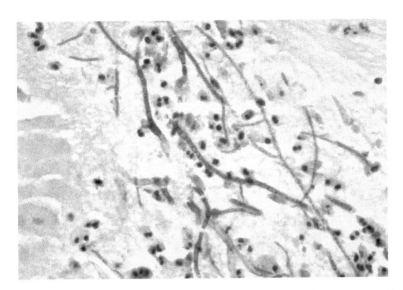

Figure 8 Hematoxylin and eosin stained nasal tissue demonstrating fungal hyphae, eosinophils and Charcot-Leyden crystals. *Source*: Diagnosis of chronic rhinosinusitis. Lanza DC. Annals of Otology, Rhinology, & Laryngology – Supplement. 2004; 193:10–14.

include the demonstration of five characteristics as defined by Bent and Kuhn: gross production of eosinophilic mucin containing non-invasive fungal hyphae, nasal polyposis, characteristic radiographic findings, immunocompetence, and allergy to fungus (83). AFS is characterized by a sustained eosinophilic inflammatory response to colonizing fungi. Mucus secretions, termed allergic mucin, in AFS are characterized as being highly viscous and contain branching non-invasive fungal hyphae within sheets of eosinophils and Charcot–Leyden crystals (84–88) (Fig. 8).

A non-IgE-dependent association of fungus with CRS has also been proposed. In 1999, Ponikau et al. reported a fungal colonization in 96% of consecutive patients with CRS, using an ultra-sensitive method of fungal identification. Additionally, certain fungi were demonstrated to elicit an upregulation of IL-5 and IL-13 and a resulting eosinophilic inflammatory response. This eosinophilic response was IgE, and therefore, allergy-independent, which was thought to indicate a broader role of fungus in CRS than previously hypothesized (89).

Allergy

Environmental allergens are frequently considered as important environmental factors in CRS, and atopy is identified as a prominent systemic host factor in CRS. However, the exact contribution of allergy to the development of CRS is still under investigation. Both pediatric and adult patients with allergic rhinitis are more commonly affected with CRS than non-allergic patients (90). Furthermore, these individuals have been reported to respond more poorly to medical management and to more frequently undergo endoscopic sinus surgery (91,92). Inflammatory changes contribute to the development of CRS in allergic patients. They are stimulated by the production of cytokines, allergic mediators, and neurogenic stimulation. More specifically, allergen stimulation of T_H2 cells leads to the production of IL-4, which in turn causes B-cell activation and IgE antibody production. Subsequent allergen exposure causes IgE cross-linking and release of inflammatory mediators, such as histamine, leukotrienes, and tryptase, and results in the later phase response–eosinophil infiltration, mucus hypersecretion, and mucosal edema. Continued allergen activation, referred to as "priming," further increases the concentration and magnitude of action of inflammatory cells such as eosinophils and neutrophils and their associated cytokines. Furthermore, an IgE response to staphylococcal antigens has been implicated in the development of NPs in CRS, and this relationship is currently under investigation (8,12,93–95).

Environmental Pollutants

A number of other environmental factors can be linked to the development of CRS. In a study of 5300 Swedish children, Andrae et al. found a significantly higher rate of asthma and hay fever in children living near polluting factories (96). Futhermore, Suonpaa reported an increased incidence of acute sinusitis and nasal polyposis in southwestern Finland over a decade, which provides additional evidence for the presence of an environmental impact in CRS (97). Dust, ozone, sulfur dioxide, volatile organic compounds, and smoke are just a few of the pollutants that have been implicated in CRS. The majority of these chemicals share a similar pathologic mechanism: they act as nasal irritants causing dryness and local inflammation with an influx of neutrophils (98,99). In addition to this mechanism, environmental tobacco smoke has been shown to cause secondary ciliary disorders, which consist primarily of microtubular defects (100). Occupational exposure to nickel, leather, or wood dust has been associated with epithelial metaplasia as well as carcinoma (101).

SUMMARY

Maintenance of key functional components—ostiomeatal patency, mucociliary clearance, and normal mucus production—of the paranasal sinus is essential for prevention and recovery from CRS. CRS is a complex disease process that can result from a single or multiple independent etiologies, as well as from multiple independent or interdependent etiologies (Fig. 9).

The factors contributing to this disease process can be divided into systemic host, local host, and environmental factors. Systemic host factors, such as genetic and autoimmune diseases, are important to identify so that appropriate treatment modifications can be made, if available. Likewise,

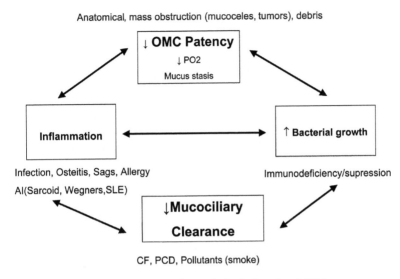

Figure 9 Etiological factors in the pathological cycle of CRS.

local host factors such as anatomic abnormalities and environmental factors such as infection, allergy, and pollution need to be recognized and appropriately managed.

There is a clear need for further research into the pathophysiology of this disorder. Current research on biofilms, sags, and osteitis will hopefully provide us with a better understanding of the role of infection in CRS. Likewise, research on allergic CRS and other noninfectious etiologies of CRS will help to better elucidate the role inflammation plays in this disorder. A better understanding of both infectious and inflammatory mechanisms of CRS will provide us with more effective and individualized therapies.

REFERENCES

1. Majima, Y. Mucoactive medication and airway disease. Paediatr Respir Rev 2002; 3:104–109.
2. Lehrer RI, Lichenstein AK, Ganz T. Defensins: antimicrobial and cytotoxic peptides of mammalian cells. Annu Rev Immunol 1993; 11:105–128.
3. Martin E, Ganz T, Lehrer RI. Defensins and other endogenous peptide antibiotics of vertebrates. J Leukoc Biol 1995; 58:128–136.
4. Lee SH, Kim JE, Lee HM, Choi JO. Antimicrobial defensin peptides of the human nasal mucosa. Ann Otol Rhino Laryngol 2002; 111(2):135–141.
5. Goldman MJ, Anderson GM, Stolzenberg ED, Kari UP, Zasloff M, Wilson JM. Human beta-defensin-1 is a salt sensitive antibiotic that is inactivated in cystic fibrosis. Cell 1997; 88:553–560.
6. Knowles MR, Bouchers RC. Mucus clearance as a primary innate defense mechanism for mammalian airways. J Clin Investig 2002; 109:571–577.

7. Lanza DC, Kennedy DW. Adult rhinosinusitis defined. Otolaryngol Head Neck Surg 1997; 117:S1–S7.
8. Benninger MS, Ferguson BJ, Hadley, JA, Hamilos DL, Jacobs M, Kennedy DW, Lanza DC, Marple BF, Osguthrope JD, Stankiewicz JA, Anon J, Denvey J, Emanuel I, Levine H. Adult chronic rhinosinusitis: definitions, diagnosis, epidemiology, and pathophysiology. Otolaryngol Head Neck Surg 2003; 129:S1–S32.
9. Wald ER, Miloe GJ, Bowen A, Ledesma-Medina J, Salamon N, Bluestone CD. Acute maxillary sinusitis in children. N Engl J Med 1981; 304:749–754.
10. Wald ER, Byers C, Guerra N, Casselbrandt M, Beste D. Subacute sinusitis in children. J Pediatr 1989; 115:28–32.
11. Wald ER, Reilly JS, Casselbrant M, Ledesma-Medina J, Milmore GJ, Bluestone CD, Chipows D. Treatment of acute maxillary sinusitis in childhood: a comparative study of amoxicillin and cefaclor. J Pediatr 1984; 104:297–302.
12. Meltzer EO, Hamilos DL, Hadley JA, Lanza DC, Marple BF, Nicklas RA. Rhinosinusitis: establishing definitions for clinical research and patient care. Otolaryngol Head Neck Surg 2004; 131:S1–S62.
13. Evans FO Jr, Sydnor JB, Moore WE, Manwariring JZL, Brill AH, Jackson RT, Hanna S, Skaar JS, Holdeman LV, Fitz-Hugh S, Sunde MA, Gwaltney JM, Jr. Sinusitis of maxillary antrum. N Engl J Med 1975; 293(15):735–739.
14. Berg O, Carenfelt C, Kronvall G. Bacteriology of maxillary sinusitis in relation to character of inflammation and prior treatment. Scand J Infect Dis 1988; 20:511–516.
15. Pederson M, Sakakura Y, Winther B, Brofeldt S, Mygind N. Nasal mucociliary transport, number of ciliated cells, and beating pattern in naturally acquired common colds. Eur J Respir Dis Suppl 1983; 128:355–365.
16. Hinni ML, McCaffrey TV, Kasperbauer JL. Early mucosal changes in experimental sinusitis. Otolaryngol Head Neck Surg 1992; 107:537–548.
17. Marks SC. Acute sinusitis in the rabbit model: histologic analysis. Laryngoscope 1998; 108:320–325.
18. Rudack C, Hauser U, Wagenmann M, Bachert C, Ganzer U. Cytokine pattern in various forms of sinusitis. Laryngorhinootologie 1998; 77:34–37.
19. Repka-Ramirez S, Naranch K, Park YJ, Clauw D, Baraniuk JN. Cytokines in nasal lavage fluids from acute sinusitis, allergic rhinitis, and chronic fatigue syndrome subjects. Allergy Asthma Proc 2002; 23:185–190.
20. Berger G, Kattan A, Bernheim J, Ophir D. Polypoid mucosa with eosinophilia and glandular hyperplasia in chronic sinusitis: a histopathological and immunohistochemical study. Laryngoscope 2002; 112:738–745.
21. Kramer MF, Ostertag P, Pfronger E, Rasp G. Nasal Interleukin-5, immunoglobin E, eosinophilic cationic protein, and soluble intercellular adhesion molecule-1 in chronic sinusitis, allergic rhinitis, and nasal polyposis. Laryngoscope 2000; 110:1056–1062.
22. Bachert C, Gevaert P, Holtappels G, Johansson SG, van Cawenberge P. Total and specific IgE in nasal polyps is related to local eosinophilic inflammation. J Allergy Clin Immunol 2001; 107:607–614.
23. Rhyoo C, Sanders SP, Leopold DA, Proud D. Sinus mucosal IL-8 gene expression in chronic rhinosinusitis. J Allergy Clin Immunol 1999; 103:395–400.

24. Nonoyama T, Harada T, Shinogi J, Yoshimura E, Sakakura Y. Immunohistochemical localization of cytokines and cell adhesion molecules in maxillary sinus mucosa in chronic sinusitis. Auris Nasis Larynx 2000; 27:51–58.

25. Bachert C, Wagemann M, Rudack C, Hopken KZ, Hillebrandt M, Wang D, van Cawenberge P. The role of cytokines in infectious sinusitis and nasal polyposis. Allergy 1998; 53:2–13.

26. Rudack C, Stoll W, Bachert C. Cytokines in nasal polyposis, acute and chronic sinusitis. Am J Rhinol 1998; 12:383–388.

27. Bachert C, Gevaert P, van Cauwenberge P. *Staphylococcus aureus* enterotoxins: a key in airway disease? Allergy 2002; 57:480–487.

28. Hamilos DL, Leung DY, Huston DP, Kamil A, Wood R, Hamid Q. GM-CSF, Il-5, and RANTES immunoreactivity and mRNA expression in chronic hyperplastic sinusitis with nasal polyposis. Clin Exp Allergy 1998; 28: 1145–1152.

29. Coste A, Girodon E, Louis S, Pruliere-Escabasse V, Goossens M, Peynegre R, Escudier E. Atypical sinusitis in adults must lead to looking for cystic fibrosis and primary ciliary dyskinesia. Laryngoscope 2004; 144:839–843.

30. Varlotta L. Management and care of the newly diagnosed patient with cystic fibrosis. Curr Opin Pulm Med 1998; 4:311–318.

31. Hulka GF. Head and neck manifestations of cystic fibrosis and ciliary dyskinesia. Otolaryngol Clin North Am 2000; 33:1333–1341.

32. Doull JM. Recent advances in cystic fibrosis. Arch Dis Child 2001; 85:62–66.

33. Gysin C, Alothman GA, Papsin BC. Sinonasal disease in cystic fibrosis: clinical characteristics, diagnosis, and management. Pediatr Pulmonol 2000; 30:481–489.

34. Tandon R, Derkay C. Contemporary management of rhinosinusitis and cystic fibrosis. Curr Opin Otolaryngol Head Neck Surg. 2003; 11:41–44.

35. Thaler ER. Postoperative care after endoscopic sinus surgery. Arch Otolaryngol Head Neck Surg 2002; 128:1204–1206.

36. Meeks M, Bush A. Primary ciliary dyskinesia. Pediatr Pulm 2000; 29:307–316.

37. Bianchi E, Savasta S, Carligaro A, Beluffi G, Poggi P, Tinelli M, Mevio E, Martinetti M. HLA haptlotype segregation and ultrastructure study in familial immotile cilia syndrome. Hum Genet 1992; 89:270–274.

38. Pan Y, McCaskill CD, Thompson K, Hicks J, Casey B, Shaffer LG, Craigen WJ. Paternal isodisomy of chromosome 7 associated with complete situs inversus and immotile cilia. Am J Hum Genet 1998; 62:1551–1555.

39. Witt M, Wang Y-F, Wang S, Sun C-E, Pawlik J, Rutkiewicz E, Zebrak J, Diehl SR. Exclusion of chromosome 7 for Kartenger syndrome but suggestion of linkage in families with other forms of primary ciliary dyskinesia. Am J Hum Genet 1998; 64:313–318.

40. Berlinger NT. Sinusitis in immunodeficient and immunosuppressed patients. Laryngoscope 1985; 95:29–33.

41. Rubin J, Honigsberg R. Sinusitis in patients with acquired immunodeficiency syndrome. Ear Nose Throat J 1990; 69:460–463.

42. Friedman M, Landsberg R, Tanyeri H, Schults RA, Kelanic S, Caldarelli DD. Endoscopic sinus surgery in patients with HIV. Laryngoscope 2000; 110: 1613–1616.

43. Long CM, Smith TL, Loehrl TA, Komorowski RA, Tookill TJ. Sinonasal disease in patients with sarcoidosis. Am J Rhinol 2001; 15:211–215.
44. Hewins P, Tervaert JW, Savage CO, Kallenberg CG. Is Wegner's granulomatosis and autoimmune disease? Curr Opin Rheumatol 2000; 12:3–10.
45. Watts RA. Wegener's granulomatosis: unusual presentations. Hosp Med 2000; 61:250–253.
46. Settipane RA, Lieberman P. Update on nonallergic rhinitis. Ann Allergy Asthma Immunol 2001; 86:494–507.
47. Beers RF. Intolerance to aspirin. Ann Intern Med 1968; 68:975–983.
48. Jones NS. CT of paranasal sinuses: a review of the correlation with clinical, surgical, and histopathologic findings. Clin Otolaryngol 2002; 27:11–17.
49. Alho OP. Paranasal sinus bony structures and sinus functioning during viral colds in subjects with and without a history of recurrent sinusitis. Laryngoscope 2003; 113:2163–2168.
50. Richtsmeier WJ. Top 10 reasons for endoscopic maxillary sinus surgery failure. Laryngoscope 2001; 111:1952–1956.
51. Som PM, Shapiro MD, Biller HF, Sasaki C, Lawson W. Sinonasal tumors and inflammatory tissue differentiation with MR imaging. Radiology 1988; 167:803–808.
52. Naranch K, Park YJ, Repka-Ramirez MS, Velarde A, Clauw D, Baranick JN. A tender sinus does not always mean rhinosinusitis. Otolaryngol Head Neck Surg 2002; 127:387–397.
53. Kennedy DW, Senior BA, Gannon FH, Montone KT, Hwang P, Lanza DC. Histology and histomorpholometry of ethmoid bone in chronic rhinosinusitis. Laryngoscope 1998; 108:502–507.
54. Perloff JR, Gannon FH, Bolger WE, Montone KT, Orlandi R, Kennedy DW. Bone involvement in sinusitis: an apparent pathway for the spread of disease. Laryngoscope 2000; 110:2095–2099.
55. Khalid AN, Hunt J, Perloff JR, Kennedy DW. The role of bone in chronic sinusitis. Laryngoscope 2002; 112(11):1951–1957.
56. Brook I. Sinusitis—overcoming bacterial resistance. Int J Pediatr Otorhinolaryngol 2001; 58:27–36.
57. Brook I, Yoeum P, Shah K. Aerobic and anaerobic bacteriology of concurrent chronic otitis media with effusion and chronic sinusitis. Arch Otolaryngol Head Neck Surg 2000; 126:174–176.
58. Doyle PW, Woodham JD. Evaluation of the microbiology of chronic ethmoid sinusitis. J Clin Microbiol 1991; 29:2396–2400.
59. Hoyt WH III. Bacterial patterns found in patients with chronic sinusitis. J Am Osteopath Assoc 1992; 92:209–212.
60. Hsu J, Lanza, DC, Kennedy DW. Antimicrobial resistance in bacterial chronic sinusitis. Am J Rhinol 1998; 12:243–248.
61. Biel MA, Brown CA, Levinson RM, Gavis GE, Paisner HM, Sigel ME, Tedford TM. Evaluation of the microbiology of chronic maxillary sinusitis. Ann Otol Rhinol Laryngol 1998: 107:942–945.
62. Brook I, Frazier EH. Correlation between microbiology and previous sinus surgery in patients with chronic maxillary sinusitis. Ann Otol Rhinol Laryngol 2001; 110:148–151.

63. Jiang RS, Lin JF, Hsu CY. Correlation between bacteriology of the middle meatus and ethmoid sinus in chronic sinusitis. J Laryngol Otol 2002; 116:443–446.
64. Finegold SM, Flynn MJ, Rose FV, et al. Bacteriologic findings associated with chronic bacterial maxillary sinusitis in adults. Clin Infect Dis 2002; 35:428–433.
65. Costerton JW, Vech R, Shirtlift M, Pasmore M, Post JC, Erlich G. The application of biofilm science to the study and control of chronic bacterial infections. J Clin Invest 2003; 112:1446–1477.
66. Stewart PS, Costerton JW. Antibiotic resistance of bacterial biofilms. Lancet 2001; 358:135–138.
67. Post CJ. Direct evidence of bacterial biofilms in otitis media. Laryngoscope 2001; 111(12):2083–2094.
68. Ehrlich GD, Vech R, Wang X, Costerton JW, Hayes JD, Hu FZ, Daigle BJ, Erlich MD, Post JC. Mucosal biofilm formation on middle-ear mucosa in the chinchilla model of otitis media. JAMA 2002; 287:1710–1715.
69. Costerton JW, Stewart PS, Greenberg EP. Bacterial biofilms: a common cause of persistent infections. Science 284:318–322.
70. Hoyle BD, Costerton WJ. Bacterial resistance to antibiotics: the role of biofilms. Prog Drug Res 1991; 37:91–105.
71. Cryer J, Schipor I, Perloff JR, Palmer JN. Evidence of bacterial biofilms in human chronic sinusitis. ORL 2004; 66:155–158.
72. Choi YW, Kotzin B, Heron L, Callahan J, Marrack P, Kappler J. Interaction of *Staphylococcus aureus* toxin "superantigen" with human T cells. Proc Natl Acad Sci USA 1989; 86:8941–8945.
73. Kappler J, Kotzin B, Herron L, Gelfand EW, Bigler RD, Boylston A, Carrel S, Posnett DN, Choi Y, Marrack P. V beta-specific stimulation of human T cells by staphylococcal toxins. Science 1989; 244:811–813.
74. Fraser JD. High-affinity binding of staphylococcal enterotoxin A activated human T cells. J Immunol 1989; 144:4663–4669.
75. Hong-Geller H, Gupta G. Therapeutic approaches to superantigen-based diseases: a review. J Mol Recogn 2003; 16:91–101.
76. Carlsson R, Sjogren HO. Kinetics of IL-2 and interferon-gamma production, expression of IL-2 receptors, and cell proliferation in human mononuclear cells exposed to staphylococcal entertoxin A. Cell Immunol 1985; 96:175–183.
77. Rodhe G, Gevaert P, Holtappels G, Borg I, Wiethege A, Arinir U, Schultze-Werninghaus G, Bachert C. Increased IgE-antibodies to *Staphylococcus aureus* enterotoxins in patients with COPD. Respir Med 2004; 98:858–864.
78. Bachert C, Gevart P, Holtappels G, Johansson SG, van Crauwenberge P. Total and specific IgE in nasal polyps is related to local eosinophilic inflammation. J Allergy Clin Immunol 2001; 107:607–614.
79. Schubet MS. A superantigen hypothesis for the pathogenesis of chronic hypertrophic rhinosinusitis, allergic fungal sinusitis, and related disorders. Ann Allergy Asthma Immunol 2001; 87:181–188.
80. deShazo RD, O'Brien M, Chapin K, Soto-Aguilar M, Gardner L, Swain R. A new classification and diagnostic criteria for invasive fungal sinusitis. Arch Otolaryngol Head Neck Surg 1997; 123:1181–1188.
81. Schell WA. Unusual fungal pathogens in fungal rhinosinusitis. Otolaryngol Clin North Am 2000; 33:375–387.

82. Stringer S, Ryan MW. Chronic invasive fungal rhinosinusitis. Otolaryngol Clin North Am 2000; 33:375–387.
83. Bent JP III, Kuhn FA. Diagnosis of allergic fungal sinusitis. Otolaryngol Head Neck Surg 1994; 111:580–588.
84. Miloshev B, Davidson CM, Gentles JC, Sandison AT. Aspergilloma of paranasal sinuses and orbit in Northern Sudanese. Lancet 1966; 1:746–747.
85. Stevenson DD, Simon RA, Mathison DA, Christiansen SC Monteleukast is only partially effective in inhibiting aspirin responses in aspirin-sensitive asthmatics. Ann Allergy Asthma Immunol 2000; 85:477–482.
86. Miller J, Johnston A, Lamb D. Allergic aspergillosis of the maxillary sinuses. Proc Scot Thor Soc 1981; 36:710–715.
87. Lamb D, Miller J, Johnston A. Allergic aspergillosis of the paranasal sinuses. J Pathol 1982; 137.
88. Katzenstein AL, Sale SR, Greenberger PA. Allergic aspergillosis sinusitis: a newly recognized form of sinusitis. J Allergy Clin Immunol 1983; 72:89–93.
89. Ponikau JU, Sherris DA, Kern EB, et al. The diagnosis and incidence of allergic fungal sinusitis (AFS). Mayo Clin Proc 1999; 74:877–884.
90. Smith LF, Brindley PC. Indications, evaluation, complications, and results of functional endoscopic sinus surgery in 200 patients. Otolaryngol Head Neck Surg 1993; 108:688–696.
91. Benninger MS. Rhinitis, sinusitis and their relationship to allergy. Am J Rhinol 1992; 6:37–43.
92. Emaneul I, Shah S. Chronic rhinosinusitis: allergy and sinus computed tomographic relationships. Otolaryngol Head Neck Surg 2000; 123:687–691.
93. Baroody FM, Suh SH, Naclerio RM. Total IgE serum levels correlate with sinus mucosal thickness on CT. J Allergy Clin Immunol 1997; 100:563–568.
94. Naclerio RM, deTineo ML, Baroody FM. Ragweed allergic rhinitis and the paranasal sinuses. A computed tomographic study. Arch Otolaryngol Head Neck Surg 1997; 123:193–196.
95. Suzuki M, Watanabe T, Suko T, Mogi G. Comparison of sinusitis with and without allergic rhinitis: characteristics of paranasal sinus effusion and mucosa. Am J Otolaryngol 1999; 20:143–150.
96. Andrae S, Axelson O, Bjorksten B, Fredriksson M, Kjellman NJ. Symptoms of bronchial hyperreactivity and asthma in relation to environmental factors. Arch Dis Child 1988; 63:473–478.
97. Suonpaa J, Antila J. Increase of acute frontal sinusitis in southwestern Finland. Scand J Infect Dis 1990; 22:563–568.
98. Bascom R. Air pollution. In: Mygind N, Naclerio RM, eds. Allergic and Nonallergic Rhinitis. Copenhagen: Munksgaard, 1993:33–86.
99. Graham D, Henderson F, House D. Neutrophil influx measured in nasal lavages of humans exposed to ozone. Arch Environ Health 1988; 43:228–233.
100. Afzlius B. Immotile cilia syndrome and ciliary abnormalities induced by infection and injury. Am Rev Respir Dis 1981; 124:107–109.
101. Zeiger RS. Differential diagnosis and classification of rhinosinusitis. In: Schatz M, Zeiger RS, Settipane GA, eds. Nasal Manifestations of Systemic Diseases. Providence, RI: Oceanside Publications, 1991.

SECTION III. MICROBIOLOGY

7

Infective Basis of Acute and Recurrent Acute Sinusitis

Ellen R. Wald

Department of Pediatrics and Otolaryngology, University of Pittsburgh School of Medicine, Allergy, Immunology, and Infectious Diseases, Pittsburgh, Pennsylvania, U.S.A.

INTRODUCTION

Sinusitis is a common complication of viral upper respiratory infection and allergic inflammation. Although the paranasal sinuses are believed to be sterile under normal circumstances, the upper respiratory tract—specifically the nose and nasopharynx—are heavily colonized by normal flora. Despite differences in normal nasal flora, the acute bacterial pathogens that cause acute sinusitis are similar in adults and children.

OBTAINING SPECIMENS

To determine the infective basis of acute or recurrent acute sinusitis, a sample of sinus secretions must be obtained from one of the paranasal sinuses without contamination by normal respiratory or oral flora (1). The maxillary sinus is the most accessible of the paranasal sinuses. There are two non-endoscopic approaches to the maxillary sinus: via either the canine fossa or the inferior meatus. Both the canine fossa and the nasal vestibule are colonized by pathogenic bacteria. Accordingly, sterilization of the nasal vestibule and the mucosa beneath the inferior nasal turbinate or of the mucosa overlying the canine fossa is recommended if an aspirate of the maxillary sinus is planned.

To avoid misinterpretation of culture results, acute infection is defined as the recovery of a bacterial species in high density, that is, a colony count of at least 10^3–10^4 colony-forming units per milliliter (cfu/mL). This quantitative definition increases the probability that organisms recovered from the maxillary sinus aspirate truly represent in situ infection and not contamination from either the mucosa overlying the canine fossa or beneath the inferior turbinate. In fact, most sinus aspirates from acutely infected sinuses are associated with colony counts in excess of 10^4 cfu/mL. If quantitative cultures cannot be performed, Gram stain of the aspirated specimens affords semiquantitative data. If bacteria are readily apparent on a Gram stain, the approximate bacterial density is 10^5 cfu/mL. The Gram stain is especially helpful if bacteria are seen on the smear and the specimen fails to grow when using standard aerobic culture techniques. Anaerobic organisms or other fastidious bacteria, such as a bacterial biofilm or partially antibiotic-treated infections, should be suspected. Performance of a Gram stain will also permit an assessment of the local inflammatory response. The presence of many white blood cells in association with a positive bacterial culture in high density makes it likely that a bacterial infection is present. Alternatively, a paucity or absence of white blood cells in association with the presence of a positive culture in low density suggests that these bacteria have contaminated the culture rather than have caused infection.

Endoscopic Cultures in Children and Adults

Recently there has been interest in and enthusiasm for obtaining cultures of the middle meatus endoscopically, as a surrogate for cultures of a sinus aspirate. The endoscopically obtained culture is less invasive and associated with less morbidity (2). In normal children, unfortunately, the middle meatus has been shown to be colonized by the same bacterial species such as *Streptococcus pneumoniae*, *Haemophilus influenzae*, and *Moraxella catarrhalis*, as are commonly recovered from children with sinus infection (3). Accordingly, middle meatus cultures are not interpretable. This technique cannot be recommended for a precise bacterial diagnosis in children with sinus infections.

In three recent studies, cultures of the middle meatus have been obtained endoscopically from normal adults. The bacterial species recovered were coagulase-negative staphylococci in 35 to 50% of cultures, *Corynebacterium* spp. in 16 to 23% and *Staphylococcus aureus* in 8 to 20% (4–6). The only overlap between commensals and potential pathogens is *S. aureus*. While several studies in adults have shown a good correlation between cultures of the middle meatus and the sinus aspirate in patients with acute sinusitis (7,8), others have not (9,10). In a retrospective review of the literature between 1950 and 2000, Benninger et al. concluded that the data were insufficient to recommend substitution of cultures of the middle meatus for maxillary sinus aspirates in patients with acute rhinosinusitis (11).

Occasionally, neither a sinus aspirate nor a specimen obtained endos-copically is sufficient for the diagnosis of a sinus infection. This is especially true of patients with very protracted symptoms. In this instance, biopsy of the sinus mucosa for culture and appropriate stains may be required.

MICROBIOLOGY OF ACUTE SINUSITIS IN CHILDREN

The microbiology of paranasal sinus infection can be anticipated according to the age of the patient, clinical presentation, and immunocompetency of the host. Despite the substantial prevalence and clinical importance of sinusitis in childhood, study of the microbiology of acute and subacute sinusitis in children has been relatively limited. Using a study design similar to the one described by investigators at the University of Virginia (12), an investigation of the microbiology of acute sinusitis in pediatric patients was reported by the Children's Hospital of Pittsburgh in 1981 (13). Patients were eligible for this study if they were between 2 and 16 years of age and presented with one of two clinical pictures: onset with either "persistent" or "severe" respiratory symptoms.

Sinus radiographs were performed on eligible children. When a maxillary sinus aspirate was performed on children presenting with clinical symptoms and significantly abnormal sinus radiographs, bacteria in high density were recovered from 70% (14). The bacterial isolates in their relative order of prevalence are shown in Table 1. *S. pneumoniae* was most common, followed closely by *H. influenzae* and *M. catarrhalis*. No staphylococci were recovered. Mixed infection with heavy growth of two bacterial species was occasionally found. In 25% of patients with bilateral maxillary sinusitis, there were discordant bacterial culture results. In some cases, one sinus aspirate was positive, while the other was negative. In the remaining cases, different bacterial species were recovered from each aspirate.

Table 1 Bacterial Species Cultured from 79 Sinus Aspirates in 50 Children

	Single isolates	Multiple isolates	Total
Streptococcus pneumoniae	14	8	22
Moraxella catarrhalis	13	2	15
Haemophilus influenzae	10	5	15
Eikenella corrodens	1	0	1
Group A streptococcus	1	0	1
Group C streptococcus	0	1	1
α-Streptococcus	1	1	2
Peptostreptococcus	0	1	1
Moraxella spp.	1	0	1

Source: Adapted from Ref. 13.

Viral cultures were also performed on the maxillary sinus aspirates. Because many children were evaluated after 10 or more days of symptoms, viruses were recovered infrequently. Adenovirus as the only isolate was grown from the aspirate of one subject; parainfluenza virus in combination with a bacterial isolate was recovered from a second (13). In studies of adults with acute sinusitis, other viruses, including influenza and rhinovirus, have been recovered from approximately 10% of sinus aspirates (12). Nucleic acid amplification technology was not available at the time of these investigations (12,13).

MICROBIOLOGY OF ACUTE COMMUNITY-ACQUIRED SINUSITIS IN ADULTS

Acute Maxillary Sinusitis

The most elegant work detailing the microbiology of acute sinusitis has been done at the University of Virginia in Charlottesvile since 1975 (12). Information is derived mainly from cultures of specimens obtained by aspiration of the maxillary sinus because of the accessibility of this particular sinus. In general, a sinus infection is caused by a single bacterial isolate in high density. In 25% of cases, two bacterial species, each in high density, will be recovered.

The two most important causes of acute community-acquired sinusitis in adults are *S. pneumoniae* and non-typeable *H. influenzae* (Table 2) (15,16). One remarkable change observed by Gwaltney et al. between 1975 and 1991 was the increase in the prevalence of beta-lactamase producing *H. influenzae* (16).

Next in frequency were anaerobic bacterial species and streptococci other than pneumococci. The role of anaerobes in acute community-acquired disease has been variable. Although anaerobic bacteria have a more remarkable role in chronic rather than acute sinus disease, they account for 7% of acute cases, some of which arise from a primary dental pathology. *Moraxella* and *S. aureus* account for 4% and 3% of cases, respectively.

Table 2 Community-Acquired Acute Sinusitis in Adults

Streptococcus pneumoniae	41%
Haemophilus influenzae	35%
Anaerobes	7%
Streptococcal species	7%
Moraxella catarrhalis	4%
Staphylococcus aureus	3%
Other	4%

Source: Adapted from Ref. 16.

Acute Sphenoid Sinusitis

Most of the study of the microbiology of acute and recurrent acute sinusitis has focused on the maxillary sinus. There have been several reports on the microbiology of sphenoid sinusitis (17,18), including a recent study of 23 patients who were cared for between 1975 and 2000 (19). Most of the patients were adults. All of the specimens for culture were obtained at the time of surgery, suggesting that the population of patients studied had serious disease. The most common aerobic isolate in patients with acute disease was *S. aureus*. *Streptococcal* species (viridans streptococci, microaerophilic streptococci, *S. pneumoniae*, Group F streptococci, and *Streptococcus pyogenes*) were next most common. The predominance of gram-positive coccal species is consistent across all reports (17–19). There were two isolates of *H. influenzae*. Anaerobes were recovered from several patients (*Peptostreptococcus* spp., *Propionibacterium acnes*, *Fusobacterium nucleatum*, and *Prevotella melaninogenica*).

Acute Frontal Sinusitis

The microbiology of frontal sinusitis has been evaluated in three studies (20–22). In a recent review of Brook's experience over a 26-year period, 28 cases of frontal sinusitis were described microbiologically (15 acute and 13 chronic) (22). The primary isolates in patients with acute frontal sinusitis were *S. pneumoniae*, *H. influenzae*, and *M. catarrhalis*. There was an occasional isolation of anaerobes. These results are similar to those described by other authors (22,21).

Recurrent Acute Bacterial Sinusitis

There has been relatively little study of the microbiology of recurrent acute sinusitis. One small series, recently published, reviewed the results for eight patients (23). Specimens were obtained via maxillary sinus endoscopy under local anesthesia, through the middle meatus, with calcium alginate–tipped microswabs. The swabs were placed in 1 mL of media and shaken vigorously for two minutes, serially diluted, and inoculated. Only bacteria found in numbers greater than 10^4/mL were considered to be pathogens. Not surprisingly, the isolates recovered were *S. pneumoniae*, *H. influenzae*, and *M. catarrhalis*. There was only a single isolate of *S. aureus*.

Viruses as a Cause of Acute sinusitis

Although we commonly consider acute sinusitis to be a complication of viral upper respiratory tract infections, several investigators have shown that radiographic and other imaging abnormalities are very common in both children and adults with the common cold, suggesting the presence of early viral sinusitis (24,25). In a study by Puhakka et al., 200 young adults with the common cold were followed for 21 days. Plain radiographs were performed on days 1, 7, and 21 of the common cold (26). Patients recorded their symptoms on a diary card for 20 days, rating symptoms such as watery rhinitis, purulent rhinitis, nasal congestion, nasal irritation, headache, cough, sputum, sore throat, and fever on a severity scale of zero to three (ranging from absent to severe). The etiologic role of 10 viruses (rhinovirus, adenovirus, coronavirus, enterovirus, influenza A and B viruses, parainfluenza virus types 1, 2, and 3, and respiratory syncytial virus) was investigated by virus culture, antigen detection, serology, and rhinovirus polymerase chain reaction (PCR). Antibody concentrations to five bacteria (*Chlamydia pneumoniae, H. influenzae, M. catarrhalis, Mycoplasma pneumoniae* and *S. pneumoniae*) were assayed. Altogether, 57% of the patients had sinus abnormalities (mucosal thickening, total opacity, air–fluid level, cyst, or polyp) during the 21 days of the common cold. This compares to 87% of adult patients with an uncomplicated common cold demonstrating significant abnormalities when evaluated by computed tomography (24). Antimicrobial treatment was not provided in this study and all patients recovered spontaneously, suggesting that there was no substantial component of bacterial superinfection (26).

The etiology of the common cold was determined in 69.5% of the subjects. Viral infection was detected in 81.6% of the patients with sinusitis and in 63.3% of the patients without sinusitis. Rhinovirus was the most frequent cause of infection, detected in 55.3% and in 48.3% of subjects, respectively. No significantly increased levels of antibodies to bacteria were detected in the sinusitis group.

Support for the likelihood that these cases of radiologic "sinusitis" represent actual virus infection of the paranasal sinuses is found in a study by Pitkaranta et al. (27). Twenty adult patients with a diagnosis of acute community-acquired sinusitis were studied between May and July of 1996. All patients had purulent rhinorrhea, nasal obstruction, and abnormal radiographs. A nasal swab was obtained from each patient at the area of puncture below the inferior turbinate. After puncture with a needle, a bronchoscope brush was passed through the needle into the sinus and rotated. Cultures and PCR for virus were performed on the nasal swab and the bronchial brush specimen. Rhinovirus was detected in specimens from 10 of the patients, including maxillary samples from eight and nasal swabs from nine by reverse transcription–PCR (RT–PCR). These findings suggest that viral invasion of the sinus cavity itself may be a common event during uncomplicated upper respiratory infections. However, a positive PCR may also have been caused by the presence of virions in the sinus or viral RNA produced by replication elsewhere in the upper respiratory tract epithelium and introduced during coughing or sneezing, or potentially even by RNA from human rhinovirus introduced into the sinus at the time of puncture.

Fungal Sinusitis

Most cases of fungal sinusitis, especially the allergic forms of fungal sinusitis, present with very protracted clinical symptoms and therefore are not considered under the heading of either acute or recurrent acute sinusitis. The only type of fungal sinusitis likely to present as acute disease is locally or systemically invasive fungal sinusitis in immunoincompetent patients.

Patients particularly prone to fungal infections of the paranasal sinuses include diabetics, patients with leukemia and solid malignancies who are febrile and neutropenic (most of whom will have received broad-spectrum antimicrobial therapy), patients on high-dose steroid therapy (e.g., for connective tissue disease, transplant recipients), and patients with severe impairment of cell-mediated immunity (e.g., transplant recipients, persons with congenital T-cell immunodeficiencies) (28).

The most common cause of fungal sinusitis in immunosuppressed patients is aspergillus. Much less commonly, acute or chronic sinusitis may be caused by *Candida* spp. or Mucor spp; the latter agent most frequently affects diabetic patients. In addition, *Pseudallescheria boydii*, *Alternaria* spp., *Exserohilum* spp., and *Bipolaris* spp. have been observed to cause sinusitis in the immunosuppressed. These infections will be covered in more detail in the chapters on sinusitis in the immunocompromised host and fungal sinusitis.

Protozoa

Although protozoan species have not been described as a cause of acute or chronic sinusitis in normal individuals, a case of acute sinusitis caused by cryptosporidium has been reported in a 17-year-old boy with congenital hypogammaglobulinemia, who presented with a three-week history of increasingly severe headaches (29). Physical examination showed turbid nasal discharge, friable nasal mucosa, and facial tenderness over the maxillary sinuses. CT revealed pansinusitis. The maxillary sinus aspirate contained a moderate number of neutrophils and rare *Cryptosporidium oocysts*. Extensive culturing for other microbiologic species was negative. The patient's headache improved after therapy with oral spiramycin and intravenous 2 difloro-methylornithine HCl-monohydrate.

CONCLUSION

Most cases of clinically important acute and recurrent acute sinusitis are caused by the bacterial species *S. pneumoniae*, *H. influenzae*, and *M. catarrhalis*. The most common predisposing event is a viral upper respiratory tract infection. Coinfection by viruses and bacteria is likely, as is self-limited viral infection alone.

REFERENCES

1. American Academy of Pediatrics. Subcommittee on Management of Sinusitis and Committee on Quality Improvement. Clinical practice guideline: management of sinusitis. Pediatrics 2001; 108:798–808.
2. Talbot GH, Kennedy DW, Scheld WM, Granito K. Rigid nasal endoscopy versus sinus puncture and aspiration for microbiologic documentation of acute bacterial maxillary sinusitis. Clin Infect Dis 2001; 33:1668–1675.
3. Gordts F, Abu Nasser I, Clement PA, Pierad D, Kaufman L. Bacteriology of the middle meatus in children. Int J Pediatr Otorhinolaryngol 1999; 48:163–167.
4. Gordts F, Harlewyck S, Pierard D, Kaufman L, Clement PA. Microbiology of the middle meatus: a comparison between normal adults and children. J Laryngol Otol 2000; 114:184–188.
5. Klossek JM, Dubreuil L, Richet H, Richet B, Sedallian A, Beutter P. Bacteriology of the adult middle meatus. J Laryngol Otol 1996; 110:847–849.
6. Nadel DM, Lanza DC, Kennedy DW. Endoscopically guided cultures in chronic sinusitis. Am J Rhinol 1998; 12:233–241.
7. Gold SM, Tami TA. Role of middle meatus aspiration culture in the diagnosis of chronic sinusitis. Laryngoscope 1997; 107:1586–1589.
8. Vogan JC, Bolger WE, Keyes AS. Endoscopically guided sinonasal cultures: a direct comparison with maxillary sinus aspirate cultures. Otolaryngol Head Neck Surg 2000; 122:370–373.
9. Winther B, Vicery CL, Gross CW, Hendley O. Microbiology of the maxillary sinus in adults with chronic sinus disease. Am J Rhinol 1996; 10:347–350.
10. Kountakis SE, Skoulas IG. Middle meatal vs. antral lavage cultures in intensive care unit patients. Otolaryngol Head Neck Surg 2002; 126:377–381.
11. Benninger MS, Appelbaum PC, Denneny JC, Osguthorpe DJ. Maxillary sinus puncture and culture in the diagnosis of acute rhinosinusitis: the case for pursuing alternative culture methods. Otolaryngol Head Neck Surg 2002; 127(1): 7–12.
12. Evans FO Jr, Sydnor JB, Moore WE, Moore GR, Manwaring JL, Brill AH, Jackson RT, Hanna S, Skaar JS, Holdeman LV, Fitz-Hugh S, Sande MA, Gwaltney JM Jr. Sinusitis of the maxillary antrum. N Engl J Med 1975; 293:735–739.
13. Wald ER, Milmoe GJ, Bowen AD, Ledesma-Medina J, Salmon N, Bluestone CD. Acute maxillary sinusitis in children. N Engl J Med 1981; 304: 749–754.
14. Wald ER, Reilly JS, Casselbrant M, Ledesma-Medina J, Milmoe GJ, Bluestone CD, Chiponis D. Treatment of acute maxillary sinusitis in childhood. A comparative study of amoxicillin and cefaclor. J Pediatr 1984; 104:297–302.
15. Anon JB, Jacobs MR, Poole MD, Ambrose PG, Benninger MS, Hadley JA, Craig WA. Sinus and allergy health partnership. Antimicrobial treatment guidelines for acute bacterial rhinosinusitis. Otolaryngol Head Neck Surg 2004; 130(suppl 1):1–45.
16. Gwaltney JM Jr. Acute community-acquired sinusitis. Clin Infect Dis 1996; 23:1209–1225.
17. Lew D, Southwick FS, Montgomery WW, Weber AL, Baker AS. Sphenoid sinusitis. A review of 30 cases. N Engl J Med 1983; 309:1149–1154.

18. Ruoppi P, Seppa J, Pukkila M, Nuutinen J. Isolated sphenoid sinus diseases: report of 39 cases. Arch Otolaryngol Head Neck Surg 2000; 126:777–781.
19. Brook I. Bacteriology of acute and chronic sphenoid sinusitis. Ann Otol Rhinol Laryngol 2002; 111:1002–1004.
20. Suonpaa J, Antila J. Increase of acute frontal sinusitis in southwestern Finland. Scand J Infect Dis 1990; 22:563–568.
21. Ruoppi P, Seppa J, Nuutinen J. Acute frontal sinusitis: etiological factors and treatment outcome. Acta Otolaryngol (Stockh) 1993; 113:201–205.
22. Brook I. Bacteriology of acute and chronic frontal sinusitis. Arch Otolaryngol Head Neck Surg 2002; 128:583–585.
23. Brook I, Frazier EH. Microbiology of recurrent acute rhinosinusitis. Laryngoscope 2004; 114:129–131.
24. Gwaltney JM Jr, Phillips CG, Miller RD, Riker DK. Computed tomographic study of the common cold. N Engl J Med 1994; 330:25–30.
25. Glasier CM, Mallory GB Jr, Steele RW. Significance of opacification of the maxillary and ethmoid sinuses in infants. J Pediatr 1989; 114:45–50.
26. Puhakka T, Makela MJ, Alanen A, Kallio T, Korsoff L, Arstila P, Leinonen M, Pulkkinen M, Suonpaa J, Mertsola J, Ruuskanen O. Sinusitis in the common cold. J Allergy Clin Immunol 1998; 102:408.
27. Pitkaranta A, Arruda E, Molinberg H, Hayden FG. Detection of rhinovirus in sinus brushings of patients with acute community-acquired sinusitis by reverse transcription-PCR. J Clin Microbiol 1997; 35:1791–1793.
28. Wald ER. Microbiology of acute and chronic sinusitis in children and adults. Am J Med Sci 1998; 31:13–20.
29. Davis JJ, Heyman MB. Cryptosporidiosis and sinusitis in an immunodeficient adolescent. J Infect Dis 1988; 158:649.

8

Infectious Causes of Sinusitis

Itzhak Brook

Departments of Pediatrics and Medicine, Georgetown University School of Medicine, Washington, D.C., U.S.A.

INTRODUCTION

The upper respiratory tract, including the nasopharynx, serves as the reservoir for pathogenic bacteria that can cause respiratory infections including sinusitis (1). During a viral respiratory infection, potential pathogens can relocate from the nasopharynx to the sinus cavity, causing sinusitis (2). Establishment of the correct microbiology of all forms of sinusitis is of primary importance as it can serve as a guide for choosing adequate antimicrobial therapy. This chapter presents the current information regarding the microbiology of all forms of sinusitis.

THE ORAL CAVITY NORMAL FLORA

The human mucosal and epithelial surfaces are covered with aerobic and anaerobic microorganisms (3). The organisms that reside at these sites are predominantly anaerobic and are actively multiplying. The trachea, bronchi, esophagus, stomach, and upper urinary tract are not normally colonized by indigenous flora. However, a limited number of transient organisms may be present at these sites from time to time. Microflora also vary in different sites within the body system, as in the oral cavity; the microorganisms present in the buccal folds differ in their concentration and types of strains from those isolated from the tongue or gingival sulci. However, the organisms that prevail in one body system tend to belong to certain major bacterial species, and their presence in that system is predictable. The relative and total counts of organisms can be affected by various factors, such as age, diet, anatomical variations, illness, hospitalization, and antimicrobial therapy. However, these sets of bacterial flora, remain stable through life, with predictable patterns, despite their subjection to perturbing factors.

Anaerobes outnumber aerobic bacteria in all mucosal surfaces, and certain organisms predominate in the different sites. The number of anaerobes at a site is generally inversely related to the oxygen tension (3). Their predominance in the skin, mouth, nose, and throat, which are exposed to oxygen, is explained by the anaerobic microenvironment generated by the facultative bacteria that consume oxygen.

Knowledge of the composition of the flora at certain sites is useful for predicting which organisms may be involved in an infection adjacent to that site and can assist in the selection of a logical antimicrobial therapy, even before the exact microbial etiology of the infection is known.

The normal flora is not just a potential hazard for the host, but also a beneficial partner. Normal body flora also serves as protector from colonization and subsequent invasion by potentially virulent bacteria. In instances where the host defenses are impaired or a breach occurs in the mucus membranes or skin, however, the members of the normal flora can cause infections.

Microbial Composition

The formation of the normal oral flora is initiated at birth. Certain organisms such as lactobacilli and anaerobic streptococci, which establish themselves at an early date, reach high numbers within a few days. *Actinomyces, Fusobacterium*, and *Nocardia* are acquired by the age of six months. Subsequently, *Prevotella, Porphyromonas* spp., *Leptotrichia, Propionibacterium*, and *Candida* also become part of the oral flora (3). *Fusobacterium* populations attain high numbers after dentition and reach maximal numbers at age one year.

The most predominant group of facultative microorganisms native to the oropharynx are the alpha-hemolytic streptococci, which include *Streptococcus mitis, Streptococcus milleri, Streptococcus sanguis, Streptococcus intermedius, Streptococcus salivarius*, and several others (4). Other groups of organisms native to the oropharynx are *Moraxella catarrhalis* and *Haemophillus influenzae* that are capable of producing beta-lactamase and may spread to adjacent sites causing otitis, sinusitis, or bronchitis. Encapsulated *H. influenzae* also induces serious infections such as meningitis and bacteremia. The oropharynx also contains *Staphylococcus aureus* and *Staphylococcus epidermidis* that can also produce beta-lactamase and take part in infections.

The normal oropharynx is seldom colonized by gram-negative enterobacteriaceae. In contrast, hospitalized patients are generally heavily colonized with these organisms. The reasons for this change in microflora are not known, but may be related to changes in the glycocalyx of the pharyngeal epithelial cells or because of selective processes that occur following the administration of antimicrobial therapy (5). The shift from predominantly gram-positive to gram-negative bacteria is thought to contribute to the high incidence of sinus infection caused by gram-negative bacteria in patients with chronic illnesses.

Anaerobic bacteria are present in large numbers in the oropharynx, particularly in patients with poor dental hygiene, caries, or periodontal disease. They outnumber their aerobic counterpart in a ratio of 10:1 to 100:1 (Fig. 1). Anaerobic bacteria can adhere to tooth surfaces and contribute, through the elaboration of metabolic by-products, to the development of both caries and periodontal disease (4). The predominant anaerobes are anaerobic streptococci, *Veillonella* spp., *Bacteroides* spp., pigmented *Prevotella*, and *Porphyromonas* spp. (previously called *Bacteroides melaninogenicus* group), and *Fusobacterium* spp. (4). These organisms are a potential source of a variety of chronic infections including otitis and sinusitis, aspiration pneumonia lung abscesses, and abscesses of the oropharynx and teeth.

The microflora of the oral cavity is complex and contains many kinds of obligate anaerobes. The distribution of bacteria within the mouth seems to be a function of their ability to adhere to the oral surfaces. The differences in numbers of the anaerobic microflora probably occur because of considerable variations in the oxygen concentration in parts of the oral cavity.

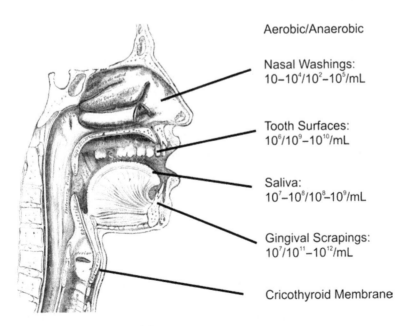

Aerobic/Anaerobic

Nasal Washings:
$10-10^4/10^2-10^5$/mL

Tooth Surfaces:
$10^6/10^9-10^{10}$/mL

Saliva:
$10^7-10^8/10^8-10^9$/mL

Gingival Scrapings:
$10^7/10^{11}-10^{12}$/mL

Cricothyroid Membrane

Figure 1 Oropharyngeal flora.

For example, the maxillary and mandibular buccal folds contain 0.4% and 0.3% oxygen, respectively, whereas the anterior and posterior tongue surfaces contain 16.4% and 12.4%. The environment of the gingival sulcus is more anaerobic than the buccal folds, and the periodontal pocket is the most anaerobic area in the oral cavity. The ratio of anaerobic bacteria to aerobic bacteria in saliva is approximately 10:1. The total count of anaerobic bacteria is $1.1 \times 10^8/\text{mL}$ (Fig. 1). The predominant anaerobic bacteria that colonize the anterior nose are *P. acnes*. *Fusobacterium nucleatum* is the main species of *Fusobacterium* present in the oral cavity. Anaerobic gram-negative bacilli found in the oral cavity include pigmented *Prevotella* and *Porphyromonas* (previously called black-pigmented *Bacteroides*), *Porphyromonas gingivalis*, *Prevotella oralis*, *Prevotella orisbuccae* (*ruminicola*), *Prevotella disiens*, and *Bacteroides ureolyticus*.

Fusobacteria are also a predominant part of the oral flora (6), as the treponemas (7). Pigmented *Prevotella* and *Porphyromonas* represent <1% of the coronal tooth surface, but constitute 4% to 8% of gingival crevice flora. Veillonellae represent 1% to 3% of the coronal tooth surface, 5% to 15% of the gingival crevice flora, and 10% to 15% of the tongue flora. Microaerophilic streptococci predominate in all areas of the oral cavity, and they reach high numbers in the tongue and cheek (8). Other anaerobes prevalent in the mouth are *Actinomyces* (9), *Peptostreptococci*, *Leptotrichia buccalis*, *Bifidobacterium*, *Eubacterium*, and *Propionibacterium* (10).

Pigmented *Prevotella*, *Porphyromonas*, and *Fusobacterium* species can also produce beta-lactamase (11). The recovery rate of aerobic and anaerobic beta-lactamase producing bacteria (BLPB) in the oropharynx has increased in recent years, and these organisms were isolated from more than half of the patients with head and neck infections including sinusitis (11). BLPB can be involved directly in the infection, protecting not only themselves from the activity of penicillins but also penicillin-susceptible organisms. This can occur when the enzyme beta-lactamase is secreted into the infected tissue or abscess fluid in sufficient quantities to break the penicillin's beta-lactam ring before it can kill the susceptible bacteria (12) (Fig. 2).

The high incidence of recovery of BLPB in upper respiratory tract infections may be because of the selection of these organisms following antimicrobial therapy with beta-lactam antibiotics. Emergence of penicillin-resistant flora can occur following only a short course of penicillin (13,14).

Obtaining Appropriate Sinus Content Cultures while Avoiding the Normal Flora

If a patient with sinusitis develops severe infection, is immunocompromised or fails to show significant improvement or shows signs of deterioration despite treatment, it is important to obtain a culture, preferably through sinus puncture, as this may reveal the presence of causative bacteria.

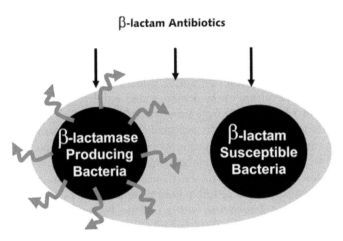

Figure 2 Protection of penicillin-susceptible bacteria from penicillin by beta-lactamase-producing bacteria.

However, obtaining a culture through sinus endoscopy is an alternative approach.

Sinus aspirates for culture must be obtained free of contamination so that saprophytic organisms or normal flora are excluded and culture results can be interpreted correctly. As indigenous aerobic and anaerobic bacteria are present on the nasopharyngeal mucous membranes in large numbers, even minimal contamination of a specimen with the normal flora can give misleading results. The use of sinus puncture is the "gold standard" method of obtaining such specimens (15). There is, however, data that supports the use of endoscopically obtained cultures in assessing the microbiology of infected sinuses (16a–23).

Sinus Puncture

Obtaining sinus aspirates by puncture is the traditional method of specimens collection. The maxillary sinus is the most accessible of all of the paranasal sinuses. There are two approaches to the maxillary sinus that use puncture: via either the canine fossa or the inferior meatus. The nasal vestibule is often heavily colonized with pathogenic bacteria, mostly *S. aureus*. Therefore, sterilization of the nasal vestibule and the area beneath the inferior nasal turbinate is suggested.

Contamination with nasal flora may, however, occur. To prevent misinterpretation of the culture results, an infection is defined as the recovery of a bacterial species in high density [i.e., a colony count of at least 10^3 to 10^4 colony forming units per milliliter (cfu/mL)]. This quantitative definition increases the probability that microorganisms isolated from the sinus aspirate truly represent in situ infection and not contamination. Most aspirates from infected sinuses contain colony counts above 10^4 cfu/mL. If quantitative cultures cannot be performed, Gram stain of aspirated specimens enables semiquantitative assessment. If bacteria are readily seen on a Gram stain preparation, the approximate bacterial density is about 10^5 cfu/mL. Of 12 cases in which an antral puncture showed at least 10^5 cfu/mL pathogens, the Gram stain demonstrated either organisms or white blood cells in all 12 cases, and organisms as well as white blood cells in 9 of 12 cases (16a). A Gram stain is especially useful if organisms are observed on smear and the specimen fails to grow using standard aerobic culture techniques, in which case anaerobic organisms or other fastidious bacteria or antibiotic-inhibited flora should be suspected. A Gram stain can also allow an assessment of the local inflammatory response. The presence of many white blood cells in association with a positive bacterial culture in high density makes it probable that a bacterial infection is present. A Gram stain does not, however, differentiate between neutrophils and eosinophils. In contrast, a paucity or absence of white blood cells in association with the presence of a positive culture in low-density suggests bacterial contamination.

Endoscopic Cultures

Recently, there has been an interest in obtaining cultures of the middle meatus endoscopically, as a substitute or surrogate for cultures of a sinus aspirate. The endoscopically obtained culture is less invasive and associated with less morbidity (16a). Unfortunately, the middle meatus in normal children is colonized with the same bacterial species, namely, *S. pneumoniae*, *H. influenzae*, and *M. catarrhalis*, as are commonly recovered from children with sinus infection (17). Accordingly, this technique cannot be recommended for precise bacterial diagnosis in children with sinus infections.

In three recent studies, the bacterial species recovered from middle meatal samples obtained from normal adults were coagulase-negative staphylococci (CNS, 35–50%), *Corynebacterium* spp. (16–23%), and *S. aureus* (8–20%) (18–20). The only overlap between commensals and potential pathogens is *S. aureus*.

Several studies in adults have shown a good correlation between cultures of the middle meatus and the sinus aspirate in patients with acute sinusitis, especially when purulence is in the middle meatus (16a,21,22,25). However, other studies have not found such a correlation (23,24).

Concordance in the types and concentrations of organisms recovered by endoscopic aspirates and those isolated during sinus surgery was found in all six cases in one study (25). Sixteen of the 18 anaerobes isolated from sinus aspirates were also found in the concomitant endoscopic sample. Five aerobic isolates were found in both sinus aspirates and endoscopic samples and their concentration was similar. However, contamination by four aerobic gram-positive bacteria (in numbers of $<10^4$ cfu/sample) were found in endoscopic samples.

CNS is usually interpreted as a nonpathogen in acute sinusitis. Talbot et al. (16a) correlated the results of endoscopically obtained cultures and the cultures obtained from maxillary sinus aspirates. They reported no situations in which the puncture demonstrated CNS in $>10^5$ cfu/mL; however, a swab of the middle meatus grew CNS in 6 of 53 patients. Interpretation of the pathogenicity of *S. aureus* is more difficult. Two of 53 patients had $>10^5$ cfu/mL, which correlated with the endoscopic swab. However, in an additional six patients, there was no agreement between sites (16a).

In rare instances, neither a sinus aspirate nor a specimen obtained endoscopically is sufficient for the diagnosis of a sinus infection. In this instance, biopsy of the sinus mucosa and broth culture and appropriate stains may be required to demonstrate the bacterial etiology.

Discrepancies in the Recovery of Bacteria from Multiple Sinuses in Sinusitis

There are differences in the distribution of organisms in a single patient who suffers from infections in multiple sinuses that emphasize the importance of obtaining cultures from all infected sinuses. A recent study has evaluated the discrepancies among infected sinuses by studying the aerobic and anaerobic microbiology of acute and chronic sinusitis in patients with involvement of multiple sinuses (16b). The 155 evaluated patients had sinusitis of either the maxillary, ethmoid, or frontal sinuses (any combination) and had organisms recovered from two to four concomitantly infected sinuses. Similar aerobic, facultative, and anaerobic organisms were recovered from all the groups of patients. In patients who had organisms isolated from two sinuses and had acute sinusitis, 31 (56%) of the 55 isolates were found only in a single sinus and 24 (44%) were recovered concomitantly from two sinuses. In those with chronic infection, 31 (34%) of the 91 isolates were recovered only from a single sinus and 60 (66%) were found concomitantly from two sinuses. Anaerobic bacteria were more often concomitantly isolated from two sinuses (50 of 70) than aerobic and facultative (10 of 21, $p < 0.05$). Similar findings were observed in patients who had organisms isolated from three or four sinuses. Beta-lactamase–producing bacteria were more often isolated from patients with chronic infection (58–83%) as compared to those with acute infections (32–43%). These findings illustrate that there are differences in the distribution of organisms in a single patient who suffers from infections in multiple sinuses, and emphasize the importance of obtaining cultures from all infected sinuses.

INTERFERING FLORA

The nasopharynx of healthy individuals is generally colonized by relatively nonpathogenic aerobic and anaerobic organisms (26), some of which

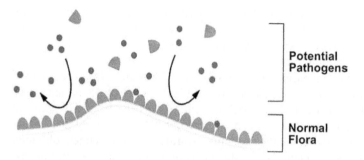

Figure 3 The role of normal flora in preventing colonization and subsequent infection by pathogenic bacteria.

possess the ability to interfere with the growth of potential pathogens (27) (Fig. 3). This phenomenon is called "bacterial interference." These organisms include the aerobic alpha-hemolytic streptococci (mostly *S. mitis* and *S. sanguis*) (28) and anaerobic bacteria (*Prevotella melaninogenica* and *Peptostreptococcus anaerobius*) (29). Many of these organisms produce bacteriocins, which are bactericidal proteins. Nasopharyngeal carriage of upper respiratory tract pathogens such as *S. pneumoniae*, *H. influenzae* and *M. catarrhalis* can, however, occur in healthy individuals, and increases significantly in the general population of young children during respiratory illness (30,31). The number of interfering organisms is lower in children prone to sinusitis (32). The absence of these organisms may explain the higher recovery of pathogens in these children. The presence of organisms with interfering potential may play a role in the prevention of colonization by pathogens and the occurrence of upper respiratory infections.

Administration of antimicrobial agents can influence the composition of nasopharyngeal flora (33). Members of the oral flora with interfering capability (e.g., aerobic and anaerobic streptococci as well as penicillin-susceptible *P. melaninogenica* strains) can become resistant to amoxicillin, but stay susceptible to amoxicillin–clavulanate. Beta-lactamase–producing *P. melaninogenica* strains are susceptible to amoxicillin–clavulanate. All these organisms are more resistant to second- and third-generation cephalosporin therapy. Therapy with oral second-generation cephalosporins does not eliminate organisms with interfering capabilities, as do amoxicillin (34) or amoxicillin–clavulanate.

NASAL FLORA

The origin of organisms that are introduced into the sinuses and may eventually cause sinusitis is the nasal cavity. The normal flora of that site is comprised of certain bacterial species, which include *S. aureus*,

S. epidermidis, alpha- and gamma-streptococci, *Propionibacterium acnes*, and aerobic diphtheroid (35–37). Potential sinus pathogens have been isolated from healthy nasal cavity but relatively rarely. These included *S. pneumoniae* (0.5–15%), *H. influenzae* (0–6%), *M. catarrhalis* (0–4%), *Streptococcus pyogenes* (0–1%), and anaerobic bacteria [*Peptostreptococcus* spp. (7–16%) and *Prevotella* spp. (6–8%)] (35–37).

The flora of the nasal cavity of patients with sinusitis is different from healthy flora. While the recovery of *Staphylococcus* spp. and diphtheroids is reduced, the isolation of pathogens increases—*S. pneumoniae* was found in 36% of patients, *H. influenzae* in over 50%, *S. pyogenes* in 6%, and *M. catarrhalis* in 4% (38–42).

In many studies of the nasal bacterial flora in sinusitis, a simultaneous sinus aspirate was not taken (40,41), whereas in other studies, the correlation was found to be poor in some (40,43) but good in others (42,44). A good correlation was, however, found in one study (38); in this study, when the sinus aspirate culture yielded a presumed sinus pathogen, the same organism was found in the nasal cavity sample in 91% of the 185 patients. The predictive value of a pathogen-positive nasal finding was high for *S. pyogenes* (94%), *H. influenzae* (78%), and *S. pneumoniae* (69%), but was low for *M. catarrhalis* (20%). Despite this encouraging data, nasopharyngeal culture is not an acceptable alternative to culture through aspiration.

NORMAL SINUS FLORA

It is known that after sinus surgery, the sinus cavities quickly become colonized with bacteria and are no longer sterile. The question of whether normal bacterial flora in the sinuses exists is controversial. The communication of the sinuses with the nasal cavity through the ostia could enable organisms that reside in the nasopharynx to spread into the sinus. Following closure of the ostium, these bacteria may become involved in the inflammation. Organisms have been recovered from uninflamed sinuses in several studies (45–48). The bacterial flora of noninflamed sinuses was studied for aerobic and anaerobic bacteria in 12 adults who underwent corrective surgery for septal deviation (45). Organisms were recovered from all aspirates with an average of four isolates per sinus aspirate. The predominant anaerobic isolates were *Prevotella*, *Porphyromonas*, *Fusobacterium*, and *Peptostreptococcus* spp. The most common aerobic bacteria were *S. pyogenes*, *S. aureus*, *S. pneumoniae*, and *H. influenzae*.

In another study, specimens were processed for aerobic bacteria only, and thus *Staphylococcus* spp. and alpha-hemolytic streptococci were isolated (46). Organisms were recovered in 20% of maxillary sinuses of patients who underwent surgical repositioning of the maxilla (47). In contrast, another report of aspirates of 12 volunteers with no sinus disease showed no bacterial growth (48). Jiang et al. evaluated (49) the bacteriology of maxillary sinuses with normal endoscopic findings. Organisms were recovered from 14 of 30 (47%) swab specimens and 7 of 17 (41%) of mucosal specimens.

Gordts et al. (50) reported the microbiology of the middle meatus in normal adults. They noted in 52 patients that 75% had the presence of bacterial isolates, most commonly CNS (35%), *Corynebacterium* spp. (23%), and *S. aureus* (8%). However, only low numbers of these species were present as compared to previous studies in children where the most common organisms were *H. influenzae* (40%), *M. catarrhalis* (34%), and *S. pneumoniae* (50%) of children. Nonhemolytic streptococci and *Moraxella* spp. were absent in adults.

MICROBIOLOGY OF SINUSITIS

The pattern of many upper respiratory infections including sinusitis evolves through several phases (Fig. 4). The early stage often is a viral infection that generally lasts up to 10 days and complete recovery occurs in most individuals (39). However, in a small number of patients (estimated at 0.5%) with viral sinusitis, a secondary acute bacterial infection may develop. This is generally caused by facultative aerobic bacteria (i.e., *S. pneumoniae*, *H. influenzae*, and *M. catarrhalis*). If resolution does not take place, anaerobic bacteria of oral flora origin become predominant over time. The dynamics of these bacterial changes were recently demonstrated by performing serial cultures in patients with maxillary sinusitis (51).

The Role of Bacterial Superantigens in Sinus Disease

Some microorganisms (bacteria, viruses, and fungi) can produce exotoxins (also called enterotoxins) that are able to nonspecifically up-regulate

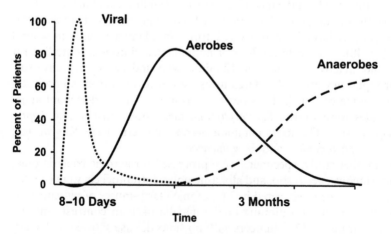

Figure 4 Microbiological dynamics of sinusitis.

T lymphocytes by cross-linking the MHC II molecule on antigen-presenting cells with the variable beta (Vβ) region of the T-cell receptor (TCR). These exotoxins are called superantigens because they activate in a nonspecific manner the subpopulations representing up to 30% of T lymphocytes in contrast to classical antigens, which activate only <0.01% of T lymphocytes. Furthermore, superantigens can also act as classical antigens-bringing about the concomitant generation of antisuperantigen antibodies that are often IgE isotypes (52).

S. aureus is a common colonizer of the nasal passage of patients with nasal polyps. *S. aureus* superantigens may play a role in nasal polyps, as 50% of polyp homogenates contained specific IgE to *S. aureus* exotoxins. Polyps associated with IgE to superantigens had significantly greater eosinophilia and markers of eosinophilic inflammation than controls (53).

Staphylococcal exotoxin-specific serum IgE was present in 5 of 10 (50%) patients with nasal polyposis and in none of 13 control patients. Patients with IgE to these superantigens have an increase in tissue eosinophilia and a higher incidence of asthma compared to control patients (54).

S. aureus was present in 7 of 13 patients with nasal polyps and all produced exotoxins, namely, staphylococcus enterotoxin A (SEA), toxic shock syndrome toxin-1 (TSS T-1), or staphylococcus enterotoxin B (SEB). A clonal expansion of Vβ specific to the isolated exotoxin was observed in the three patients studied (55).

Viral Infections

Viral illness is the most common predisposing factor for upper respiratory tract infections, including sinusitis (56). Rhino- and para-influenzae viruses are the most common causes of sinusitis (57,58). It is uncertain whether the viral infection precedes or is concurrent with the bacterial infection. The actual mechanisms by which a virus causes sinus disease are unknown. The mechanism whereby viruses predispose to sinusitis may involve microbial synergy, induction of local inflammation that blocks the sinus ostia, increase of bacterial attachment to the epithelial cells, and disruption of the local immune defense (Fig. 5).

Epithelial cells are often infected with the common respiratory viruses, which can induce the production of several cytokines (56,59,60). In the case of rhinoviruses, the virus is transported to the posterior nasopharynx after deposition in the nose (59,61) and attaches to a specific rhinovirus receptor (62). Following initiation of the infection, several inflammatory pathways and the sympathetic nervous system, which generates the classic symptoms of a cold, are stimulated (63). The common cold involves not only the nasal passages but also the paranasal sinuses. Sinus computed tomography (CT) scans of 31 young adults with early common colds

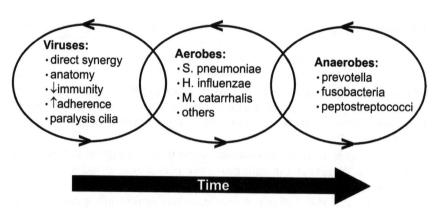

Figure 5 Dynamics of upper respiratory tract infection.

showed frequent abnormalities in the sinus cavity (64). Mucosal thickening is observed in radiographs of 87% of patients with colds (64), probably because of excess amounts of mucus discharged from goblet cells. These were observed in the maxillary, ethmoid, frontal, and sphenoid sinuses in 87, 65, 32, and 39% of the cases, respectively. Similar sinus abnormalities during colds were also observed in adults and children (65,66).

Activation of the inflammatory pathways results in engorgement of the venous erectile tissue in the nasal turbinates, which leads to leakage of plasma into the nose and sinuses, discharge of goblet cells and seromucous glands, sneezing, and sensation of pain.

CT scans show occlusion of the infundibulum in 77% of patients with viral rhinosinusitis (64). A malfunction in the ability of cilia to move material deposits towards the ostia because of the increased amount of viscous material and their induced slowing and paralysis is also observed (67). The adverse effect of this dysfunction is compounded by infundibular and osteomeatal obstruction from mucosal swelling. Some viral infections, such as influenza, can cause destructive epithelial damage, which enhances bacterial adherence.

During a cold, nasal fluid containing viruses, bacteria, and inflammatory mediators is suctioned into the sinus cavities where it produces inflammation and/or infection and is thickened by exocytosis of mucin from the numerous goblet cells in the sinus epithelium. The CT abnormalities observed in viral sinusitis could, therefore, be because of an inflammation alone or a viral infection of sinus epithelium cells. In sinus puncture studies in patients with acute community acquired rhinosinusitis, 15% of the sinus aspirates yielded rhinovirus, 5% influenza virus, 3% parainfluenza virus, and 2% adenovirus (68). Some of the sinus aspirates yielded both viruses and bacteria.

Bacteria in Acute Sinusitis

Bacteria can be isolated from two-thirds of patients with acute infection of the maxillary, ethmoid, frontal, and sphenoid sinuses (69). The microbiology of acute sinusitis is presented in greater details in Chapter 7. The bacteria recovered from pediatric and adult patients with community-acquired acute purulent sinusitis, using sinus aspiration by puncture or surgery, are the common respiratory pathogens (*S. pneumoniae, M. catarrhalis, H. influenzae*, and beta-hemolytic streptococci) and are considered as part of the normal flora of the nose (*S. aureus*) (Table 1) (70–72). *S. aureus* is a common pathogen in sphenoid sinusitis (72), whereas the other organisms are common in other sinuses.

The bacteria that cause the infection in children are generally the same as those found in acute otitis media. *S. pneumoniae* was isolated in 28% of 50 children with acute sinusitis, and both *H. influenzae* as well as *M. catarrhalis* were isolated in 19% of the aspirates. Beta-lactamase–producing strains of *H. influenzae* and *M. catarrhalis* were found in 20% and 27% of the cases, respectively.

The infection is polymicrobial in about a third of the cases. Enteric bacteria are recovered less commonly, and anaerobes were recovered from only a few cases with acute sinusitis. However, appropriate methods for their recovery were rarely employed in most studies of acute sinusitis. Anaerobic bacteria are commonly recovered from acute sinusitis associated with dental disease, mostly as an extension of the infection from the roots of the premolar or molar teeth (73,74) (see Chap. 19).

Pseudomonas aeruginosa and other gram-negative rods are common in sinusitis of nosocomial origin (especially in patients who have nasal tubes or catheters), the immunocompromised patients with human immune-deficiency virus (HIV) infection, and patients who suffer from cystic fibrosis (75).

Bacteria in Chronic Sinusitis

Although the exact etiology of the inflammation associated with this chronic sinusitis is uncertain, the presence of bacteria within the sinuses in this patient population has been well documented (76,77). Most clinicians believe that bacteria play a major role in the etiology and pathogenesis of most cases of chronic sinusitis and prescribe antimicrobials therapy for its treatment.

In contrast to the agreement regarding the microbiology of acute sinusitis, there is disagreement regarding the microbiology of chronic sinusitis. Unfortunately, there are several issues that confound the reliability of many of these studies and, therefore, contribute to the disparity of their results. These issues include: various methods used to sample the sinus cavity (i.e., aspiration, irrigation, Calginate swab, or biopsy); failure to sterilize the area

Table 1 Microbiology of Sinusitis (% of Patients)

Bacteria	Maxillary		Ethmoid		Frontal		Splenoid	
	Acute	Chronic N=66	Acute N=26	Chronic N=17	Acute N=15	Chronic N=13	Acute N=16	Chronic N=7
Aerobic								
S. aureus	4	14	15	24	–	15	56	14
S. pyogenes	2	8	8	6	3	–	6	–
S. pneumoniae	31	6	35	6	33	–	6	–
H. influenzae	21	5	27	6	40	15	12	14
M. catarrhalis	8	6	8	–	20	–	–	–
Enterobactiaceae	7	6	–	47	–	8	–	28
P. aeruginosa	2	3	–	6	–	8	6	14
Anaerobic								
Peptostreptococcus sp.	2	56	15	59	3	38	19	57
P. acnes		29	12	18	3	8	12	29
Fusobacterium sp.	2	17	4	47	3	31	6	54
Prevotella and Porphyromonas sp.	2	47	8	82	3	62	6	86
B. fragilis		6	–	–	–	15	–	–

Source: From Refs. 16b, 68, 85, 90, 125–127.

through which the trocar or endoscope is passed; different sinuses or areas that are sampled (i.e., ethmoid bulla or maxillary antrum or middle meatus); lack of assessment of the inflammatory response; lack of quantitation of bacteria; previous or current use of antibiotics; variable patient selection (i.e., age, duration, extent of disease, surgical, or nonsurgical subjects), presence of nasal polyps and time of culture transport and method of culture.

Numerous studies have examined the bacterial pathogens associated with chronic sinusitis. However, most of these studies did not employ methods that are adequate for the recovery of anaerobic bacteria. Studies have described significant differences in the microbial pathogens present in chronic sinusitis as compared with acute sinusitis. *S. aureus, S. epidermidis*, and anaerobic gram-negative bacteria predominate in chronic sinusitis. The pathogenicity of some of the low virulence organisms such as *S. epidermidis*, a colonizer of the nasal cavity, is questionable (50,78). The absence of quantitation or performance of Gram stains in most studies prevents an assessment of both the density of organisms and the accompaniment of an inflammatory response. The common resistance of *S. epidermidis* to antimicrobials does not prove its pathogenicity. Although *S. epidermidis* is discounted as a pathogen in sinusitis, its role as a pathogen in other body sites has been well documented (i.e., neutropenic sepsis, infections of indwelling catheters, and in burn patients) (79). Their frequent recovery from swabs obtained from the middle meatus of normal subjects marks them as commensals and likely contaminants. In the unusual situation in which a large number of white blood cells and gram-positive cocci were present on Gram stain there was heavy growth of *S. epidermidis*, proper anaerobic cultures showed no growth of other organisms, and the possibility of a true infection by *S. epidermidis* should be entertained (80).

Gram-negative enteric rods were also reported in recent studies (79–82). These included *P. aeruginosa, Klebsiella pneumoniae, Proteus mirabilis, Enterobacter* spp., and *Escherichia coli*. As these organisms are rarely found in cultures of the middle meatus obtained from normal individuals, their isolation from these symptomatic patients may suggest their pathogenic role. These organisms may have been selected out following administration of antimicrobial therapy in patients with chronic sinusitis.

The pathophysiology of chronic sinusitis often differs from that of acute sinusitis. The exact events leading to chronic sinusitis have been difficult to identify or prove (83). It has been proposed that chronic sinusitis is an extension of unresolved acute sinusitis. As mentioned previously, the etiology of acute sinusitis frequently is viral, which can establish an environment that is synergistic with the growth of other organisms, both aerobic and anaerobic. If the infection is not properly treated, the inflammatory process can persist, which, over time, fosters the growth of anaerobic bacteria. Thus, the pathogens in sinusitis appear to evolve over the course of infection—from viruses to aerobic to anaerobic bacterial growth—as the symptoms and pathology persist over a period of weeks to months. (Figs. 4 and 5)

The microbiology of chronic sinusitis differs from that of acute sinusitis (Table 1) (84–87). The transition from acute to chronic sinusitis by repeated aspiration of sinus secretions using endoscopy was illustrated in five patients who presented with acute maxillary sinusitis that did not respond to antimicrobial therapy (51). Most bacteria isolated from the first culture were aerobic or facultative bacteria—*S. pneumoniae, H. influenzae,* and *M. catarrhalis.* Failure to respond to therapy was associated with the emergence of resistant aerobic and anaerobic bacteria in subsequent aspirates. These organisms included *F. nucleatum,* pigmented *Prevotella, Porphyromonas* spp., and *Peptostreptococcus* spp. (Fig. 6). Eradication of the infection was finally achieved by administration of effective antimicrobial agents and in three cases by surgical drainage.

This study illustrates that as chronicity develops, the aerobic and facultative species are gradually replaced by anaerobes (51). This may result from the selective pressure of antimicrobial agents that enable resistant organisms to survive and from the development of conditions appropriate for anaerobic growth, which include the reduction in oxygen tension and an increase in acidity within the sinus (88). These are caused by the persistent edema and swelling, which reduce blood supply, and by the consumption of oxygen by the aerobic bacteria (88). Other factors are the emergence over time or selection of anaerobes that possess virulence factors such as capsule (89).

In chronic infections, when adequate methods are used, anaerobes can be recovered in more than half of all cases; the usual pathogens in acute

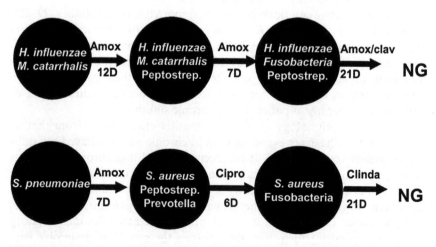

Figure 6 Dynamics of sinusitis. Changes in the microbiology of sinusitis in 2 patients treated with antibiotics. *Source*: From Ref. 51.

sinusitis (e.g., *S. pneumoniae*, *H. influenzae*, and *M. catarrhalis*) are found with lower frequency (84–87,90). Polymicrobial infection is common in chronic sinusitis, which is a synergistic infection (89) and may therefore be more difficult to eradicate with narrow-spectrum antimicrobial agents. Chronic sinusitis caused by anaerobes is of particular concern, clinically, because many of the complications associated with this condition (e.g., mucocele formation, osteomyelitis, local and intracranial abscess) are caused by these organisms (91).

That anaerobes play a role in chronic sinusitis is supported by the ability to induce chronic sinusitis in a rabbit by intrasinus inoculation of *Bacteroides fragilis* (92) and the rapid production of serum IgG antibodies against this organism in the infected animals (93). The pathogenic role of these organisms is also supported by the detection of antibodies (IgG) to two anaerobic organisms commonly recovered from sinus aspirates (*F. nucleatum* and *P. intermedia*) (94). Antibody levels to these organisms declined in the patients who responded to therapy and were cured, but not in those who failed therapy (Fig. 7).

Aside from their role as pathogens, the production of beta-lactamases among many gram-negative anaerobes (e.g., *Prevotella*, *Porphyromonas*, and *Fusobacterium* spp.) can shield or protect other organisms, including aerobic pathogens, from beta-lactam antibiotics (12,95) (Fig. 2).

Studies in Children

There have been 10 studies of the microbiology of chronic rhinosinusitis in children between 1981 and 2000 (86,96–104). Four of these studies were

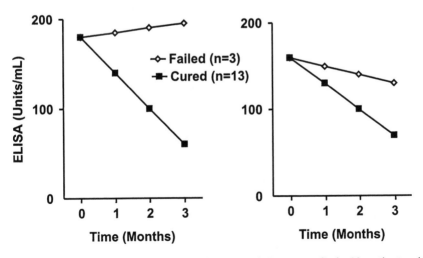

Figure 7 Serum antibodies to *F. nucleatum* and *P. intermedia* in 23 patients with chronic sinusitis. *Source*: From Ref. 94.

prospective (96,97,101,103) and six were retrospective. In all but two studies, the maxillary sinus was sampled by transnasal aspiration. The most common criteria for evaluation were the symptoms that lasted over 90 days. An attempt was made to sterilize the nose prior to obtaining the culture only in five studies, and bacterial quantitation was rarely done. In two of the studies, normal nasal flora (i.e., *S. epidermidis* and alpha-hemolytic strepto-cocci) was recovered. It is difficult to know what pathologic significance to ascribe to these organisms. In the remaining studies, the usual sinus pathogens (i.e., *H. influenzae*, *S. pneumoniae*, and *M. catarrhalis*) were recovered in about 60% of cases. This was especially true when the criteria for entry included purulent secretions. In the remaining 30 to 40% of children, contaminants were recovered. Anaerobes were recovered in three studies, the only one that employed methods for their isolation (86,96,103).

S. *aureus* (19%) and alpha-hemolytic streptococci (23%) were the predominant isolates in ethmoid sinusitis in one study (99), and S. *epidermidis* and alpha-hemolytic streptococci were the major ones in another (97). *M. catarrhalis* was the most common isolate in a study of children with allergies, although 25% of the patients had polymicrobial flora (105). *S. pneumoniae* and *H. influenzae* predominated in children with acute exacerbations (106).

Brook and Yocum (107) studied 40 children with chronic sinusitis. The sinuses infected were the maxillary (15 cases), ethmoid (13), and frontal (7). Pansinusitis was present in five patients. A total of 121 isolates (97 anaerobic and 24 aerobic) were recovered. Anaerobes were recovered from all 37 culture-positive specimens, and in 14 cases (38%) they were mixed with aero-bes. The predominant anaerobic organisms were gram-negative bacilli (36 isolates), anaerobic gram-positive cocci (28), and *Fusobacterium* spp. (13). The predominant aerobic isolates were alpha-hemolytic streptococci (7), S. *aureus* (7), and *Haemophilus* spp. (4).

Brook et al. (96) correlated the microbiology of concurrent chronic otitis media with effusion and chronic maxillary sinusitis in 32 children. Two-third of the patients had a bacterial etiology. The most common isolates were *H. influenzae* (9 isolates), *S. pneumoniae* (7), *Prevotella* spp. (8), and *Peptostreptococcus* spp. (6). Microbiological concordance between the ear and sinus was found in 22 (69%) of culture-positive patients.

Erkan et al. (103) studied 93 chronically inflamed maxillary sinuses in children. Anaerobic bacteria were isolated in 81of 87 (93%) culture-positive specimens, recovered alone in 61 (70%) cases, and mixed with aerobic or facultative bacteria in 20 (23%). Aerobic or facultative bacteria were present alone in six cases (7%). A total of 261 isolates, 19 anaerobes, and 69 aerobes or facultatives were isolated. The predominant anaerobic organisms were *Bacteroides* spp. and anaerobic cocci; the predominant aerobes or faculta-tives were *Streptococcus* spp. and S. *aureus*.

Studies in Adults

The presence of anaerobic bacteria in chronic sinusitis in adults was found to be clinically significant (108,109). In a study of chronic maxillary sinusitis Finegold et al. (87) found recurrence of signs and symptoms twice as frequent when cultures showed anaerobic bacterial counts above 10^3 cfu/mL.

Anaerobes were identified in chronic sinusitis whenever techniques for their cultivation were employed. The predominant isolates were pigmented *Prevotella, Fusobacterium,* and *Peptostreptococcus* spp. The predominant aerobic bacteria were *S. aureus, M. catarrhalis,* and *Haemophilus* spp. Aerobic and anaerobic BLPB were isolated from over one-third of these patients (80,84,85,90,109,110). These BLPB were *S. aureus, Haemophilus, Prevotella, Porphyromonas,* and *Fusobacterium* spp.

A summary of 17 studies of chronic sinusitis done since 1974, including 1758 patients (133 were children), is shown in Table 2 (85–87,103,110–123). Anaerobes were recovered in 12% to 93% of patients. The variability in recovery may result from differences in the methodologies used for transportation and cultivation, patient population, geography, and previous antimicrobial therapy.

Brook and Frazier (124), who correlated the microbiology with the history of sinus surgery in 108 patients with chronic maxillary sinusitis, found a higher rate of isolation of *P. aeruginosa* and other gram-negative bacilli in patients with previous sinus surgery. Anaerobes were, however, isolated more frequently in patients who did not have prior surgery.

Brook et al. (125) evaluated the microbiology of 13 chronically infected frontal, seven sphenoid (126), and 17 ethmoid sinuses (127) (Table 1). Anaerobic bacteria were recovered in over two-thirds of the patients. The predominant anaerobes included *Prevotella, Peptostreptococcus,* and *Fusobacterium* spp. The main aerobic organisms were gram-negative bacilli (*H. influenzae, K. pneumoniae, E. coli, and P. aeruginosa*).

Nadel et al. (80) also recovered gram-negative rods more commonly in previous surgery patients or those who had sinus irrigation. *P. aeruginosa* was more common in patients who received systemic steroids. Other studies have also noted this shift toward gram-negative organisms in patients who have been extensively and repeatedly treated (79,82,128a). The bacterial flora includes *Pseudomonas* spp., *Enterobacter* spp., methicillin-resistant *S. aureus, H. influenzae,* and *M. catarrhalis.*

Bacteria in Chronic Maxillary Sinusitis Associated with Nasal Polyposis

Nasal polyps can impair paranasal sinus ventilation and drainage by blockage of the ostiomeatal complex. Several studies have shown that in the majority of cases of chronic sinusitis where nasal polyps are present, bacterial cultures are negative. Even polymerase chain reaction (PCR)

Table 2 Summary of 18 Studies on the Role of Anaerobes in Chronic Bacterial Sinusitis

Ref.	No. of patients	Condition	Patients from whom anaerobic organisms were isolated (%)	Organisms that were anaerobes (%)
Frederick and Braude (111)	83	Chronic sinusitis	75	52
Van Cauwenberge et al. (112)	66	Acute and chronic sinusitis	39	39
Karma et al. (113)	40 adults	Chronic sinusitis	100	19
Berg et al. (114)	54 adults	Chronic sinusitis	33	42
Fiscella and Chow (115)	15 adults	Chronic sinusitis	38	48
Sedallian et al. (116)	40	Chronic sinusitis	69	46
Simoncelli et al. (117)	132 adults	Chronic sinusitis	NS	22
Tabaqchali (118)	35	Chronic sinusitis	70	39
Brook (86)	40 children	Chronic sinusitis	100	80
Hartog et al. (119)	90	Chronic sinusitis	81	29
Ito et al. (120)	10	Chronic maxillary sinusitis	100	60
Erkan et al. (103)	93 children	Chronic maxillary sinusitis	93	93
Erkan et al. (121)	126 adults	Chronic maxillary sinusitis	90	88
Brook et al. (85)	68 adults	Chronic maxillary sinusitis	100	82
Edelstein et al. (122)	114 adults	Acute and chronic sinusitis	NS	12
Klossek et al. (123)	412	Chronic sinusitis	NS	26
Finegold et al. (87)	150 adults	Chronic maxillary sinusitis	54	49

Abbreviation: NS, not specified.

techniques have failed to demonstrate bacterial infection in most cases (128b). Hamilos et al. (128c) obtained antral culture in 12 subjects with chronic maxillary sinusitis with nasal polyps and isolated organisms in only three patients. However, none of these studies employed methods that were adequate for the recovery of anaerobic bacteria.

We evaluated aspirates of 48 chronically inflamed maxillary sinuses from patients who had nasal polyposis that were cultured for aerobic and anaerobic bacteria (128d). Bacterial growth was present in 46 (96%) specimens. Aerobic or facultative bacteria were present in 6 (13%) specimens, anaerobic bacteria alone in 18 (39%), and mixed aerobic and anaerobic bacteria in 22 (48%). There were 110 bacterial isolates (2.4 per specimen).

Thirty-nine of the isolates were aerobic or facultative organisms (0.85 per specimen). The predominant aerobic or facultative organisms were *S. aureus*, microaerophilic streptococci, *H. influenzae*, and *M. catarrhalis*. There were 71 anaerobes isolated (1.5 per specimen). The predominant anaerobes were *Peptostreptococcus* spp., *Prevotella* spp., *P. asaccharolytica*, *Fusobacterium* spp., and *P. acnes*. These findings suggest that the microbiology of the maxillary sinus of patients with chronic sinusitis with polyposis is not different than those who develop chronic sinusitis without this condition, as the major isolates are polymicrobial aerobic–anaerobic flora.

Bacteria in Acute Exacerbation of Chronic Sinusitis

Acute exacerbation of chronic sinusitis (AECS) represents a sudden worsening of the baseline chronic sinusitis with either worsening or new symptoms. Typically, the acute (not chronic) symptoms resolve completely between occurrences (129). We evaluated the microbiology of acute AECS (130) by performing repeated endoscopic sinus aspirations in seven patients over a period of 125 to 242 days. Bacteria were recovered from all 22 aspirates and the number of isolates varied between two and four. A total of 54 isolates were isolated, 16 aerobic as well as facultatives and 38 anaerobic bacteria. The aerobic bacteria were seven *H. influenzae*, three *S. pneumoniae*, three *M. catarrhalis*, two *S. aureus*, and one *K. pneumoniae*. The anaerobic bacteria included pigmented *Prevotella* and *Porphyromonas* spp. (19 isolates), *Peptostreptococcus* spp. (9), *Fusobacterium* spp. (8), and *acnes* (2). A change in the types of isolates was noted in all consecutive cultures obtained from the same patients as different organisms emerged and previously isolated bacteria were no longer recovered. An increase in antimicrobial resistance was noted in six instances. These findings illustrate the microbial dynamics of AECS where anaerobic and aerobic bacteria prevail and highlight the importance of obtaining cultures from patients with this infection for guidance in selection of proper antimicrobial therapy.

Brook (131) compared the aerobic and anaerobic microbiology of maxillary AECS with the microbiology of chronic maxillary sinusitis.

Included in the study were 32 cases with chronic sinusitis and 30 with AECS. A total of 81 isolates were recovered from the 32 cases (2.5 per specimen) with chronic sinusitis, 33 aerobic, and 48 anaerobic. Aerobes alone were recovered in eight specimens (25%), anaerobes only were isolated in 11 (34%), and mixed aerobes and anaerobes were recovered in 13 (41%). The predominant aerobic and facultatives were Enterobacteriacaeae and *S. aureus*. The predominant anaerobic bacteria were *Peptostreptococcus* spp., *Fusobacterium* spp., anaerobic gram-negative bacilli, and *P. acnes*. A total of 89 isolates were recovered from the 30 cases (3.0 per specimen) with AECS, 40 aerobic and facultatives, and 49 anaerobic. Aerobes were recovered in eight instances (27%), anaerobes only in 11 (37%), and mixed aerobes and anaerobes were recovered in 11 (37%). The predominant aerobes were *S. pneumoniae*, Enterobacteriaceae, and *S. aureus*. The prominante anaerobes were *Peptostreptococcus* spp., *Fusobacterium* spp., gram-negative bacilli, and *P. acnes*. This study illustrates that the organisms isolated from patients with AECS were predominantly anaerobic and were similar to those generally recovered in chronic sinusitis. However, aerobic bacteria that are usually found in acute infections (e.g., *S. pneumoniae*, *H. influenzae*, and *M. catarrhalis*) can also emerge in some of the episodes of AECS.

Nosocomial Rhinosinusitis

Patients with nosocomial sinusitis are usually those who require extended periods of intensive care (postoperative patients, burn victims, and patients with severe trauma) involving prolonged endotracheal or nasogastric intubation (132). Nasotracheal intubation places the patient at a substantially higher risk for nosocomial sinusitis than orotracheal intubation (133). Approximately 25% of patients requiring nasotracheal intubation for more than five days develop nosocomial sinusitis (134). In contrast to community-acquired sinusitis, the usual pathogens are gram-negative enterics (e,g., *P. aeruginosa*, *K. pneumoniae*, *Enterobacter* spp., *P. mirabilis*, and *Serratia marcescens*) and gram-positive cocci (occasionally streptococci and staphylococci) (chap. 16) (133–137). Whether these organisms are actually pathogenic is unclear, and they usually represent colonization of an environment with impaired mucociliary transport and foreign body presence in the nasal cavity.

Evaluation of the microbiology of nosocomial sinusitis in nine children with neurologic impairment revealed anaerobic bacteria, always mixed with aerobic and facultative bacteria in 6 (67%) sinus aspirates and aerobic bacteria only in 3 (33%) (138). There were 24 bacterial isolates, 12 aerobic or facultative and 12 anaerobic. The predominant aerobic isolates were *K. pneumoniae*, *E. coli*, and *S. aureus* (two each) and *P. mirabilis*, *P. aeruginosa*, *H. influenzae*, *M. catarrhalis*, and *S. pneumoniae* (one each). The predominant anaerobes were *Prevotella* spp. (5), *Peptostreptococcus* spp. (4), *F. nucleatum* (2), and *B. fragilis* (1). Organisms similar to those recovered from the sinuses were also isolated from tracheostomy site and gastrostomy wound aspirates in five of seven instances. This study demonstrates the uniqueness of the microbiologic features of sinusitis in neurologically impaired children in which, in addition to the organisms known to cause infection in normal children, facultative and anaerobic gram-negative organisms that can colonize other body sites are predominant.

Atypical Organisms

Chlamydia pneumoniae has been isolated from patients with respiratory infection that included clinical features of sinusitis (139), and serological evidence of its presence in patients with sinusitis was found in only 2% of 103 patients (140). However, as it was only isolated in one case from sinus aspirate (141), its exact role in sinusitis is uncertain.

Mycoplasma pneumoniae has been suspect as a cause of acute sinusitis, but no attempts have been made so far to recover it from infected sinuses. However, serological evidence of an increase in antibody titres suggests a link between sinusitis and *M. pneumoniae* infection (142) in purulent bacterial and nonpurulent nonbacterial sinusitis.

One study identified *M. pneumoniae*–specific DNA in a small group of subjects with sinusitis and/or nasal polyposis (143). However, a more recent study failed to confirm the presence of bacterial-specific DNA sequences for 16S ribosomal RNA (144).

THE ROLE OF FUNGI IN SINUSITIS

Fungal "colonization" of the nose and paranasal sinuses is common in the normal and inflamed sinuses because of the ubiquitous nature of the organisms (145–148). Under certain conditions, however, clinically significant growth of fungus balls (also called mycetomas) or saprophytic growth of fungus may occur. This can cause the formation and accumulation of fungal mycelia within the nose and paranasal sinuses without significant mucosal inflammation. In such cases, extirpation of the offending fungal growth is generally sufficient. However, in other forms, the inflammatory response to the fungi may result in clinically significant disease.

Fungal sinusitis can be either noninvasive or invasive (chap. 20). Invasive involvement is generally considered as an acute and fulminant disease. In immunologically deficient patients, however, the invasive fungal sinusitis is mild or not apparent, and can have a long and chronic course. Diagnosis is confirmed by histological evidence of nasal or sinus invasive fungal involvement lasting longer than 12 weeks.

Management of the disease necessitates correction of immunological deficiency, surgical debridements, and long-term systemic and topical antifungal treatment. The disease can progress and recur despite aggressive therapy, and can occasionally be fatal.

Fungi can occasionally cause commonly acquired sinusitis (149). They are especially common in patients with uncontrolled diabetes, HIV disease, and those on prolonged immunosuppression therapy (especially transplant recipients) and courses of antimicrobial therapy. *Aspergillus fumigatus* is the most common fungus associated with sinusitis (150), and it can cause disease in normal as well as the immunocompromised hosts. The organism is a saprophyte of soil, dust, and decaying organic material. It has an invasive and a noninvasive form; its portal of entry is the respiratory tract. Sinusitis caused by *aspergillus* has been associated with the smoking of marijuana, as it contaminates the leaves. The organism has a noninvasive, an invasive, and a disseminated form. The noninvasive form causes chronic rhinitis and nasal obstruction, and if untreated, can spread to the blood stream, seeding numerous sites.

Other *Aspergillus* species have also caused sinusitis in normal hosts and include *Aspergillus flavus* and *Aspergillus niger* (151,152).

Chronic invasive fungal sinusitis is divided into granulomatous and nongranulomatous subtypes based on histopathology. Chronic invasive fungal rhinosinusitis has been associated with *Mucor, Alternaria, Curvularia, Bipolaris, Candida, Sporothrix schenckii,* and *Pseudallescheria boydii.* Other fungi that can cause sinus infection include *Schizophyllum commune* (153), *Emericella nidulans* (154), *Pseudoallescheria boydii* (155), *Paecilomyces* spp., *Cryptococcus neoformans, Penicillium melinii, Scedosporium (monosporium), Apiospermum,* and *Blastomycocis dermatitides* (156). Saprophytic fungi causing infections are O*reschslera* spp., *Alternaria* spp., *Curvularia lunata, and Exserohilum* spp. (157). Mucomycosis is caused by fungi of the Mucurales order. The sinusitis induced occurs mainly in diabetic and immunocompromised patients.

Allergic sinusitis has been associated with *Alternaria, Aspergillus, Bipolaris, Chrysporium, Dreschlera,* and *Exserohilum* (158). Allergic fungal sinusitis from *Aspergillus* spp. is similar to allergic bronchopulmonary aspergillus with secretions containing eosinophils, Charcot–Leyden crystals, and fungal hyphe (159). Patients usually have evidence of atopy or asthma. The sinusitis is protracted and generally involves multiple sinuses. *Myriodontium keratinophelum* produces also allergic-like fungal sinusitis (160). The patients generally suffer from chronic sinusitis, nasal polyps, and proptosis owing to orbital and ethmoid cell invasion. Allergic fungal sinusitis was also described to be associated with *Dreschslera* (161), *Alternaria,* and *Curvularia* (162).

Chronic invasive fungal sinusitis is divided into granulomatous and nongranulomatous subtypes based on histopathology. Chronic invasive fungal rhinosinusitis has been associated with *Mucor, Alternaria, Curvularia, Bipolaris, Candida, S. schenckii,* and *P. boydii* (152).

CONCLUSION

Sinusitis generally develops as a complication of viral or allergic inflammation of the upper respiratory tract. The bacterial pathogens in acute sinusitis are *S. pneumoniae*, *H. influenzae*, and *M. catarrhalis*, whereas anaerobic bacteria and *S. aureus* are predominant in chronic sinusitis. *P. aeruginosa* has emerged as a potential pathogen in the immunocompromised patients and in those who have nasal tubes or catheters, or are intubated.

REFERENCES

1. Faden H, Stanievich J, Brodsky L, Benstein J, Ogra PL. Changes in the nasopharyngeal flora during otitis media of childhood. Pediatr Infect Dis 1990; 9:623–626.
2. Del Beccaro MA, Mendelman PM, Inglis AF, Richardson MA, Duncan NO, Clausen CR, Stull TL. Bacteriology of acute otitis media: a new perspective. J Pediatr 1992; 120:856–862.
3. Socransky SS, Manganiello SD. The oral microflora of man from birth to senility. J Periodontol 1971; 42:485–496.
4. Gibbons RJ, Socransky SS, Dearaujo WC, Varihoute J. Studies of the predominant cultivable microbiota of dental plaque. Arch Oral Biol 1964; 9: 365–370.
5. Valenti WM, Trudell RG, Bentley DW. Factors predisposing to oropharyngeal colonization with gram-negative bacilli in the aged. N Engl J Med 1978; 298:1108–1110.
6. Baird-Parker AC. The classification of fusobacteria from the human mouth. J Genet Microbiol 1960; 22:458–469.
7. Smibert RM. Spirochaetales: a review. CRC Crit Rev Microbiol 1973; 2:491.
8. Gibbons RJ. Aspects of the pathogenicity and ecology of the indigenous oral flora of man. In: Balows A, et al. eds. Anaerobic Bacteria, Role in Disease, Springfield, IL: Charles C Thomas, 1974.
9. Rasmussen EG, Gibbons RJ, Socransky SS. A taxonomic study of fifty grampositive anaerobic diphtheroides isolated from the oral cavity of man. Arch Oral Biol 1966; 11:573–579.
10. Gibbons RJ, Socransky SS, Sawyer S, Kapsimalii B, MacDonald JB. The microbiota of the gingival crevice of man: II. The predominant cultivable organisms. Arch Oral Biol 1963; 8:281–289.
11. Brook I. Beta-lactamase producing bacteria in head and neck infection. Larynscope 1988; 98:428–431.
12. Brook, I. The role of beta-lactamase-producing bacterial in the persistence of streptococcal tonsillar infection. Rev Infect Dis 1984; 6:601–607.
13. Brook I, Gober AE. Emergence of beta-lactamase-producing aerobic and anaerobic bacteria in the oropharynx of children following penicillin chemotherapy. Clin Pediatr 1984; 23:338–341.

14. Tuner K, Nord CE. Emergence of beta-lactamase-producing microorganisms in the tonsils during penicillin treatment. Eur J Clin Microbiol 1986; 5: 399–404.

15. American Academy of Pediatrics. Subcommittee on management of sinusitis and committee on quality improvement. Clinical practice guideline: management of sinusitis. Pediatrics 2001; 108:798–808.

16a. Talbot GH, Kennedy DW, Scheld WM, Granito K. Rigid nasal endoscopy versus sinus puncture and aspiration for microbiologic documentation of acute bacterial maxillary sinusitis. Clin Infect Dis 2001; 33: 1668–1675.

16b. Brook I. Discrepancies in the recovery of bacteria from multiple sinuses in acute and chronic sinusitis. J Med Microbiol 2004; 53:879–885.

17. Gordts F, Abu Nasser I, Clement PA, Pierad D, Kaufman L. Bacteriology of the middle meatus in children. Int J Pediatr Otorhinolaryngol 1999; 48: 163–167.

18. Gordts F, Harlewyck S, Pierard D, Kaufman L, Clement PA. Microbiology of the middle meatus: a comparison between normal adults and children. J Laryngol Otol 2000; 114:184–188.

19. Klossek JM, Dubreuil L, Richet H, Richet B, Sedallian A, Beutter P. Bacteriology of the adult middle meatus. J Laryngol Otol 1996; 110:847–849.

20. Nadel DM, Lanza DC, Kennedy DW. Endoscopically guided cultures in chronic sinusitis. Am J Rhinol 1998; 12:233–241.

21. Gold SM, Tami TA. Role of middle meatus aspiration culture in the diagnosis of chronic sinusitis. Laryngoscope 1997; 107:1586–1589.

22. Vogen JC, Bolger WE, Keyes AS. Endoscopically guided cultures: a direct comparison with maxillary sinus aspirate cultures. Oto-HNS 2000; 122: 370–373.

23. Winther B, Vicery CL, Gross CW, Hendley O. Microbiology of the maxillary sinus in adults with chronic sinus disease. Am J Rhinol 1996; 10:347–350.

24. Kountakis SE, Skoulas IG. Middle meatal vs. antral lavage cultures in intensive care unit patients. Otolaryngol Head Neck Surg 2002; 126: 377–381.

25. Brook I, Frazier EH, Foote PA. Microbiology of chronic maxillary sinusitis: comparison between specimens obtained by sinus endoscopy and by surgical drainage. J Med Microbiol 1997; 46:430–432.

26. Mackowiak PA. The normal flora. N Engl J Med 1983; 307:83–93.

27. Sprunt K, Redman W. Evidence suggesting importance of role of interbacterial inhibition in maintaining balance of normal flora. Ann Intern Med 1968; 68:579–590.

28. Bernstein JM, Sagahtaheri-Altaie S, Dryjd DM, Vactawski-Wende J. Bacterial interference in nasopharyngeal bacterial flora of otitis-prone and non-otitis-prone children. Acta Otol Rhinol Laryngol Belg 1994; 48:1–9.

29. Murray PR, Rosenblatt JE. Bacterial interference by oropharyngeal and clinical isolates of anaerobic bacteria. J Infect Dis 1976; 134:281–285.

30. Faden H, Zaz MJ, Bernstein JM, Brodsky L, Stamievich J, Ogru PL. Nasopharyngeal flora in the first three years of life in normal and otitis-prone children. Ann Otol Rhinol Laryngol 1991; 100:612–615.

31. Brook I, Gober A. Bacterial interference in the nasopharynx of otitis media prone and not otitis media prone children. Arch Otolaryngol Head Neck Surg 2000; 126:1011–1013.

32. Brook I, Gober AE. Bacterial interference in the nasopharynx and nasal cavity of sinusitis prone and non-sinusitis prone children. Acta Otolaryngol 1999; 119:832–836.

33. Foote PA Jr, Brook I. Penicillin and clindamycin therapy in recurrent tonsillitis. Effect of microbial flora. Arch Otolaryngol Head Neck Surg 1989; 15: 856–859.

34. Brook I, Foote PA. Effect of antimicrobial therapy with amoxicillin and cefprozil on bacterial interference and beta-lactamase production in the adenoids. Ann Otol Rhinol Laryngol 2004; 113:902–905.

35. Brook I. Aerobic and anaerobic bacteriology of purulent nasopharyngitis in children. J Clin Microbiol 1988; 26:592–594.

36. Savolainen S, Ylikoski J, Jousimies-Somer H. The bacterial flora of the nasal cavity in healthy young men. Rhinology 1986; 24:249–255.

37. Winther B, Brofeldt S, Gronborg H, Mygind N, Pedersen M, Vejlsgaard R. Study of bacteria in the nasal cavity and nasopharynx during naturally acquired common colds. Acta Otolaryngol 1984; 98:315–320.

38. Jousimies-Somer HR, Savolainen S, Ylikoski JS. Comparison of the nasal bacterial floras in two groups of healthy subjects and in patients with acute maxillary sinusitis. J Clin Microbiol 1989; 27:2736–2743.

39. Gwaltney JM Jr, Sydnor A, Sande MA. Etiology and antimicrobial treatment of acute sinusitis. Ann Otol Rhinol Laryngol 1981; 90(suppl 84):68–71.

40. Lystad A, Berdal P, Lund-Iversen L. The bacterial flora of sinusitis with an in vitro study of the bacterial resistance to antibiotics. Acta Otolaryngol Suppl 1964; 188:390–400.

41. Nylen O, Jeppsson P-H, Branefors-Helander P. Acute sinusitis. A clinical, bacteriological and serological study with special reference to *Haemophilus influenzae*. Scand J Infect Dis 1972; 4:43–48.

42. Björkwall T. Bacteriological examination in maxillary sinusitis: bacterial flora of the nasal meatus. Acta Otolaryngol Suppl 1950; 83:1–32.

43. Catlin FI, Cluff LE, Reynolds RC. The bacteriology of acute and chronic sinusitis. South Med J 1965; 58:1497–1502.

44. Savolainen S, Ylikoski J, Jousimies-Somer H. Predictive value of nasal bacterial culture for etiological agents in acute maxillary sinusitis. Rhinology 1987; 25:49–55.

45. Brook I. Aerobic and anaerobic bacterial flora of normal maxillary sinuses. Laryngoscopy 1981; 91:372–376.

46. Su WY, Liu CR, Hung SY, Tsai WF. Bacteriological studies in chronic maxillary sinusitis. Laryngoscope 1983; 93:931–934.

47. Cook HE, Haber J. Bacteriology of the maxillary sinus. J Oral Maxillofac Surg 1987; 45:1011–1014.

48. Sobin J, Engquist S, Nord CE. Bacteriology of the maxillary sinus in healthy volunteers. Scand J Infect Dis 1992; 24:633–635.

49. Jiang RS, Liang KL, Jang JW, Hsu CY. Bacteriology of endoscopically normal maxillary sinuses. J Laryngol Otol 1999; 113:825–828.

50. Gordts F, Halewyck S, Pierard D, Kaufman L, Clement PA. Microbiology of the middle meatus: a comparison between normal adults and children. J Laryngol Otol 2000; 114:184–188.
51. Brook I, Frazier EH, Foote PA. Microbiology of the transition from acute to chronic maxillary sinusitis. J Med Microbiol 1996; 45:372–375.
52. Schubert MS. A superantigen hypothesis for the pathogenesis of chronic hypertrophic rhinosinusitis, allergic fungal sinusitis, and related disorders. Ann Allergy Asthma Immunol 2001; 87:181–188.
53. Bachert C, Gevaert P, Holtappels G, Johansson SG, van Cauwenberge P. Total and specific IgE in nasal polyps is related to local eosinophilic inflammation. J Allergy Clin Immunol 2001; 107:607–614.
54. Conley DB, Tripathi A, Ditto AM, Grammer LC, Kern RC. Chronic sinusitis with nasal polyps: staphylococcal exotoxin immunoglobulin E and cellular inflammation. Am J Rhinol 2004; 18:273–278.
55. Bernstein JM, Ballow M, Schlievert PM, Rich G, Allen C, Dryja D. A superantigen hypothesis for the pathogenesis of chronic hyperplastic sinusitis with massive nasal polyposis. Am J Rhinol 2003; 17:321–326.
56. Subausie MC, Jacoby DB, Richards SM, Proud D. Infection of a human respiratory epithelial cell line with rhinovirus: induction of cytokine release and modulation of susceptibility to infection by cytokine exposure. J Clin Invest 1995; 96:549–557.
57. Evans FO Jr, Sydnor JB, Moore WEC, Moore GT, Manwaning Z, Brill AH, Jackson RT, Hanna S, Skaar JS, Holdeman LV, Fritz-Hugh S, Sande MA, Gwaltney JM Jr. Sinusitis of the maxillary antrum. N Engl J Med 1975; 293:735–739.
58. Hamory BH, Sande MA, Sydnor A Jr, Seale DL, Gwaltney JM Jr. Etiology and antimicrobial therapy of acute maxillary sinusitis. J Infect Dis 1979; 139:197–202.
59. Osur SL. Viral respiratory infections in association with asthma and sinusitis: a review. Ann Allergy Asthma Immunol 2002; 89:553–560.
60. Elias JA, Zheng T, Einarsson O, Landry M, Trow T, Robert N, Panuska J. Epithelial interleukin-11: regulation by cytokines, respiratory syncytial virus, and retinoic acid. J Biol Chem 1994; 269:22261–22268.
61. Winther B, Gwaltney JM Jr, Mygind N, Turner RB, Hendley JO. Sites of rhinovirus recovery after point inoculation of the upper airway. JAMA 1986; 256:1763–1767.
62. Greve JM, Davis G, Meyer AM, Forte CP, Yost SC, Marbov CW, Kamarik ME, McClelland A. The major human rhinovirus receptor is ICAM-1. Cell 1989; 56:839–847.
63. Gwaltney JM Jr. Rhinovirus infection of the normal human airway. Am J Respir Crit Care Med 1995; 152:S36–S39.
64. Gwaltney JM Jr, Phillips CD, Miller RD, Riker DK. Computed tomographic study of the common cold. N Engl J Med 1994; 330:25–30.
65. Puhakka T, Mäkelä MJ, Alanen A, Kallio T, Korsoff L, Arstila P, Leinonen M, Pulkkinen M, Suonpää J, Mertsola J, Ruuskanen O. Sinusitis in the common cold. J Allergy Clin Immunol 1998; 102:403–408.

66. Kristo A, Uhari M, Luotonen J, Koivunen P, Ilkko E, Tapiainen T, Alho O-P. Paranasal. Sinus findings in children during respiratory infection evaluated with magnetic resonance imaging. Pediatrics 2003; 111:e586–e589.

67. Sasaki Y, Togo Y, Wagner HN Jr, Hornick RB, Schwartz AR, Proctor DF. Mucociliary function during experimentally induced rhinovirus infection in man. Ann Otol Rhinol Laryngol 1973; 82:203–211.

68. Gwaltney JM Jr. Acute community-acquired sinusitis. Clin Infect Dis 1996; 23:1209–1225.

69. Gwaltney JM Jr, Scheld WM, Sande MA, Sydnor A. The microbial etiology and antimicrobial therapy of adults with acute community-acquired sinusitis: a fifteen-year experience at the University of Virginia and review of other selected studies. J Allergy Clin Immunol 1992; 90:457–462.

70. Wald ER, Milmore GJ, Bowen AD, Ledema-Medina J, Salamon N, Bluestone CD. Acute maxillary sinusitis in children. N Engl J Med 1981; 304:749–754.

71. Wald ER, Guerra N, Byers C. Upper respiratory tract infections in young children: duration of and frequency of complications. Pediatrics 1991; 87: 129–133.

72. Lew D, Southwick FS, Montgomery WW, Weber AL, Baker AS. Sphenoid sinusitis. A review of 30 cases. N Engl J Med 1983; 309:1149–1154.

73. Brook I, Frazier EH, Gher ME Jr. Microbiology of periapical abscesses and associated maxillary sinusitis. J Periodontal 1996; 67:608–610.

74. Brook I, Friedman EM. Intracranial complications of sinusitis in children. A sequela of periapical abscess. Ann Otol Rhinol Laryngol 1982; 91:41–43.

75. Shapiro ED, Milmoe GJ, Wald ER, Rodnan JB, Bowen AD. Bacteriology of the maxillary sinuses in patients with cystic fibrosis. J Infect Dis 1982; 146: 589–593.

76. Wald ER. Microbiology of acute and chronic sinusitis in children and adults. Am J Med Sci 1998; 316:13–20.

77. Biel MA, Brown CA, Levinson RM, Gravis GE, Paisner HM, Siegil ME, Tedford TM. Evaluation of the microbiology of chronic maxillary sinusitis. Ann Otol Laryngol Rhinol 1998; 107:942–945.

78. Jiang RS, Hsu CY, Jang JW. Bacteriology of the maxillary and ethmoid sinuses in chronic sinusitis. J Laryngol Otol 1998; 112:845–848.

79. Hsu J, Lanza DC, Kennedy DW. Antimicrobial resistance in bacterial chronic sinusitis. Am J Rhinol 1998; 12:243–248.

80. Nadel DM, Lanza DC, Kennedy DW. Endoscopically guided cultures in chronic sinusitis. Am J Rhinol 1998; 12:233–241.

81. Bahattacharyya N, Kepnes LJ. The microbiology of recurrent rhinosinusitis after endoscopic sinus surgery. Arch Otolaryngol Head Neck Surg 1999; 125:1117–1120.

82. Bolger WE. Gram negative sinusitis: emerging clinical entity. Am J Rhinol 1994; 8:279–283.

83. Kaliner M, Osguthorpe J, Fireman P, Anon J, Georgitis J, Davis ML, Naclerio R, Kennedy D. Sinusitis: bench to bedside. Otolaryngol Head Neck Surg 1997; 116(suppl):S1–S20.

84. Nord CE. The role of anaerobic bacteria in recurrent episodes of sinusitis and tonsillitis. Clin Infect Dis 1995; 20:1512–1524.

85. Brook I, Thompson D, Frazier E. Microbiology and management of chronic maxillary sinusitis. Arch Otolaryngol Head Neck Surg 1994; 120: 1317–1320.
86. Brook I. Bacteriologic features of chronic sinusitis in children. JAMA 1981; 246:967–969.
87. Finegold SM, Flynn MJ, Rose FV, Jousimies-Somer H, Jakielaszek C, McTeague M, Wexler HM, Berkowitz E, Wynne B. Bacteriologic findings associated with chronic bacterial maxillary sinusitis in adults. Clin Infect Dis 2002; 35:428–433.
88. Carenfelt C, Lundberg C. Purulent and non-purulent maxillary sinus secretions with respect to PO_2, PCO_2 and pH. Acta Otolaryngol 1977; 84:138–144.
89. Brook I. Role of encapsulated anaerobic bacteria in synergistic infections. Crit Rev Microbiol 1987; 14:171–193.
90. Brook I. Bacteriology of chronic maxillary sinusitis in adults. Ann Otol Rhinol Laryngol 1989; 98:426–428.
91. Brook I. Brain abscess in children: microbiology and management. Child Neurol 1995; 10:283–288.
92. Westrin KM, Stierna P, Carlsoo B, Hellstrom S. Mucosal fine structure in experimental sinusitis. Ann Otol Rhinol Laryngol 1993; 102(8 Pt 1): 639–645.
93. Jyonouchi H, Sun S, Kennedy CA, Roche AK, Kajander KC, Miller JR, Germaine GR, Rimell FL. Localized sinus inflammation in a rabbit sinusitis model induced by *Bacteroides fragilis* is accompanied by rigorous immune responses. Otolaryngol Head Neck Surg 1999; 120:869–875.
94. Brook I, Yocum P. Immune response to *Fusobacterium nucleatum* and *Prevotella intermedia* in patients with chronic maxillary sinusitis. Ann Otol Rhinol Laryngol 1999; 108:293–295.
95. Brook I, Yocum P, Frazier EH. Bacteriology and beta-lactamase activity in acute and chronic maxillary sinusitis. Arch Otolaryngol Head Neck Surg 1996; 122:418–422.
96. Brook I, Yocum P, Shah K. Aerobic and anaerobic bacteriology of concurrent chronic otitis media with effusion and chronic sinusitis in children. Arch Otolaryngol Head Neck Surg 2000; 126:174–176.
97. Orobello PW Jr, Park RI, Belcher L, et al. Microbiology of chronic sinusitis in children. Arch Otolaryngol Head Neck Surg 1991; 117:980–983.
98. Tinkleman DG, Silk HJ. Clinical and bacteriologic features of chronic sinusitis in children. Am J Dis Child 1989; 143:938–941.
99. Muntz HR, Lusk RP. Bacteriology of the ethmoid bullae in children with chronic sinusitis. Arch Otolaryngol Head Neck Surg 1991; 117:179–181.
100. Otten FWA, Grote JJ. Treatment of chronic maxillary sinusitis in children. Int J Pediatr Otorhinolaryngol 1988; 15:269–278.
101. Otten FWA. Conservative treatment of chronic maxillary sinusitis in children. Long term follow-up. Acta Otol Rhinol Laryngol Belg 1997; 51:173–175.
102. Don D, Yellon RF, Casselbrant M, Bluestone CD. Efficacy of stepwise protocol that includes intravenous antibiotic treatment for the management of chronic sinusitis in children and adolescents. Otolaryngol Head Neck Surg 2001; 127:1093–1098.

103. Erkan M, Ozcan M, Arslan S, Soysal V, Bozdemir K, Haghighi N. Bacteriology of antrum in children with chronic maxillary sinusitis. Scand J Infect Dis 1996; 28:283–285.
104. Slack CL, Dahn KA, Abzug MJ, Chan KH. Antibiotic-resistant bacteria in pediatric chronic sinusitis. Pediatr Infect Dis J 2001; 20:247–250.
105. Goldenhersh MJ, Rachelefsky GS, Dudley J, Brill J, Katz RM, Rohr AS, Spector SL, Siegel SC, Summanen P, Baron EJ. The microbiology of chronic sinus disease in children with respiratory allergy. J Allergy Clin Immunol 1990; 85:1030–1039.
106. Wald ER, Byers C, Guerra N, et al. Subacute sinusitis in children. J Pediatr 1989; 115:28–32.
107. Brook I, Yocum P. Antimicrobial management of chronic sinusitis in children. J Laryngol Otol 1995; 109:1159–1162.
108. Finegold SM. Anaerobic bacteria in human disease. Orlando, FL: Academic Press, Inc., 1977.
109. Brook I. Pediatric Anaerobic Infections. 3rd. NY: Marcel Dekker Inc, 2002.
110. Mustafa E, Tahsin A, Mustafa Ö, Nedret K. Bacteriology of antrum in adults with chronic maxillary sinusitis. Laryngoscope 1994; 104:321–324.
111. Frederick J, Braude AI. Anaerobic infections of the paranasal sinuses. N Engl J Med 1974; 290:135–137.
112. Van Cauwenberge P, Verschraegen G, Van Renterghem L. Bacteriological findings in sinusitis (1963–1975). Scand J Infect Dis Suppl 1976; 9:72–77.
113. Karma P, Jokipii L, Sipila P, Luotonen J, Jokipii AM. Bacteria in chronic maxillary sinusitis. Arch Otolaryngol 1979; 105:386–390.
114. Berg O, Carenfelt C, Kronvall G. Bacteriology of maxillary sinusitis in relation to character of inflammation and prior treatment. Scand J Infect Dis 1988; 20(5):511–516.
115. Fiscella RG, Chow JM. Cefixime for the treatment of maxillary sinusitis. Am J Rhinol 1991(2,5):193–197.
116. Sedallian AB, Bru JP, Gaillat J. Bacteriologic finding of chronic sinusitis. (Abstr no. P2.71). The 17th International Congress of the Management of Infection. Berlin, 1992.
117. Simoncelli C, Ricci G, Molini E, von Garrel C, Capolunghi B, Giommetti S. Bacteriology of chronic maxillary sinusitis. HNO 1992; 40:16–18.
118. Tabaqchali S. Anaerobic infections in the head and neck region. Scand J Infect Dis Suppl 1988; 57:24–34.
119. Hartog B, Degener JE, Van Benthem PP, Hordijk GJ. Microbiology of chronic maxillary sinusitis in adults: isolated aerobic and anaerobic bacteria and their susceptibility to twenty antibiotics. Acta Otolaryngol 1995; 115:672–677.
120. Ito K, Ito Y, Mizuta K, Ogawa H, Suzuki T, Miyata H, Kato N, Watanabe K, Ueno K. Bacteriology of chronic otitis media, chronic sinusitis, and paranasal mucopyocele in Japan. Clin Infect Dis 1995; 20(suppl 2):S214–S219.
121. Erkan M, Aslan T, Ozcan M, Koc N. Bacteriology of antrum in adults with chronic maxillary sinusitis. Laryngoscope 1994; 104(3 Pt 1):321–324.
122. Edelstein DR, Avner SE, Chow JM, Ouerksen RL, Johnson J, Ronis M, Rybak LP, Bierman WC, Matthews BL. Once-a-day therapy for sinusitis:

a comparison study of cefixime and amoxicillin. Laryngoscope 1993; 103:33–41.

123. Klossek JM, Dubreuil L, Richet H, Richet B, Beutter P. Bacteriology of chronic purulent secretions in chronic rhinosinusitis. J Laryngol Otol 1998; 112:1162–1166.

124. Brook I, Frazier EH. Correlation between microbiology and previous sinus surgery in patients with chronic maxillary sinusitis. Ann Otol Rhinol Laryngol 2001; 110:148–151.

125. Brook I. Bacteriology of acute and chronic frontal sinusitis. Arch Otolaryngol Head Neck Surg 2002; 128:583–585.

126. Brook I. Bacteriology of acute and chronic sphenoid sinusitis. Ann Otol Rhinol Laryngol 2002; 111:1002–1004.

127. Brook I. Bacteriology of acute and chronic ethmoid sinusitis. J Clin Microb 2005; 43:3479–3480.

128a. Bhattacharyya N, Kepnes LJ. The microbiology of recurrent rhinosinusitis after endoscopic sinus surgery. Arch Otolaryngol Head Neck Surg 1999; 125:1117–1120.

128b. Bucholtz GA, Salzman SA, Bersalona FB, Boyle TR, Ejercito VS, Penno L, Peterson DW, Stone GE, Urquhart A, Shukla SK, Burmester JK. PCR analysis of nasal polyps, chronic sinusitis, and hypertrophied turbinates for DNA encoding bacterial 16S rRNA. Am J Rhinol 2002; 16:169–173.

128c. Hamilos DL, Leung DYM, Wood R, Meyers A, Stephens JK, Barkans J, Bean DK, Kay AB, Hamid Q. Association of tissue eosinophilia and cytokine mRNA expression of granulocyte-macrophage colony-stimulating factor and interleukin-3. J Allergy Clin Immunol 1993; 91:39–48.

128d. Brook I, Frazier EH. Bacteriology of chronic maxillary sinusitis associated with nasal polyposis. J Med Microbiol 2005; 54:595–597.

129. Clement PA, Bluestone CD, Gordts F, Lusk RP, Otten FW, Goossens H, Scadding GK, Takahashi H, van Buchem FL, Van Cauwenberge P, Wald ER. Management of rhinosinusitis in children: consensus meeting, Brussels, Belgium, September 13, 1996. Arch Otolaryngol Head Neck Surg 1998; 124:31–34.

130. Brook I, Foote PA, Frazier EH. Microbiology of acute exacerbation of chronic sinusitis. Laryngoscope 2004; 114:129–131.

131. Brook I. Bacteriology of chronic sinusitis and acute exacerbation of chronic sinusitis. Annals Otolary Head Neck Surg.

132. Bach A, Boehrer H, Schmidt H, Geiss HK. Nosocomial sinusitis in ventilated patients: nasotracheal versus orotracheal intubation. Anaesthesia 1992; 47:335–339.

133. O'Reilly MJ, Reddick EJ, Black W, Carter PL, Erhardt J, Fill W, Maughn D, Sado A, Klatt GR. Sepsis from sinusitis in nasotracheally intubated patients: a diagnostic dilemma. Am J Surg 1984; 147:601–604.

134. Mevio E, Benazzo M, Quaglieri S, Mencherini S. Sinus infection in intensive care patients. Rhinology 1996; 34:232–236.

135. Caplan ES, Hoyt NJ. Nosocomial sinusitis. JAMA 1982; 247:639–641.

136. Kronberg FG, Goodwin WJ. Sinusitis in intensive care unit patients. Laryngoscope 1985; 95:936–938.

137. Arens JF, LeJeune FE Jr, Webre DR. Maxillary sinusitis, a complication of nasotracheal intubation. Anesthesiology 1974; 40:415–416.
138. Brook I, Shah K. Sinusitis in neurologically impaired children. Otolaryngol Head Neck Surg 1998; 119:357–360.
139. Hahn DL, Dodge RW, Golubjatnikov R. Association of *Chlamydia pneumoniae* (strain TWAR) infection with wheezing, asthmatic bronchitis, and adult-onset asthma. JAMA 1991; 266:225–230.
140. Thom DH, Grayston JT, Campbell LA, Kuo CC, Diwan VK, Wang SP. Respiratory infection with *Chlamydia pneumoniae* in middle-aged and older adult outpatients. Eur J Clin Microbiol Infect Dis 1994; 13:785–792.
141. Hashigucci K, Ogawa H, Suzuki T, Kazuyama Y. Isolation of *Chlamydia pneumoniae* from the maxillary sinus of a patient with purulent sinusitis. Clin Infect Dis 1992; 15:570–571.
142. Savolainen S, Jousimies-Somer H, Kleemola M, Ylikoski J. Serological evidence of viral or *Mycoplasma pneumoniae* infection in acute maxillary sinusitis. Eur J Clin Microbiol Infect Dis 1989; 8:131–135.
143. Gurr PA, Chakraverty A, Callanan V, Gurr SJ. The detection of *M. pneumoniae* in nasal polyps. Clin Otolaryngol 1996; 21:269–273.
144. Bucholtz GA, Salzman SA, Bersalona FB, Boyle TR, Ejercito VS, Pinno L, Peterson DW, Stone GE, Urguhart A. PCR analysis of nasal polyps, chronic sinusitis, and hypertrophied turbinates for DNA encoding bacterial 16S rRNA. Am J Rhinol 2002; 16:169–173.
145. Vennewald I, Henker M, Klemm E, Seebacher C. Fungal colonization of the paranasal sinuses. Mycosis 1999; 42(suppl 2):33–36.
146. Ponikau JU, Sherris DA, Kern EB, Homburger HA, Frigas E, Gaffey TA, Roberts GD. The diagnosis and incidence of allergic fungal sinusitis. Mayo Clin Proc 1999; 74:877–884.
147. Catten MD, Murr AH, Goldstein JA, Miatre AN, Lalwani AK. Detection of fungi in the nasal mucosal using polymerase chain reaction. Laryngoscope 2001; 111:399–403.
148. Stringer SP, Ryan MW. Chronic invasive fungal rhinosinusitis. Otolaryngol Clin North Am 2000; 33:375–387.
149. Ferguson BJ. Definitions of fungal rhinosinusitis. Otolaryngol Clin North Am 2000; 33:227–235.
150. Gwaltney JM Jr. Microbiology of sinusitis. In: Druce HM, ed. Sinusitis: Pathophysiology and Treatment. New York: Marcel Dekker, 1994:41–56.
151. Morgan MA, Wilson WR, Neil HB III, Roberts GD. Fungal sinusitis in healthy and immunocompromised individuals. Am J Clin Pathol 1984; 82:597–601.
152. Jahrsdoerfer RA, Ejercito VS, Johns MME, Cantrell RW, Sydnor JE. Aspergillosis of the nose and paranasal sinuses. Am J Otolaryngol 1979; 1:1–14.
153. Kern ME, Uecker FA. Maxillary sinus infection caused by the Homobasidiomycetous fungus Schizophyllum commune. J Clin Microbiol 1986; 23:1001–1005.
154. Mitchell RG, Chaplin AJ, MacKenzie DWR. *Emericella nidulans* in a maxillary sinus fungal mass. J Med Vet Mycol 1987; 25:339–341.
155. Winn RE, Ramsey PD, McDonald JC, Dunlop KJ. Maxillary sinusitis from Pseudoalles-cheria boydii. Efficacy of surgical therapy. Arch Otolaryngol 1983; 109:123–125.

156. Adam RD, Paquin ML, Petersen EA, Saubolle MA, Rinaldi MG, Corcoran JN, Solaonya RE. Phaeohyphomycosis caused by the fungal general Bipolaris and Exserohilum. Medicine 1986; 65:203–217.
157. Zieske LA, Kople RD, Hamill R. Dermataceous fungal sinusitis. Otolaryngol Head Neck Surg 1991; 105:567–577.
158. Goldstein MF, Dvorin DJ, Dunsky EH, Lesser RW, Heuman PJ, Loose JH. Allergic rhizomucor sinusitis. J Allergy Immun 1992; 90:394–404.
159. Katzenstein A, Sale SR, Greenberger PA. Pathologic findings in allergic Aspergillus sinusitis. Am J Surg Pathol 1983; 7:439–443.
160. Maran ACD, Kwong K, Mine LJR, Lamb D. Frontal sinusitis caused by *Myriodontium keratinophilum*. Br Med J 1985; 290:207.
161. Friedman GC, Hartwick RW, Ro JY, et al. Allergic fungal sinusitis. Report of three cases associated with dermataceous fungi. Am J Clin Pathol 1991; 96:368–372.
162. Bartynski JM, McCaffrey TV, Frigas E. Allergic fungal sinusitis secondary to dermataceous fungi—*Curvularia lunata* and Alternaria. Otolaryngol Head Neck Surg 1990; 103:32–39.

9

Antimicrobial Management of Sinusitis

Itzhak Brook

Departments of Pediatrics and Medicine, Georgetown University School of Medicine, Washington, D.C., U.S.A.

INTRODUCTION

The growing resistance to antimicrobial agents of all respiratory tract bacterial pathogens has made the management of sinusitis more difficult. This chapter presents the current information regarding the antimicrobial resistance of the organisms involved in sinusitis and the approaches to antimicrobial therapy.

ANTIMICROBIAL RESISTANCE

To manage bacterial sinusitis is often a challenging endeavor in which selection of the most appropriate antimicrobial agents remains a key decision. This has become more difficult in recent years as all the predominant bacterial pathogens have gradually developed resistance to most of the commonly used antibiotics.

The observed increase in bacterial resistance to antibiotics is related to their frequent use. Previous therapy can increase the prevalence of beta-lactamase-producing bacteria (BLPB). In a study of 26 children who had received seven days of therapy with penicillin, 12% harbored BLPB in their oropharyngeal flora prior to therapy (1). This increased to 46% at the conclusion of therapy, and the incidence was 27% after three months. The incidence of BLPB was high in siblings and parents of patients treated with penicillin, who probably acquired these organisms from the patient (2).

A greater prevalence of recovery of BLPB in the oropharynx of children occurs in the winter and a lower one in the summer (3). These changes correlated with the intake of beta-lactam antibiotics. To monitor the local seasonal variations in the rate of recovery of BLPB in the community may help the empirical choice of antimicrobial agents, the proper and judicious use of which may help to control the increase of BLPB.

Risk factors for the development of resistance to antimicrobial agents include prior antibiotic exposure, day care attendance, age under two years, recent hospitalization, and recurrent infection (especially in those who are very young or very old) (4,5).

The variety of organisms involved in sinusitis, increasing levels of resistance to antibiotic agents, and the phenomenon of beta-lactamase "shielding" from antibiotic agents all contribute to the therapeutic challenges associated with the management of acute and chronic sinusitis. Brook and Gober (5) identified the antimicrobial susceptibility of the pathogens isolated from patients with maxillary sinusitis who failed to respond to antimicrobial therapy and correlates it with previous antimicrobial therapy and smoking. The data illustrated a relationship between resistance to antimicrobials and failure of patients with sinusitis to improve. A statistically significant higher recovery of resistant organisms was noted in those treated two to six months previously, and in those who smoked.

Three major mechanisms of resistance to penicillins occur:

1. Porin channel blockage (e.g., used by *Pseudomonas* spp. to resist carbapenems)
2. Production of the enzyme beta-lactamase (e.g., utilized by *Haemophilus influenzae* and *Moraxella catarrhalis*).
3. Alterations in the penicillin-binding protein (e.g., used by *Streptococcus pneumoniae*).

BETA-LACTAMASE PRODUCTION

Bacterial resistance to the antibiotics used for the treatment of sinusitis has been increased consistently in recent years. Production of the enzyme beta-lactamase is one of the most important mechanisms of penicillin resistance.

The production of the enzyme beta-lactamase is an important mechanism of virulence of anaerobic gram-negative bacilli as well as other aerobic and anaerobic bacteria. The production of beta-lactamase can have wider implication than just protecting the bacteria that produces the enzyme. In polymicrobial infections BLPB can "shield" other co-pathogens that are penicillin-susceptible (6,7) (Fig. 2 in Chap. 8). It has been hypothesized that this protection can occur when the enzyme beta-lactamase is secreted into the infected tissues or sinus fluids in sufficient quantities to break the penicillin's beta-lactam ring before it can kill the susceptible bacteria, thus contributing to treatment failure.

The emergence and persistence of BLPB after antibiotic therapy has implications for antimicrobial selection for in treatment of sinusitis as well as other infections of the upper respiratory tract, particularly chronic conditions in which patients are likely to have had recent antibiotic exposure.

Clinical and laboratory studies provide support for this hypothesis. Animal studies demonstrated the ability of the enzyme beta-lactamase to influence polymicrobial infections. Hackman and Wilkins (8) showed that penicillin-resistant strains of *Bacteroides fragilis*, pigmented *Prevotella* and *Porphyromonas* spp., and *Prevotella oralis* protected a penicillin-sensitive *Fusobacterium necrophorum* from penicillin therapy in mice. Using a subcutaneous abscess model in mice, Brook et al. (9) demonstrated protection of group A beta-hemolytic streptococci (GABHS) from penicillin by *B. fragilis* and *Prevotella melaninogenica*. Clindamycin or the combination of penicillin and clavulanic acid (a beta-lactamase inhibitor), which are active against both GABHS and anaerobic gram-negative bacilli, were effective in eradicating the infection. Similarly, beta-lactamase–producing facultative bacteria protected a penicillin-susceptible *P. melaninogenica* from penicillin (10).

In vitro studies have also demonstrated this phenomenon. A 200-fold increase in resistance of GABHS to penicillin was observed when it was inoculated with *Staphylococcus aureus* (11). An increase in resistance was also noted when GABHS was grown with *Haemophilus parainfluenzae* (12). When mixed with cultures of *B. fragilis*, the resistance of GABHS to penicillin increased 8500-fold (13).

Several species of BLPB occur in sinusitis (Table 1). BLPB have been recovered from over one-third of patients with sinusitis (14,15). *H. influenzae* and *M. catarrhalis* are the predominant BLPB in acute sinusitis, and *S. aureus*, pigmented *Prevotella*, *Porphyromonas*, and *Fusobacterium* spp. predominate in chronic sinusitis.

Table 1 Resistance to Antimicrobial Agents in Bacterial Sinusitis

Bacteria	Incidence (%)	Resistance to penicillin (%)
Acute sinusitis		
S. pneumoniae	30–40	20–40
H. influenzae[a]	25–30	30–40
M. catarrhalis[a]	10–15	95
Chronic sinusitis		
S. aureus[a]	10–35	95
Pigmented *Prevotella*[a] and *Porphyromonas*[a] spp.	15–30	10–60
Fusobacterium[a] spp.	15–40	10–60

[a]Resistance due to beta-lactamase production.

Table 2 Beta-Lactamase Detected in Four Acute Bacterial Sinusitis Aspirates Obtained from Patients Treated with Amoxicillin

	Patient			
Organism	1[a]	2[a]	3	4
S. pneumoniae	+	+		
M. catarrhalis (beta-lactamase positive)	+		+	
H. influenzae (beta-lactamase positive)		+		+
Beta-lactamase activity in pus	+	+	−	+

[a]"Shielding" of S. pneumoniae by beta-lactamase producers is evident in patients 1 and 2.
Source: Data from Ref. 7.

The actual activity of the enzyme beta-lactamase and the potential of the presence of the phenomenon of "shielding" were demonstrated in acutely and chronically inflamed sinus fluids (7). BLPB were isolated in four of 10 acute sinusitis aspirates and in 10 of 13 chronic sinusitis aspirates (Tables 2 and 3). The predominant BLPB isolated in acute sinusitis were *H. influenzae* and *M. catarrhalis*, and those found in chronic sinusitis were *S. aureus*, *B. fragilis*, and *Prevotella* and *Fusobacterium* spp. (7). "Free" beta-lactamase was detected in 86% of aspirates that contained these organisms,

Table 3 Beta-Lactamase Detected in Four Chronic Bacterial Sinusitis Aspirates Obtained from Patients Treated with Amoxicillin

	Patient			
Organism	1	2	3	4
S. aureus BL (+)		+		+
S. pneumoniae	+			
Peptostreptococcus spp.	+			+
Propionibacterium acnes	+			
Fusobacterium spp. BL (+)		+		+
Fusobacterium spp. BL (−)		+		+
Prevotella spp. BL (+)			+	
Prevotella spp. BL (−)	+	+	+	
Bacteroides fragilis group BL (+)	+			+
Beta-Lactamase activity in pus	+	+	+	+

[a]"Shielding" is present in all cases.
Abbreviation: BL (+), beta-lactamase–producing organism.
Source: Data from Ref. 7.

and was associated with persistence of even penicillin-susceptible pathogens despite antimicrobial therapy.

Haemophilus influenzae Resistance to Antimicrobials

Resistance to beta-lactams among strains of *H. influenzae* has increased throughout the past three decades. In the 1980s, the prevalence of beta-lactamase–producing *H. influenzae* was between 10% and 15% (16,17). Resistance among strains of *H. influenzae* increased steadily throughout the 1990s, and presently approximately 40% of *H. influenzae* strains are beta-lactamase producers. Beta-lactamase–producing strains of *H. influenzae* are most prevalent in the northcentral, northeast, and southcentral regions of the United States (18). Generally, higher doses of beta-lactams are not effective in overcoming this mechanism of resistance; however, the addition of a beta-lactamase inhibitor (e.g., clavulanic acid) shifts *H. influenzae* strains to the susceptible range [e.g., minimal inhibitory concentration (MIC) $\leq 4\,\mu g/mL$], transforming the susceptibilities to those of beta-lactamase–negative strains. Agents that are stable in the presence of beta-lactamases are another option for treating infections caused by this pathogen.

Among the oral beta-lactam antibiotics, amoxicillin/clavulanate (because of the beta-lactamase inhibitor), cefixime, ceftibuten, cefdinir, and cefpodoxime are highly active against beta-lactamase–producing *H. influenzae* (19). Macrolides in general have limited activity against *H. influenzae*; among the three agents (i.e., erythromycin, clarithromycin, and azithromycin), clarithromycin is least active against *H. influenzae* (20). Inhibition of *H. influenzae* by macrolides is dependent on the ability to achieve concentrations above the MICs at the site of infection. Based on pharmacokinetic/pharmacodynamic (PK/PD) breakpoints, the MICs of virtually all *H. influenzae* strains in the 1998 surveillance study were below PK/PD breakpoints (i.e., resistant) for erythromycin, clarithromycin, and azithromycin. Furthermore, azithromycin failed to eradicate 61% of *H. influenzae* from the middle ear of children with otitis media (21). Resistance to trimethoprim-sulfamethoxazole (TMP/SMX) was exhibited among 24% of isolates. Fluoroquinolones, particularly the newer agents, are very active against *H. influenzae*, with relatively no resistance according to the recent surveillance data (20).

Moraxella catarrhalis Resistance to Antimicrobials

Virtually all strains of *M. catarrhalis* produce beta-lactamase. The 1998 prevalence among outpatient isolates for beta-lactamase–producing *M. catarrhalis* was 98% (19). At PK/PD breakpoints, 100% of strains were susceptible to amoxicillin/clavulanate, fluoroquinolones, macrolides, doxycycline, and cefixime. High levels of resistance were exhibited toward TMP/SMX, cefaclor, loracarbef, cefprozil, and amoxicillin.

Streptococcus pneumoniae Resistance to Antimicrobials

Penicillin Resistance

Resistance among *S. pneumoniae* strains has been monitored in the United States since 1979. Prior to the 1990s, resistance to penicillin was not considered a clinical problem in the United States. Throughout the past decade, the prevalence of *S. pneumoniae* isolates that are either intermediate (i.e., penicillin MICs 0.12–1.0 μg/mL) or resistant to penicillin (i.e., MICs≥2.0 μg/mL) has increased, with dramatic increases within the past few years (22). The incidence of penicillin-resistance in strains of *S. pneumoniae* approaches 40% in some areas of the United States, and the incidence of high-level resistance has increased by 60-fold during the past 10 years. The mechanism of beta-lactam-resistance of *S. pneumoniae* involves genetic mutations that alter penicillin-binding protein structure, resulting in a decreased affinity for all beta-lactam antibiotics. About half of the penicillin-resistant strains are currently intermediately resistant [minimal inhibitory concentration (MIC) of 0.1–1.0 mg/mL] and the rest are highly resistant (MIC > 2.0 mg/mL).

It is important to note, however, that this change in MIC does not confer absolute resistance to all beta-lactams because the pharmacokinetics of each agent need to be considered. Thus, strains of *S. pneumoniae* with penicillin MICs ≥2 μg/mL (i.e., resistant) are not necessarily resistant to other beta-lactams (e.g., amoxicillin). Resistance to beta-lactams represents a pharmacokinetic challenge that can be overcome if a high enough concentration of beta-lactam can be achieved at the site of infection.

Penicillin-resistant strains are often also resistant to other antimicrobial agents commonly used to treat sinusitis (Table 4). The term drug-resistant *S. pneumoniae* refers to strains with penicillin MICs ≥ 0.12 μg/mL that also exhibit resistance to at least two other antimicrobial classes. The susceptibility of *S. pneumoniae* isolates to other antimicrobials is closely correlated to its susceptibility to penicillin. However, these strains are susceptible to parenteral third-generation cephalosporins (i.e., cefotaxime, ceftriaxone), the fluoroquinolones (levofloxacin, gatifloxacin, moxifloxacin, gemifloxacin), vancomycin, quinupristin with dalfopristin, telithromycin and linezolid. Intermediately resistant *S. pneumoniae* are still susceptible in vitro to high doses of penicillin or amoxicillin (23). Clindamycin and the oral second-generation cephalosporins, especially cefuroxime axetil and cefprozil, are also effective in vitro against over 95% of intermediately penicillin-resistant strains (24).

The regions of the United States with the highest proportion of penicillin-, macrolide-, and trimethoprim/sulfamethoxazole-resistant *S. pneumoniae* strains are the southcentral and southeast. The reason for increased resistance in these regions is not currently known, and the variation is not significant enough to warrant different antimicrobial recommendations for each region. Although penicillin-resistant strains are common in all age groups, the highest proportions of resistant strains are collected from

Table 4　Cross-Resistance of Penicillin-Resistant *S. pneumoniae*

Antimicrobial agent	Cross-resistance (%)	
	Intermediately resistant[a]	Highly resistant[b]
Trimethoprim-sulfamethoxazole	52	91.9
Tetracycline	22.8	47.4
Macrolides	49.8	80.4
Clindamycin	13.1	25.3
Third-generation cephalosporins:		
Oral (cefixime, ceftibuten)	60	95
Parenteral (ceftriaxone)	5	10
Rifampin	10	20
Levofloxacin	2.2	2.2
Gatifloxacin	2.1	1.9
Telithromyicn	0.1	0.6

[a]MIC 0.12–1.0 mg/mL.
[b]MIC $\geq$ 2.0 mg/mL.

children younger than two years. In addition, resistant strains are most likely to be isolated from middle ear (approximately 58% of all *S. pneumoniae* isolates), sinus (approximately 60% of all *S. pneumoniae* isolates), and nasopharyngeal specimens (approximately 55% of all *S. pneumoniae* isolates) (25). Many of these cultures were obtained from treatment failures, however, and the true prevalence of resistance in specimens isolated from these sites may be somewhat lower.

Macrolide-Resistance

Macrolide-resistance among *S. pneumoniae* has escalated at alarming rates in North America and worldwide. Macrolide-resistance among pneumococci is primarily due to genetic mutations affecting the ribosomal target site (ermAM) or active drug efflux (mefE). Ribosomal mutations that confer high-grade resistance are also cross-resistant to clindamycin, whereas efflux mutations can likely be overridden in vivo (26). Currently, about a third of macrolide-resistant strains in North America possess the efflux mutations mechanism of resistance, and the rest exhibit the ribosomal mutations. This relationship is reversed in Europe and the Far East, where most resistance is conveyed through the ribosomal mutations mechanism. Pneumococci resistant to erythromycin (by either mechanism) are also resistant to azithromycin, clarithromycin, and roxithromycin (27). Prior antibiotic exposure is the major risk factor for amplification and perpetuation of resistance. Clonal spread facilitates dissemination of drug-resistant strains. Several population-based studies noted correlations between the prevalence of macrolide resistance among *S. pneumoniae* and overall macrolide consumption in the region or country (28,29).

Fluoroquinolone-Resistance

The main resistance mechanisms to fluoroquinolones are the efflux pump system and specific point mutations. The efflux pump is a mechanism that expels the antimicrobial agent across the cell membrane, thus reducing the intracellular concentrations to sublethal levels. The pump's action is dependent on the antimicrobial's ability to bind to the bacterial efflux protein and to be exported. Some fluoroquinolones, such as moxifloxacin and trovafloxacin, are not as affected by bacterial efflux mechanisms because of their bulky side-chain moiety at position 7, which prevents export (30).

The other resistance mechanism involves specific point mutations that reduce the binding of the antimicrobial to specific enzymatic sites by altering the target site. In this regard, fluoroquinolones bind to enzymes involved in DNA replication, including DNA gyrase and DNA topoisomerase IV. Specific mutations in the genes that code for these enzymes can result in reduced binding and activity of the fluoroquinolones (31). Different fluoroquinolones exhibit weaker or stronger affinity to these enzyme-binding sites. First- and second-generation fluoroquinolones bind primarily to DNA gyrase or DNA topoisomerase IV, whereas the third-generation fluoroquinolones generally bind strongly to both DNA gyrase and DNA topoisomerase IV. Thus, a single point mutation in DNA gyrase or DNA topoisomerase IV generally affects first- and second-generation fluoroquinolones to a greater extent than third-generation fluoroquinolones. Furthermore, the third-generation C-8 methoxyfluoroquinolones, moxifloxacin and gatifloxacin, appear to bind different molecular sites within these enzymes, thereby decreasing the cross-resistance between these agents and the older fluoroquinolones (32).

Microbial resistance to the newer fluoroquinolones (levofloxacin, gatifloxacin, moxifloxacin and gemifloxacin) is relatively uncommon, currently occurring in approximately 1% of clinical isolates in North America. However, increased resistance has been observed in the some countries (33). These agents can be useful for treatment of bacterial sinusitis, but caution must be exercised to avoid the potential for selection of widespread resistance, which may occur with indiscriminate use (34).

ANTIMICROBIAL AGENTS

The antimicrobial agents most commonly used to treat acute sinusitis include amoxicillin (with and without clavulanic acid), oral and parenteral cephalosporins, macrolides, and "newer" quinolones (Tables 5 and 6).

Table 5 Antibiotics Used for Bacterial Sinusitis (PO)

Antibiotic	Adult dosage	Pediatric dosage (mg/kg)	Duration of therapy for acute sinusitis (days)
Beta-lactams			
Cefprozil (Cefzil)	250–500 mg bid	7.5–15 bid	10
Cefuroxime axetil (Ceftin)	250–500 mg bid	10–15 bid	10
Cefpodoxime (Vantin)	200–400 mg bid	5 bid	10
Cefdinir (Omnicef)	300 mg bid	7 bid/14 qd	10
Amoxicillin (Amoxil, Trimox, Wymox)	500 mg tid or 875 mg bid	20–45 bid	14
Amoxicillin-clavulanate (Augmentin)	500 mg tid[a] or 875 mg or 2000 mg (XR) bid[a]	22.5 or 45 (ES600) bid	10
Ketolides			
Telithromycin (Ketek)	800 mg qd	NA	5
Macrolides			
Azithromycin (Zithromax)	250 mg qd	10 day 1, then 5 qd	3 or 5
Clarithromycin (Biaxin)	500 mg bid	7.5 bid	14
Fluoroquinolones			
Levofloxacin (Levaquin)	500 mg qd	NA	10
Gatifloxacin (Tequin)	500 mg qd	NA	10
Moxifloxacin (Avelox)	400 mg qd	NA	10
Others			
Clindamycin (Cleocin)	150–450 mg tid or qid	7.5 qid or 6 tid	10
TMP-SMX (Bactrim, Septra)	160 mg/800 mg bid	8–12 bid	10

[a]Based on amoxicillin component.
Abbreviation: NA, not approved for patients <18 years of age.

Amoxicillin is often used for sinusitis therapy and is safe and inexpensive, and when given in a high dose, it is still the drug of choice for intermediately penicillin-susceptible *S. pneumoniae*. However, the growing resistance of *H. influenzae* and *M. catarrhalis* to amoxicillin through the production of beta-lactamase increases the risk that it will fail to clear the infection. However, the addition of clavulanic acid (a beta-lactamase inhibitor) to amoxicillin or the use of antimicrobial agents resistant to beta-lactamase activity is effective against resistant organisms.

Using higher doses of amoxicillin ± clavulanate (i.e., 4.0 g/day in adults or 90 mg/kg/day in children based on amoxicillin component) will help to

Table 6 In Vitro Efficacy of Antimicrobial Agents Used in Bacterial Sinusitis Therapy

Antimicrobial agent	S. pneumoniae		H. influenzae		M. catarrhalis	Anaerobes		S. aureus	
	Pen-S	Pen-IR	BL−	BL+	BL+	Pen-S	Pen-R	Pen-R	Pen-R[a]
Amoxicillin	+	+	+	−	−	+	−	−	−
Amoxicillin-clavulanate	+	+	+	+	+	+	+	+	+
Cephalexin (first-generation)	+	−	±	−	−	+	−	+	+
Cefactor (second-generation)	±	−	+	±	±	+	−	+	+
Cefprozil (second-generation)	+	+	+	±	+	+	−	+	+
Cefuroxime axetil (second-generation)	+	±	+	+	+	+	−	+	+
Cefpodoxime (second-generation)	+	±	+	+	+	±	−	+	+
Cefdinir (second-generation)	+	−	+	+	+	±	−	+	+
Cefixime (third-generation)	+	−	+	+	+	+	−	−	−
Ceftibuten (third-generation)	±	−	+	+	+	+	−	−	−
Loracarbef	±	−	+	±	+	±	−	+	+
Ceftriaxone[b]	+	+	+	+	+	+	−	+	±
Erythromycin-sulfisoxazole	±	−	+	±	±	±	−	+	±
Trimethoprim-sulfamethoxazole	±	−	+	±	±	−	−	±	±

Erythromycin	+	±	−	±	±	−	±
Azithromycin	+	±	±	+	±	−	±
Clarithromycin	+	±	±	±	±	−	+
Telithromycin	+	+	+	+	+	−	+
Clindamycin	±	−	−	+	+	+	±
Ciprofloxacin	+	+	+	+	+	+	−
Levofloxacin	+	+	+	+	+	−	−
Gatifloxacin	+	+	+	+	+	−	−
Moxifloxacin	+	+	+	+	+	±	±
Carbapenems[b]	+	+	+	+	+	+	+

[a] +, very susceptible; ±, minimal susceptibility; −, not susceptible. Methicillin susceptible.
[b] Available in parental form only.
[c] Available (also) in parenteral form.
[d] Imipenem–cilastatin, meropenem, ertapenem.
Abbreviations: BL−, beta-lactamase non-producers; BL+, beta-lactamase producers; Pen-S, penicillin susceptible; Pen-R, penicillin resistance; Pen-IR, penicillin intermediate resistance.

ensure adequate eradication of penicillin-resistant *S. pneumoniae* organisms (34). Amoxicillin/clavulanate is also active against anaerobic bacteria, which is an important consideration in patients with chronic sinusitis.

First-generation cephalosporins lack sufficient efficacy against *H. influenzae* and many *S. pneumoniae* strains. Generally, cefaclor and loracarbef are not considered effective for the treatment of acute sinusitis because of the limited activity of these agents. The second-generation cephalosporins (cefuroxime axetil, cefdinir, cefpodoxime, and cefprozil) are more effective because of their activity against penicillin-resistant *Haemophilus* and *Moraxella* spp. and intermediately penicillin-resistant *S. pneumoniae* (24).

Oral third-generation cephalosporins (cefixime and ceftibuten) are most effective against penicillin-resistant *Haemophilus* and *Moraxella* spp., but they are less effective against *S. pneumoniae* resistant to penicillin. Parenteral third-generation cephalosporins (cefotaxime or ceftriaxone) are effective against *H. influenzae* and *M. catarrhalis* that produce beta-lactamase, as well as over 95% of intermediately resistant *S. pneumoniae*. No oral cephalosporin is active against anaerobes, which is an important consideration for the treatment of chronic sinusitis.

TMP/SMX has lost efficacy against all major pathogens, including *S. pneumoniae* and GABHS. The sulfa component can cause hypersensitivity reactions.

Of the macrolides, erythromycin is inactive against *H. influenzae* and some GABHS. Resistance of GABHS to erythromycin and other macrolides occurs in countries where these agents were overused (e.g., Japan, Finland, Spain, Taiwan and Turkey) (35). Cross-resistance of GABHS is common among all macrolides. Azithromycin has improved efficacy against aerobic gram-negative organisms (*H. influenzae* and *M. catarrhalis*), while clarithromycin is more efficient than erythromycin against aerobic gram-positive organisms (36). Recent studies show, however, increased resistance of *S. pneumoniae* to all macrolides (up to 35%), and survival of azithromycin-susceptible *H. influenzae* in the middle ear and sinuses (21, 37). The persistence of the organism in otitis media is believed to result from accumulation of azithromycin mainly inside the middle ear white cells, and not in the middle ear fluid where most of the organisms grow.

Clindamycin is effective against anaerobes and aerobic gram-positive organisms, including most penicillin-resistant *S. pneumoniae*; however, it is not effective against aerobic gram-negative pathogens. Vancomycin (a glycopeptide) and linezolid are effective against penicillin-resistant *S. pneumoniae* and methicillin-resistant *S. aureus*. However, they are not effective against *H. influenzae* or *M. catarrhalis*.

Telithromycin is the first ketolide antibacterial to be approved for clinical use. It is structurally related to the macrolides, but has a low propensity to select for or induce resistance to macrolide-lincosamide-streptogramin antibacterials (38). In vitro, telithromycin is effective against multi-drug-resistant *S. pneumoniae* (regardless of the presence of macrolide-resistant determinants [*erm*(B), *mef*(A)]), GABHS, *M. catarrhalis*, and *H. influenzae*. In clinical trials, it has demonstrated clinical and bacteriological efficacy in the treatment of acute sinusitis due to penicillin and/or macrolide (erythromycin) resistant *S. pneumoniae* as well as *H. influenzae* or *M. catarrhalis* (39).

The first-generation fluoroquinolones (e.g., ciprofloxacin, ofloxacin) provide inadequate *S. pneumoniae* coverage and are primarily active against aerobic gram-negative bacilli (including *H. influenzae* and *M. catarrhalis*). The second-generation fluoroquinolone, levofloxacin, is the L-isomer of ofloxacin and demonstrates somewhat-improved gram-positive activity. However, susceptibility data show levofloxacin to be less potent than ciprofloxacin against such gram-negative pathogens as *Pseudomonas aeruginosa* and certain enterobacteriaceae. The third-generation fluoroquinolones include moxifloxacin, gemifloxacin, and gatifloxacin and have improved gram-positive and atypical bacteria coverage compared with first- and second-generation fluoroquinolones. Some of the newer fluoroquinolones (e.g., gatifloxacin, moxifloxacin, trovafloxacin) have activity against oral anaerobes, but their efficacy in chronic sinusitis has not been proven. In particular, these newer representatives of the fluoroquinolone class manifest greater activity against *S. pneumoniae* (40). A major concern with the use of these agents, however, is the selection of class resistance to gram-negative organisms, staphylococci, and pneumococci (19,20). None of the newer fluoroquinolones is currently approved for use in children.

Pharmacokinetics and Pharmacodynamics (PK/PD) of Antimicrobials

The goal of antibiotic therapy is to eradicate the causative organism from the sinus cavity. To achieve this goal, the antibiotic must be active in vitro against the targeted organisms and must penetrate the sinus cavity in sufficient concentrations. The effect of antibiotics in eliminating the organisms is an added effect over the natural eradication achieved in time by the host. The host defenses that participate in this process include activity of inflammatory cells, antibody, complement, and other host defense mechanisms.

The environment at the infected sinus never corresponds to the laboratory in vitro susceptibility testing conditions. The actual performance of an antibiotic in vivo depends on variables that include the oxygen tension, pH, and protein binding of an antibiotic.

Several methods are utilized to evaluate the in vitro activity of an antibiotic. Most often a MIC or a minimum bactericidal concentration (MBC) is determined to assess antibiotic activity. The utility and limitations of these tests should be appreciated. The MIC and MBC are values characterizing an antibiotic under strict test tube conditions, and clinical interpretation also requires the consideration of PK/PD issues.

Although standard parameters of antimicrobial activity such as MIC and minimal bactericidal concentration are helpful, they do not provide information about the time course or rate of kill relative to concentration or whether post-antibiotic effects contribute to activity (41). The pharmacology of antimicrobial chemotherapy in sinusitis can be divided into two components (41):

1. *pharmacokinetic component*—this pertains to the dosing regimen, drug absorption, distribution, protein binding, bioavailability, half-life, metabolism, and elimination, which determine the time course of the drug concentrations in serum, sinus fluid, and sinus mucosal tissues
2. *pharmacodynamic component*—this deals with the association between concentrations of the drug at the site of infection and its antimicrobial effect

Antibiotics can be divided into two major groups: those that exhibit concentration-dependent killing and prolonged persistent effects and those that exhibit time-dependent killing and minimal-to-moderate persistent effects (41). With drugs that fall into the former group, the area under the concentration–time curve (AUC) (i.e., quinolones) and peak levels (aminoglycosides) are the major parameters that correlate with efficacy (Fig. 1). The ratio of peak concentration to MIC is a measure of potency that also indicates the efficacy of the drug in these agents. With drugs that exhibit time-dependent killing and minimal-to-moderate persistent effects, time above MIC is the major parameter-determining efficacy. Beta-lactam and macrolide antibiotics belong to this second group.

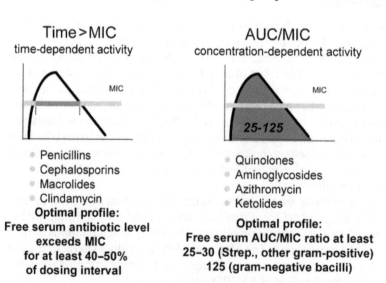

Figure 1 Predictors of bacterial eradication: pharmacokinetic/pharmacodynamic profiles.

Studies in otitis media show that there appears to be a relationship between the time above MIC in serum and in middle ear fluid (MEF) for beta-lactam antibiotics. It is predicted that to achieve at least 80% to 85% bacteriologic cure in otitis media, serum concentrations should exceed the MIC of pathogens for at least 40% of the dosing interval (42). For the same cure rate, the peak MEF to MIC ratio should be in the range of 3 to 6. If the MICs for pathogens are known, it will be possible to predict those agents for which adequate concentrations can be achieved.

Despite substantial MEF concentrations, some drugs such as the macrolides (i.e., erythromycin, azithromycin and clarithromycin) are clinically less reliable against *H. influenzae* because the MICs for this organism frequently exceed the achievable MEF concentrations. In contrast, other drugs such as the oral third-generation cephalosporins (i.e., cefixime, ceftibuten) that reach more modest absolute MEF concentrations, but have such low $MIC_{90}s$ for *H. influenzae* and *M. catarrhalis* may be more effective in eradicating this pathogen. However, these agents are ineffective against penicillin-resistant *S. pneumoniae* (41).

Fluoroquinolones demonstrate concentration-dependent killing. The ratio of the peak concentration (C_{max}) to the MIC and of the area under the curve (AUC) to the MIC appear to be the parameters that best correlate with clinical efficacy. If the free-drug AUC/MIC ratio is >25–30, the probability of a favorable clinical outcome is quite high (>100%) for patients infected with gram-positive organisms (43). Using this cutoff criterion (AUC/MIC ratio, >25–30), ciprofloxacin fares poorly against gram-positive organisms, whereas gatifloxacin, gemifloxacin, levofloxacin, and moxifloxacin all exceed this threshold. However, levofloxacin barely achieves the goal, and for isolates with MICs of $\geq 2.0\,\mu g/mL$, levofloxacin is inadequate.

PRINCIPLES OF THERAPY

Selection of the appropriate agent(s) is generally made on an empirical basis, and the agents should be effective against any potential organisms that may cause the infection (44). In the empirical choice of antimicrobial therapy for sinuses, several balances between narrow- and wide-spectrum antimicrobial agents must be made. If the patient fails to show significant improvement or shows signs of deterioration despite treatment, it is important to obtain a culture, preferably through sinus puncture, as this may reveal the presence of resistant bacteria. Further antimicrobial treatment is based, whenever possible, on results of the culture. Obtaining a culture through endoscopy is an alternative approach (45). However, the specimen may be contaminated with nasal flora. Surgical drainage may be extremely important at that time. Culture of nasal pus or of sinus exudate obtained by rinsing through the sinus ostium can give unreliable information because of contamination by the resident bacterial nasal flora.

Table 7 Causes for Failure in the Treatment of Bacterial Sinusitis

Viral infection
Noncompliance
Resistant organism(s) as a result of:
  Recent treatment with antibiotic agents
  Acquisition of resistant organisms (community, day care, school, or nosocomial)
  Emergence of resistance during therapy
Inadequate penetration of antibiotics to site
Lack of drainage (anatomical blockage or due to medication)
Persistence of predisposing risk factors
Impaired host defenses

Factors within the sinus cavity that may enable organisms to survive antimicrobial therapy are inadequate penetration of antimicrobial agents, a high protein concentration (can bind antimicrobial agents), a high content of enzymes that inactivate antimicrobial agents (i.e., beta-lactamase), decreased multiplication rate of organisms that interfere with the activity of bacteriostatic agents, and reduction in pH and oxygen partial pressure, which reduces the efficacy of some antimicrobial agents (e.g., aminoglycosides and quinolones) (46) (Table 7).

Failure to improve on completion of appropriate antibiotic therapy should prompt consideration of bacterial resistance, noncompliance, or complicated sinusitis. Antimicrobial agents that achieve good intrasinus concentrations can, however, fail to eradicate the pathogen(s) if there is impairment of local defenses (e.g., phagocytosis, ciliary motility) within the sinus environment.

Treatment of Acute Sinusitis

Amoxicillin can be appropriate for the initial treatment of acute uncomplicated mild sinusitis (Table 8). However, antimicrobials that are more effective against the major bacterial pathogens (including those that are resistant to multiple antibiotics) may be indicated (Table 9) as initial therapy and for the retreatment of those who have risk factors prompting a need for more

Table 8 Indications for Amoxicillin Therapy (high dose)

Mild illness
No history of recurrent acute sinusitis
During summer months
When no recent antimicrobial therapy has been used
When patient has had no recent contact with patient(s) on antimicrobial therapy
When community experience shows high success rate of amoxicillin

Table 9 Recommended Antibacterial Agents for Initial Treatment of Acute Sinusitis or After No Improvement

Factors prompting more effective antibiotics[a]	At diagnosis	Clinically treatment failure at 48–72 hr after starting treatment
No	High-dose amoxicillin	High-dose amoxicillin/ clavulanate or a "new" quinolone[b] or telithromycin[b] or cefuroxime or cefdinir or cefpodoxime proxetil
Yes	High-dose amoxicillin/ clavulanate or a "new" quinolone[b] or telithromycin[b] or cefuroxime-axetil or cefdinir or cefpodoxime proxetil	High-dose amoxicillin/ clavulanate or a "new" quinolone[b] or telithromycin[b] or cefuroxime-axetil or cefdinir or cefpodoxime proxetil

[a]See Table 7.
[b]Not approved for children (<18 years).

effective antimicrobials (Table 10) and those who had failed amoxicillin therapy.

These agents include amoxicillin and clavulanic acid, the "newer" quinolones (e.g., levofloxacin, gatifloxacin, moxifloxacin), telithromycin, and some second- and third-generation cephalosporins (cefdinir, cefuroxime-axetil, and cefpodoxime proxetil).

These agents should be administered to patients when bacterial resistance is likely (i.e., recent antibiotic therapy, winter season, increased resistance in the community), the presence of a moderate to severe infection, the presence of comorbidity (diabetes, chronic renal, hepatic, or cardiac pathology), and when penicillin allergy is present (Tables 9 and 10). Agents that are less effective because of growing bacterial resistance may, however, be considered for patients with antimicrobial allergy. These include the macrolides, TMP-SMX, tetracyclines, and clindamycin (47).

A number of antimicrobial agents have been studied in the therapy of acute sinusitis over the past 25 years, with the use of pre- and post-treatment aspirate cultures. Those studied were ampicillin, amoxicillin, amoxicillin–clavulanic acid, cefuroxime axetil, cefprozil, loracarbef, levofloxacin, gatifloxacin, moxifloxacin, and gemifloxacin. For a 10-day course of therapy, the success rate was a bacteriological cure over of 80% to 90%. Appropriate antibiotic therapy is of paramount importance, even though it is estimated that spontaneous recovery occurs in about half of patients (19,48).

Table 10   Risk Factors Prompting a Need for More Effective Antimicrobials[a]

Bacterial resistance is likely
   Antibiotic use in the past month, or close contact with a treated individual(s)
   Resistance common in community
   Failure of previous antimicrobial therapy
   Infection in spite of prophylactic treatment
   Child in day care facility
   Winter season
   Smoker or smoker in family
Presence of moderate to severe infection
   Presentation with protracted (>30 days) or moderate to severe symptoms
   Complicated ethmoidal sinusitis
   Frontal or sphenoidal sinusitis
   Patient history of recurrent acute sinusitis
Presence of comorbidity and extremes of life
   Comorbidity (i.e., chronic cardiac, hepatic, or renal disease, diabetes)
   Immunocompromised patient
   Younger than two years of age or older than 55 years
   Allergy to penicillin
   Allergy to amoxicillin

---

[a]Amoxicillin and clavulanic acid, second- and third-generation cephalosporins, telithromycin, and the "respiratory" quinolones.

Antimicrobial therapy is beneficial and effective in the prevention of septic complications (48). The recommended length of therapy for acute sinusitis is at least 14 days or seven days beyond the resolution of symptoms, whichever is longer. However, no controlled studies have proved the length of therapy sufficient to resolve the infection.

Within the last two years, six panels of experts recently presented reviews and rendered their recommendations on how to diagnose and manage sinusitis (19,49–53). The recommendations of three of these guidelines are summarized in Chapter 10.

Treatment of Chronic Sinusitis

Many of the pathogens isolated from chronically inflamed sinuses are resistant to penicillins through the production of beta-lactamase (7,54). These include both aerobic (*S. aureus*, *H. influenzae*, and *M. catarrhalis*) and gram-negative bacilli anaerobic isolates (all *B. fragilis* and over half of the *Prevotella*, *Porphyromonas*, and *Fusobacterium* spp.).

Retrospective studies illustrate the superiority of therapy effective against both aerobic and anaerobic BLPB in chronic sinusitis (54,55). Amoxicillin-clavulanate (54) or clindamycin (55), both effective against both aerobic and anaerobic bacteria, were superior to antimicrobials, but were not active against these organisms.

The choice of antimicrobial agent in chronic sinusitis should provide coverage for the usual pathogens in acute sinusitis (e.g., *S. pneumoniae*, *H. influenzae*, and *M. catarrhalis*) as well as beta-lactamase–producing aerobic and anaerobic organisms. Therefore, treatment with a broad-spectrum antibiotic that is stable against beta-lactamases and active against penicillin-resistant *S. pneumoniae* with anaerobic coverage may be optimal for the treatment of chronic sinusitis. Antimicrobial agents used for chronic sinusitis therapy should therefore be effective against both aerobic and anaerobic BLPB; these include the combination of a penicillin (e.g., amoxicillin) and a beta-lactamase inhibitor (e.g., clavulanic acid), clindamycin, chloramphenicol, the combination of metronidazole and a macrolide, and the "newer" quinolones (e.g., trovafloxacin). All of these agents (or similar ones) are available in oral and parenteral forms. Other effective agents that are available only in parenteral form are some of the second-generation cephalosporins (e.g., cefoxitin, cefotetan and cefmetazole), combination of a penicillin (e.g., ticarcillin, piperacillin, ampicillin) and a beta-lactamase inhibitor (e.g., clavulanic acid, tazobactam, sulbactam), and the carbapenems (i.e., imipenem, meropenem). If aerobic gram-negative organisms such as *P. aeruginosa* are involved, parenteral therapy with an aminoglycosides, a fourth-generation cephalosporin (cefepime or ceftazidime), or oral or parenteral treatment with a fluoroquinolone (only in postpubertal patients) is added. Parenteral therapy with a carbapenem (e.g., imipenem) is more expensive, but provides coverage for most potential pathogens, both anaerobes and aerobes.

From a practical point of view, it is not generally recommended or necessary for clinicians to perform a culture for anaerobic bacteria in these patients. The tests are very expensive and timely, and most clinicians do not have access to materials that are necessary to properly culture anaerobic organisms. They should however, rely, on the data that have demonstrated the existence of anaerobes (discussed above) in chronic sinusitis. Culture for anaerobes should, however, be performed in those that do not respond to therapy and/or develope a complication. Clinicians should consider the anaerobic activity for the various antimicrobials before selecting an antibiotic agent for the treatment of chronic sinusitis.

The length of therapy is at least 21 days, and may be extended up to 10 weeks. Fungal sinusitis can be treated with surgical debridement of the affected sinuses and antifungal therapy (56). In contrast to acute sinusitis, which is generally treated vigorously with antibiotics, many physicians believe that surgical drainage is the mainstay of therapy in chronic sinusitis. When the patient does not respond to medical therapy, the physician should consider surgical drainage. Impaired drainage may be a major contribution to the development of chronic sinusitis, and correction of the obstruction helps to alleviate the infection and prevent recurrence. The use of antimicrobial therapy alone, without surgical drainage of collected pus, may not result in clearance of the infection. The chronically inflamed sinus membranes with diminished vascularity may be a poor means of carrying an adequate antibiotic level to the infected tissue, even though the blood level may be therapeutic. Furthermore, the reduction in the pH and oxygen tension within the inflamed sinus may interfere further with the activity of the antimicrobial agents, which can result in bacterial survival despite a high antibiotic concentration (46).

CONCLUSIONS

Many of the organisms recovered from sinusitis are resistant to penicillins, either through the production of beta-lactamase (*H. influenzae*, *M. catarrhalis*, *S. aureus*, *Fusobacterium* spp., and *Prevotella* spp.) or through changes in the penicillin-binding protein (*S. pneumoniae*). The pathogenicity of beta-lactamase–producing bacteria is expressed directly through their ability to cause infections, and indirectly through the production of beta-lactamase. The indirect pathogenicity is conveyed not only by surviving penicillin therapy, but also by "shielding" penicillin-susceptible pathogens from the drug. The direct and indirect virulent characteristics of these bacteria require the administration of appropriate antimicrobial therapy directed against all pathogens in mixed infections. The oral antimicrobials that are the most effective in management of acute sinusitis are amoxicillin-clavulanate (given in a high dose), the newer quinolones (gatifloxacin, moxifloxacin) and the second-generation cephalosporins (cefuroxime, cefpodoxime, cefprozil, or cefdinir). The oral antimicrobials that are the most effective in management of chronic sinusitis are amoxicillin-clavulanate, clindamycin, and the combination of metonidazole and a penicillin.

REFERENCES

1. Brook I. Emergence and persistence of beta-lactamase-producing bacteria in the oropharynx following penicillin treatment. Arch Otolaryngol Head Neck Surg 1988; 114:667–670.
2. Brook I, Gober AE. Emergence of beta-lactamase-producing aerobic and anaerobic bacteria in oro-pharynx of children following penicillin chemotherapy. Clin Pediatr (Phila) 1984; 23:338–341.
3. Brook I, Gober AE. Monthly changes in the rate of recovery of penicillin-resistant organisms from children. Pediatr Infect Dis J 1997; 16:255–256.
4. McCracken GH Jr. Considerations in selecting an antibiotic for treatment of acute otitis media. Pediatr Infect Dis J 1994; 13:1054–1057.
5. Brook I, Gober AE. Resistance to antimicrobials used for therapy of otitis media and sinusitis: effect of previous antimicrobial therapy and smoking. Ann Otol Rhinol Laryngol 1999; 108:645–647.
6. Brook I. The role of beta-lactamase-producing bacteria in the persistence of streptococcal tonsillar infection. Rev Infect Dis 1984; 6:601–607.

7. Brook I, Yocum P, Frazier EH. Bacteriology and β-lactamase activity in acute and chronic maxillary sinusitis. Arch Otolaryngol Head Neck Surg 1996; 122:418–423.
8. Hackman AS, Wilkins TD. In vivo protection of *Fusobacterium necrophorum* from penicillin by *Bacteroides fragilis*. Antimicrob Agents Chemotherapy 1975; 7:698–703.
9. Brook I, Pazzaglia G, Coolbaugh JC, Walker RI. In vivo protection of group A beta-hemolytic streptococci by beta-lactamase producing *Bacteroides* species. J Antimicrob Chemother 1983; 12:599–606.
10. Brook I, Pazzaglia G, Coolbaugh JC, Walker RI. In vivo protection of penicillin susceptible *Bacteroides melaninogenicus* from penicillin by facultative bacteria which produce beta-lactamase. Can J Microbiol 1984; 30:98–104.
11. Simon HM, Sakai W. Staphylococcal anatagosim to penicillin group therapy of hemolytic streptococcal pharyngeal infection: effect of oxacillin. Pediatrics 1963; 31:463–469.
12. Scheifele DW, Fussell SJ. Frequency of ampicillin resistant *Haemophilus parainfluenzae* in children. J Infect Dis 1981; 143:495–498.
13. Brook I, Yocum P. In vitro protection of group A beta-hemolytic streptococci from penicillin and cephalothin by *Bacteroides fragilis*. Chemotheraphy 1983; 29:18–23.
14. Wald ER, Milmore GJ, Bowen AD, Ledema-Medina J, Salamon N, Bluestone CD. Acute maxillary sinusitis in children. N Engl J Med 1981; 304:749–54.
15. Mustafa E, Tahsin A, Mustafa O, Nedret K. Bacteriology of antrum in adults with chronic maxillary sinusitis. Laryngoscope 1994; 104:321–324.
16. Doern GV, Jorgensen JH, Thornsberry C, Preston DA, Tubert T, Redding JS, Maher LA. National collaborative study of the prevalence of antimicrobial resistance among clinical isolates of *Haemophilus influenzae*. Antimicrob Agents Chemother 1988; 32:180–185.
17. Jorgensen JH, Doern GV, Maher LA, Howell AW, Redding JS. Antimicrobial resistance among respiratory isolates of *Haemophilus influenzae*, *Moraxella catarrhalis*, and *Streptococcus pneumoniae* in the United States. Antimicrob Agents Chemother 1990; 34:2075–2080.
18. Jacobs MR. Worldwide trends in antimicrobial resistance among common respiratory tract pathogens in children. Pediatr Infect Dis J 2003; 22(suppl 8): S109–S1019.
19. Sinus and Allergy Health Partnership: Antimicrobial treatment guidelines for acute bacterial rhinosinusitis. Otolaryngol Head Neck Surg 2004; 130(suppl 1):1S.
20. Jacobs MR, Felmingham D, Appelbaum PC, Gruneberg RN, The Alexander Project Group. The Alexander Project 1998–2000: susceptibility of pathogens isolated from community-acquired respiratory tract infection to commonly used antimicrobial agents. J Antimicrob Chemother 2003; 52:229–246.
21. Dagan R, Johnson CE, McLinn S, Abughali N, Feris J, Leibovitz E, Burch DJ, Jacobs MR. Bacteriologic and clinical efficacy of amoxicillin/clavulanate vs. azithromycin in acute otitis media. Pediatr Infect Dis J 2000; 19:95–104.
22. Doern GV. Antimicrobial resistance with *Streptococcus pneumoniae*: much ado about nothing? Semin Respir Infect 2001; 16:177–185.
23. Dominguez MA, Pallares R. Antibiotic resistance in respiratory pathogens. Curr Opin Pulmonary Med 1998; 4:173–179.

24. Fung-Tomc JC, Huczko E, Stickle T, et al. Antibacterial activity of cefprozil compared with those of 13 oral cephems and 3 macrolides. Antimicrob Agent Chemother 1995; 39:533–538.
25. Jacobs MR, Bajaksouzian S, Zilles A, Lin GR, Pankuch GA, Appelbaum PC. Susceptibilities of *Streptococcus pneumoniae* and *Haemophilus influenzae* to 10 oral antimicrobial agents based on pharmacodynamic parameters: 1997 U. S. surveillance study. Antimicrob Agents Chemother 1999; 43:1901–1908.
26. Lynch JP III, Martinez FJ. Clinical relevance of macrolide-resistant *Streptococcus pneumoniae* for community-acquired pneumonia. Clin Infect Dis 2002 Mar 1; 34(suppl 1):S27–S46.
27. Klugman KP, Capper T, Widdowson CA, Koornhof HJ, Moser W. Increased activity of 16-membered lactone ring macrolides against erythromycin-resistant *Streptococcus pyogenes* and *Streptococcus pneumoniae*: characterization of South African isolates. J Antimicrob Chemother 1998; 42:729–734.
28. Granizo JJ, Aguilar L, Casal J, Dal-Re R, Baquero F. *Streptococcus pneumoniae* resistance to erythromycin and penicillin in relation to macrolide and b-lactam consumption in Spain (1979–1997). J Antimicrob Chemother 2000; 46:767–773.
29. Cizman M, Pokorn M, Seme K, Paragi A, Orazem A. Influence of increased macrolide consumption on macrolide resistance of common respiratory pathogens. Eur J Clin Microbiol Infect Dis 1999; 18:522–524.
30. Peterson LR. Quinolone molecular structure–activity relationships: what have we learned about improving antibacterial activity. Clin Infect Dis 2001; 33(suppl 3):S180–S186.
31. Pestova E, Beyer R, Cianciotto NP, Noskin GA, Peterson LR. Contribution of topoisomerase IV and DNA gyrase mutations in *Streptococcus pneumoniae* for resistance to novel fluoroquinolones. Antimicrob Agents Chemother 1999; 43:2000–2004.
32. Lu T, Zhao X, Drlica K. Gatifloxacin activity against quinolone-resistant gyrase: allele-specific enhancement of bacteriostatic and bactericidal activities by the C-8 methoxy group. Antimicrob Agents Chemother 1999; 43:2969–2974.
33. Scheld WM. Maintaining fluoroquinolone class efficacy: review of influencing factors. Emerg Infect Dis 2003; 9:1–9.
34. Saravolatz LD, Leggett J. Gatifloxacin, gemifloxacin, and moxifloxacin: the role of 3 newer fluoroquinolones. Clin Infect Dis 2003; 37(1):1210–1215.
35. Orden B, Perez Trallero E, Montes M, Martinez R. Erythromycin resistance of *Streptococcus pyogenes* in Madrid. Pediatr Infect Dis J 1998; 17:470–473.
36. Spangler SK, Jacobs MR, Pankuch GA, Appelbaum PC. Susceptibility of 170 penicillin-susceptible and -resistant pneumococci to six oral cephalosporins, four quinolones, desacetylcefotaxime, Ro 23–9424 and RP 67829. J Antimicrob Chemother 1993; 31:273–280.
37. Brook I, Gober AE. Resistance to antimicrobials used for therapy of otitis media and sinusitis: effect of previous antimicrobials therapy and smoking. Ann Otol Rhinol Laryngol 1999; 108:645–647.
38. Clark JP, Langston E. Ketolides: a new class of antibacterial agents for treatment of community-acquired respiratory tract infections in a primary care setting. Mayo Clin Proc 2003; 78:1113–1124.
39. Balfour JA, Figgitt DP. Telithromycin. Drugs 2001; 61:815–829.

40. Phillips I, King A, Shannon K. Comparative in-vitro properties of the quinolones. In: Andriole VT, ed. The Quinolones. 3rd ed. San Diego: Academic Press, 2000:99–137.

41. Craig WA. Pharmacokinetic/pharmacodynamic parameters: rationale for antibacterial dosing of mice and men. Clin Infect Dis 1998; 26:1–10.

42. Craig WA, Andes D. Pharmacokinetics and pharmacodynamics of antibiotics in otitis media. Pediatr Infect Dis J 1996; 15:255–259.

43. Schentag JJ, Gilliland KK, Paladino JA. What have we learned from pharmacokinetic and pharmacodynamic theories? Clin Infect Dis 2001; 32(suppl 1): S39–S46.

44. Brook I, Frazier EH, Foote PA. Microbiology of the transition from acute to chronic maxillary sinusitis. J Med Microbiol 1996; 45:372–375.

45. Brook I, Frazier EH, Foote PA. Microbiology of chronic maxillary sinusitis: comparison between specimens obtained by sinus endoscopy and by surgical drainage. J Med Microbiol 1997; 46:430–432.

46. Carenfelt C, Eneroth CM, Lundberg C, Wretlind B. Evaluation of the antibiotic effect of treatment of maxillary sinusitis. Scand J Infect Dis 1975; 7: 259–264.

47. Gwaltney JM Jr. Acute community-acquired sinusitis. Clin Infect Dis 1996; 23:209–225.

48. Wald ER, Chiponis D, Leclesma-Medina J. Comparative effectiveness of amoxicillin and amoxicillin–clavulanate potassium in acute paranasal sinus infection in children: a double-blind, placebo-controlled trial. Pediatrics 1998; 77:795–800.

49. Spector SL, Bernstein IL. Parameters for the diagnosis and management of sinusitis. J Allergy Clin Immunol 1998; 102(suppl):S107–S144.

50. Williams JW Jr, Aguilar C, Makela M, Cornell J, Holleman D, Chiquette E, Simel DL. Antibiotics for acute maxillary sinusitis. 1:Cochrane Database Syst Rev 2000; (2):CD000243.

51. Benninger MS, Holzer SES, Lau J. Diagnosis and treatment of uncomplicated acute bacterial rhinosinusitis: summary of the agency for health care policy and research evidence-based report. Otolaryngol Head Neck Surg 2000; 122:1–7.

52. Brook I, Gooch WM III, Jenkins SG, Pichichero ME, Reiner SA, Sher L, Yamauchi T. Medical management of acute bacterial sinusitis. Recommendations of a clinical advisory committee on pediatric and adult sinusitis. Ann Otol Rhinol Laryngol 2000; 109:1–20.

53. Clinical Practice Guidelines: Managemement of Sinusitis. Pediatrics 2001; 108:798–807.

54. Brook I, Thompson DH, Frazier EH. Microbiology and management of chronic maxillary sinusitis. Arch Otolaryngol Head Neck Surg 1994; 120:1317–1320.

55. Brook I, Yocum P. Management of chronic sinusitis in children. J Laryngol Otol 1995; 109:1159–1162.

56. Decker CF. Sinusitis in the immunocompromised host. Curr Infect Dis Rep 1999; 1:27–32.

10

Medical Management of Acute Sinusitis

Dennis A. Conrad

Division of Infectious Diseases, Department of Pediatrics, University of Texas Health Science Center at San Antonio, San Antonio, Texas, U.S.A.

INTRODUCTION

The medical management of acute sinusitis remains problematic due to the inherent contradictions concerning diagnosis and treatment. Although a significant number of upper respiratory tract infections (URTIs) requiring evaluation by health care providers occur annually, the ability to precisely distinguish bacterial sinusitis from viral rhinosinusitis by clinical criteria still does not exist. Even though the majority of cases of acute bacterial sinusitis will resolve spontaneously without specific anti-infective therapy, antimicrobial treatment shortens the duration of illness and lessens the severity of symptoms. An increasing prevalence of respiratory pathogens resistant to traditionally prescribed antibiotics has been documented during the last decade, yet standard antibacterial regimens still result in acceptably high cure rates despite probable microbial resistance in vitro.

Current opinion on the management of acute bacterial sinusitis embracing the principles of best practice is to establish the diagnosis of acute bacterial sinusitis as accurately as is possible by utilizing clinical information, and to prescribe and treat the patient with an antibiotic chosen for predicted probability of success and reduced potential for selection of antimicrobial resistance (1). In addition, several important analyses of the management of acute sinusitis have been published within the last seven years that specifically address the evidentiary basis for best clinical practices; synthesis of this information provides the framework for the management recommendations contained in this chapter. As has been true for previously published recommendations, these current recommendations will arise from interpretation of results achieved in clinical trials and from best estimates where definitive information is lacking.

RATIONALE FOR THE RECOMMENDED MANAGEMENT OF ACUTE BACTERIAL SINUSITIS

American Academy of Pediatrics

The principles for the judicious use of antimicrobial agents that should be used to treat acute sinusitis in children were published in 1998 (2). The authors recommended that the clinical diagnosis of acute bacterial sinusitis in children required the presence of mild nonspecific symptoms and signs of URTI, such as purulent rhinitis or cough, which persisted for 10 to 14 days, or the presence of more severe symptoms and signs, such as high fever and facial fullness or pain, which were more specific for sinus mucosal inflammation.

The diagnosis of acute sinusitis should be based on clinical finding; the use of radiographic evaluation was to be limited to episodes of recurrent sinus disease, when complications of acute sinusitis were suspected, or if the presumptive clinical diagnosis of bacterial sinusitis was in doubt.

Amoxicillin was appropriate for the initial treatment of acute uncomplicated sinusitis, whereas a β-lactamase-stable β-lactam antibiotic would be appropriate to treat recurrent infection and amoxicillin therapeutic-failures. These recommendations remain useful to date as a guide for current clinical practice.

American Academy of Allergy and Clinical Immunology

Comprehensive practice parameters on sinusitis addressing diagnosis, antimicrobial therapy, and adjunctive treatments were published in 1998 (3). Selected conclusions were that diagnosis of bacterial sinusitis should be established by a combination of clinical history with physical examination, nasal cytology, and/or imagining studies, that antibiotics were the primary therapy for bacterial sinusitis, and that treatment choice should be based on predicted effectiveness, costs, and potential adverse drug effects.

Critical analyses of the use of the adjunctive therapies of antihistamines, α-adrenergic decongestants, topical and systemic glucocorticosteroids, saline lavage, mucolytics, expectorants, and nasal endoscopic surgical intervention were also provided and detailed to a degree that merits specific attention in terms of current clinical practice as regards the non-antibiotic-therapy aspects of disease management (Table 1).

Table 1 Adjunctive Therapy in the Management of Acute Sinusitis

Adjunctive therapy	Evidence for efficacy	Potential utility
Antihistamines	None in acute sinusitis	Chronic sinusitis associated with allergic rhinitis
α-Adrenergic decongestants	Prospective studies absent	May reduce mucosal edema and improve ostial patency
Topical glucocorticosteroids	Useful in reducing mucosal inflammation and edema	Treatment of rhinitis accompanying sinusitis
Systemic glucocorticosteroids	Not adequately studied	Topical agents preferred due to reduced risk of adverse drug effects
Saline lavage,mucolytics, expectorants	No confirmation of specific efficacy	Wetting agents may provide symptomatic relief
Nasal endoscopy	Subjective improvement in patients undergoing procedure	Useful for recurrent sinusitis due to ostial obstruction

Source: From Ref. 3.

Agency for Health Care Policy and Research

In 1999, the Agency for Health Care Policy and Research published a comprehensive analysis of medical literature evidence concerning the diagnosis and treatment of community-acquired acute bacterial rhinosinusitis in children and adults (4). Utilizing a MEDLINE search of human studies of sinusitis published between 1966 and May 1998, meta-analyses were performed to evaluate clinical management strategies.

Of the eight research questions posed and subsequently answered by the review, the observations pertaining to four of the questions are particularly germane to the current medical management of acute sinusitis (Table 2). The authors of the report concluded that either symptomatic treatment or the use of clinical criteria to select patients to be treated with antibiotics were the most cost-effective strategies to manage patients with uncomplicated acute bacterial sinusitis, and that the use of either amoxicillin or trimethoprim–sulfamethoxazole should be the initial therapeutic consideration due to probable efficacy, adverse events profiles, and treatment cost.

Subcommittee on Management of Sinusitis and the Committee on Quality Improvement

Due to the limited number of randomized studies of acute bacterial sinusitis evaluated by the Agency for Health Care Policy and Research, the Subcommittee on Management of Sinusitis and the Committee on Quality

Table 2 Results of Meta-Analysis Evaluating Management of Acute Sinusitis

I. What are the values of clinical criteria and imaging for diagnosis of acute bacterial sinusitis?
  A. Clinical criteria may have a diagnostic equivalence to sinus radiography.
II. Are antibiotics effective in resolving the symptoms of acute bacterial sinusitis?
  A. Approximately 67% of patients receiving placebo recovered without antibiotic therapy.
  B. Antibiotic therapy increased the number of patients cured and shortened the duration of symptoms.
III. What is the efficacy and safety of antibiotics in treatment of acute bacterial sinusitis?
  A. Antibiotic treatment reduced the clinical failure rate by one-half when compared to placebo.
  B. Amoxicillin and trimethoprim–sulfamethoxazole were as effective as newer and more expensive antibiotics.
  C. Approximately 4% of patients receiving amoxicillin had adverse effects causing cessation of therapy; no statistical difference in this percentage was observed for patients receiving other antibiotics.
IV. Do ancillary therapies benefit the treatment of acute bacterial sinusitis?
  A. Difference in the design of individual studies prevented independent analysis of the benefit of decongestants, antihistamines, topical and systemic steroids, and surgical drainage and irrigation.

Source: From Ref. 4.

Improvement of the American Academy of Pediatrics partnered with the Agency for Health Care Policy and Research and family practice and otolaryngology colleague organizations to provide a supplement specifically for the management of acute bacterial sinusitis in children. Utilizing information gleaned from nonrandomized pediatric treatment trials that were published between 1966 and March 1999, in conjunction with the randomized trials that had been reviewed during the Agency for Health Care Policy and Research study, a technical report (5) and a clinical practice guideline for the management of sinusitis pertinent to childhood infections (6) were generated and published in 2001.

Of the four clinical practice guideline recommendations that were formulated following review of these additional studies, three of these recommendations specifically address the medical management of acute bacterial sinusitis occurring in children (Table 3).

International Journal of Pediatric Otorhinolaryngology Consensus Opinion

A consensus opinion that was published in 1999 concerning the management of rhinosinusitis in children is noteworthy for providing recommendations concerning the place for surgery in the management of sinusitis (7).

Table 3 Management of Acute Sinusitis in Children

The diagnosis of acute bacterial sinusitis in children is clinical, and is based on either persistence or severity of upper respiratory tract symptoms.

Imaging studies are not necessary to confirm a clinical diagnosis of sinusitis; computed tomography of the paranasal sinuses should be reserved for preoperative evaluation.

Antibiotic therapy is recommended for management of acute bacterial sinusitis; no recommendations can be made concerning adjuvant therapies, antimicrobial prophylaxis to prevent recurrent infection, and the use of complementary or alternative medicine to treat or prevent sinusitis.

Source: From Ref. 6.

The recommended uses of adenoidectomy and antral lavage were limited to selected cases that could not be characterized as uncomplicated acute bacterial sinusitis, and recommendations concerning the absolute and possible indications for endoscopic sinus surgery were provided (Table 4).

American College of Radiology

The American College of Radiology developed appropriateness criteria for the evaluation of sinusitis in the pediatric population that were published in 1999 (8). The recommendations that were contained in the report provided useful guidance concerning the selective use of imaging studies in the management of acute sinusitis (Table 5).

Table 4 Indications for Surgery in the Management of Acute Sinusitis

Absolute indications	Possible indications
Complete nasal obstruction in cystic fibrosis patients	Persistence of chronic rhinosinusitis failing medical management
Antrachoanal polyp	
Intracranial complication	
Mucocele/mucopyocele	
Orbital abscess	
Traumatic injury of optic canal	
Dacryocystorhinitis resistant to medical therapy	
Fungal sinusitis	
Meningoencephalocele	
Neoplasm	

Source: From Ref. 7.

Table 5 Use of Radiographic Evaluation in the Management of Acute Sinusitis

The diagnosis of acute and chronic sinusitis is based on clinical finding and not
  solely on the basis of imaging studies.
Imaging studies are not indicated for successfully treated acute sinusitis.
Coronal cranial computed tomography should be done if the symptoms of acute
  sinusitis persist beyond 10 days of appropriate therapy, and in cases of chronic
  sinusitis where imaging evaluation is desired.
Plain radiography in the evaluation of sinusitis is generally unwarranted.

Source: From Ref. 8.

Sinus and Allergy Health Partnership (2000)

In 2000, the Sinus and Allergy Health Partnership published evidence-based
recommendations for the diagnosis and treatment of acute bacterial rhinosinusitis (9).

Based on acknowledged limited information available concerning comparative clinical trials evaluating diagnostic criteria and antibiotic choices
for the management of sinusitis, the partnership recommended that the
diagnosis of disease was clinical and could be based on the persistence
of upper respiratory tract symptoms that did not improve after a 10-day
duration or worsened during a five to seven-day interval.

Recommended treatment of adult patients with mild disease who were
not exposed to antibacterial therapy in the prior four to six weeks were amoxicillin (lower dose), amoxicillin/clavulanate, cefpodoxime, or cefuroxime. Adult
patients with mild disease who had been exposed to antibacterials within the
prior four to six weeks and those patients with moderate disease should be treated with amoxicillin (higher dose), amoxicillin/clavulanate, cefpodoxime, or
cefuroxime. Adult patients with moderate disease who had been exposed to antibacterials within the prior four to six weeks should be treated with amoxicillin/
clavulanate, gatifloxacin, levofloxacin, moxifloxacin, or a combination of either
amoxicillin or clindamycin with either cefpodoxime or cefixime. Recommendations for children with sinusitis paralleled those recommendations for adult
patients, both in terms of prior antibiotic exposure and severity of disease, with
the exception of exclusion of use of fluoroquinolones in this pediatric population.

The sinusitis management recommendations offered by the partnership
were based on predicted efficacy rates that had been mathematically calculated using in vitro susceptibility data, mechanisms of bacterial killing characteristics for the different antibacterial classes, and predicted pharmacokinetics
of the individual drugs. Limited clinical trail results were available that could
actually substantiate many of the recommendations, although a concern for
the increased prevalence of bacteria which caused URTIs and were resistant
to amoxicillin and trimethoprim–sulfamethoxazole prompted recommendations to consider broader-spectrum antimicrobials for initial therapy.

Clinical Advisory Committee on Pediatric and Adult Sinusitis

A clinical advisory committee on pediatric and adult sinusitis also published recommendations for the medical management of acute bacterial sinusitis in 2000 (10). This committee evaluated the importance of individual variables of patient history, clinical assessment, and diagnostic tests for the initial diagnosis of acute sinusitis.

The elements of the patient history that were deemed significantly important to establish the diagnosis of bacterial sinusitis were a "cold" that had been present for more than 7 to 10 days, "unusually" severe upper respiratory tract complaints, fever, mucopurulent discharge of greater than seven-days duration, pain referred to maxillary teeth, and no appreciable response to decongestant therapy.

Significantly important clinical findings were facial and midface tenderness, the appearance of the nasal mucosal surface, intranasal pus, and the presence of purulent postnasal mucus in the pharynx.

Of the diagnostic tests evaluated, only anterior rhinoscopy, direct aspiration of the sinus, and bacterial cultures of aspirated material following sinus puncture were considered significantly important, with the latter two procedures limited to specific indications.

Antimicrobial therapy recommendations were ranked in a tripartite hierarchy; agents of first choice were amoxicillin and trimethoprim-sulfamethoxazole and second-line agents included cefpodoxime, cefprozil, cefuroxime, cefdinir, and amoxicillin–clavulanate. Recommended third-line agents were azithromycin, clarithromycin, ciprofloxacin, levofloxacin, gatifloxacin, moxifloxacin, and clindamycin.

In terms of adjunctive therapies, the committee endorsed the restricted use of topical decongestants limited to three days, and the use of systemic decongestants in adult patients.

The committee acknowledged that the optimum management of acute sinusitis was controversial, but that the primary care physician should recognize the condition and treat aggressively due to disease impact on the quality of life for patients with active disease.

American College of Physicians—American Society for Internal Medicine

The American College of Physicians—American Society for Internal Medicine published clinical practice guidelines in 2001 that outlined the principles of appropriate antibiotic use to treat acute sinusitis occurring in adults (11); background information that supported these recommendations was published at the same time (12).

Three recommendations concerning management of acute sinusitis were offered: sinus radiography is not recommended for the diagnosis of uncomplicated sinusitis; acute bacterial sinusitis does not require antibiotic treatment, especially when symptoms are either mild or moderate; and patients with severe symptoms or those with persistent moderate symptoms who have specific finding of bacterial infection should receive anti-infective therapy, preferentially with a narrow-spectrum agent (11).

The companion article provided the rationale that supported the three recommendations contained in the clinical guidelines, and further observed that analgesia was an important aspect of management of acute sinusitis and that topical and oral decongestants may ameliorate some of the nasal symptoms associated with infection (12).

Sinus and Allergy Health Partnership (2004)

In 2004, the Sinus and Allergy Health Partnership published antimicrobial treatment guidelines for acute bacterial rhinosinusitis (13) that updated the original that were published in 2000 (9). The more recent guidelines largely reflected those of the original publication; the areas of significant update included diagnostic modalities, contemporary antibacterial susceptibility profiles, addition of newer antimicrobial agents as recommended therapy, and expansion of the various pharmacodymanic/pharmacokinetic principles and therapeutic outcomes model (14) used to predict potential success of the individual agents.

The anti-infective agents recommended for use to treat pediatric and adult patients with mildly symptomatic sinusitis who had not been exposed to an antibiotic in the preceding four to six weeks were amoxicillin, amoxicillin–clavulanate, cefpodoxime, cefuroxime, and cefdinir. Treatment options for those adult patients with mild sinusitis who had been exposed to an antibiotic in the previous four to six weeks and those adult patients with moderately symptomatic sinusitis were gatifloxacin, levofloxacin, moxifloxacin, amoxicillin–clavulanate, ceftriaxone, or a combination of either amoxicillin or clindamycin and either cefixime or rifampin.

Treatment options for those pediatric patients with mild sinusitis who had been exposed to an antibiotic in the previous four to six weeks and those pediatric patients with moderately symptomatic sinusitis were amoxicillin–clavulanate, cefpodoxime, cefuroxime, cefdinir, ceftriaxone, or a combination of either amoxicillin or clindamycin and either cefixime or rifampin.

Summary of Varying Recommendations for the Management of Acute Bacterial Sinusitis

Despite subtle variations in the recently published recommendations for the management of acute bacterial sinusitis, consistent principles are apparent. The diagnosis of acute bacterial sinusitis should be made after consideration of the presence and persistence of symptoms and signs of an URTI without the use of radiographic or microbiologic evaluation for the majority of patients, those antimicrobial agents most commonly used to treat respiratory tract infections are also generally effective in the treatment of acute bacterial sinusitis as evidenced by clinical trials and treatment experience, selected adjunctive medicinal therapies may improve symptoms but are not critical to achieve successful outcome, and surgical intervention is appropriately restricted to complicated infections. Therefore, current recommendations for the management of acute bacterial sinusitis may legitimately be an extension of recent prior recommendations generated by individual investigators, health care partnerships, and consensus of medical experts on behalf of practitioners, professional societies, and governmental agencies.

CURRENT RECOMMENDATIONS FOR THE MANAGEMENT OF ACUTE BACTERIAL SINUSITIS

Symptomatic Treatment of URTIs

Children and adults who have a viral URTI may benefit from symptomatic therapy, largely to improve the quality of life during the acute illness. The use of normal saline as a spray or lavage may provide symptomatic improvement by liquefying secretions to encourage drainage. The short-term (three-day) use of topical α-adrenergic decongestants can also provide symptomatic relief, but use should be restricted to older children and adults due to the potential for undesirable systemic effects in infants and young children. Topical glucocorticosteroids may also be useful in reducing nasal mucosal edema, especially in those cases where a patient who has seasonal allergic rhinitis develops the complication of an acute URTI. The antipyretic and analgesic effects of nonsteroidal anti-inflammatory agents may relieve or ameliorate the associated symptoms of fever, headache, generalized malaise, and facial tenderness.

Until the clinical diagnosis of acute bacterial sinusitis is established, management of an URTI should be restricted to either no therapy or symptomatic care alone. Moreover, symptomatic care may prove useful in the management of acute bacterial sinusitis as adjunctive therapy, but no adjunct has been shown essential in improving the outcome achieved by antimicrobial therapy or effective in preventing the development of acute bacterial sinusitis in persons who have a viral URTI or allergic rhinitis.

Clinical Diagnosis of Acute Bacterial Sinusitis

The presence and persistence of mucopurulent nasal drainage for a minimum duration of time in a person who has an URTI is the most consistent feature that can establish the diagnosis of acute bacterial sinusitis by clinical criteria. An adult or a child who has an URTI and who also has persistent mucopurulent nasal drainage that has not improved during a symptomatic course of 10-days duration may be considered to have acute bacterial sinusitis for the purposes of initiating anti-infective therapy (Fig. 1).

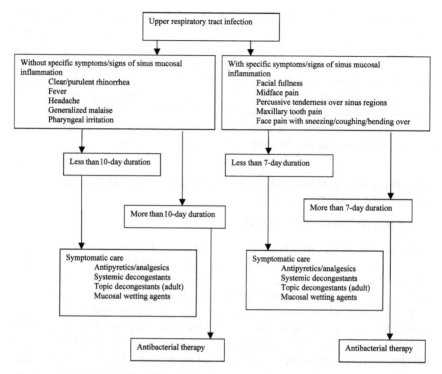

Figure 1   Diagnosis and initial management of acute sinusitis.

The presence of associated symptoms and signs that are suggestive of sinus mucosal inflammation further supports the clinical diagnosis of acute bacterial sinusitis. Unilateral or bilateral midfacial tenderness or maxillary pain, the subjective sensations of facial fullness or nasal congestion, fever, a persistent cough worsening when the patient is supine, maxillary or peri-orbital swelling, postnasal drainage, headache, and hyposmia or anosmia are symptoms and signs that are often associated with acute bacterial sinusitis. In those children and adults who have an URTI and who also have localizing symptoms and signs of sinus mucosal inflammation, the diagnosis of acute bacterial sinusitis may be made with reasonable certainty if those localized findings are present on the seventh day of symptoms of an URTI as measured from the time of initial onset.

Radiographic Diagnosis of Acute Bacterial Sinusitis

Radiographic evaluation of uncomplicated acute bacterial sinusitis is unnecessary to confirm the clinical diagnosis or direct antimicrobial therapy. Imaging studies should be restricted to patients with symptoms and signs of URTI who appear acutely ill and in whom the diagnosis of acute bacterial sinusitis is unclear, patients who have evidence of having an intracranial or intraorbital complication of acute bacterial sinusitis, patients who fail to respond appropriately despite broad-spectrum antimicrobial therapy, patients with recurrent or chronic sinusitis, and for assessment in anticipation of endoscopic sinus surgery. In these special circumstances, coronal sinus computed tomography is the evaluation of choice.

Antimicrobial Therapy

Amoxicillin and trimethoprim–sulfamethoxazole still remain the most cost-effective antimicrobial agents for the initial treatment of acute bacterial sinusitis. Recent analyses of the appropriate management of acute bacterial sinusitis have acknowledged the concern for the increasing prevalence of bacterial resistance to antimicrobial agents. This increased antibacterial resistance would have a potentially negative impact on reducing the clinical efficacy of amoxicillin or trimethoprim–sulfamethoxazole, so recent therapeutic recommendations for treatment of acute bacterial sinusitis have been expanded to include amoxicillin/clavulanate, cefpodoxime, cefuroxime, cefdinir, and, for adult patients, ceftidoren, gatifloxacin, levofloxacin, and moxifloxacin (Table 6). If the patient has a history of significant allergy to β-lactam antibiotics and is not a candidate for fluoroquinolone therapy,

Table 6 Antibacterial Regimens for Treatment of Acute Sinusitis

Antibiotic	Pediatric regimen	Adult regimen
Amoxicillin	90 mg/kg/day bid	3.5 gm/day bid
Amoxicillin/clavulanate ES-600	90 mg amoxicillin/kg/day bid	–
Amoxicillin/clavulanate XL	–	4 gm/day bid
Cefdinir	14 mg/kg/day qd-bid	600 mg/day qd-bid
Cefixime	8 mg/kg/day qd-bid	400 mg/day qd-bid
Cefpodoxime	10 mg/kg/day bid	400 mg/day bid
Ceftibuten	9 mg/kg/day qd	400 mg/day qd
Ceftidoren	–	800 mg/day bid
Cefuroxime	30 mg/kg/day bid	2 gm/day bid
Azithromycin	10 mg/kg/day qd	500 mg/day qd
Clarithromycin	15 mg/kg/day bid	1 gm/day bid
Telithromycin	–	800 mg/day qd
Clindamycin	20 mg/kg/day tid-qid	1.8 gm/day tid-qid
Gatifloxacin	–	400 mg/day qd
Gemifloxacin	–	320 mg/day qd
Levofloxacin	–	500 mg/day qd
Moxifloxacin	–	400 mg/day qd
Trimethoprim/sulfamethoxazole	12 mg/60 mg/kg/day bid	320 mg/1.6 gm/day bid

then azithromycin or clarithromycin has been proposed as alternative choices. Even though these recommendations have been validated by different mathematical and therapeutic models that have been used to predict the relative efficacy of these newer antibiotics, no clinical study has yet been performed that demonstrates the superiority of the extended-spectrum antimicrobials for the treatment of acute bacterial sinusitis due to penicillin-resistant *Streptococcus pneumoniae* and β-lactamase-producing *Haemophilus influenzae* and *Moraxella catarrhalis*. Therefore, a reasonable approach to management would be an initial use of amoxicillin in higher dose or trimethoprim–sulfamethoxazole for penicillin-allergic patients, reserving the use of extended-spectrum antimicrobial agents to those patients who fail initial therapy (Fig. 2).

Patients who have failed initial amoxicillin or trimethoprim–sulfamethoxazole therapy should be treated with an extended-spectrum antibiotic. If no appreciable improvement in symptoms has been noted after three days of the initial therapy, an anti-infective agent with an enhanced antibacterial spectrum should be substituted. For pediatric patients, amoxicillin/clavulanate, cefpodoxime, cefuroxime, or cefdinir would be a reasonable choice. These antimicrobials would also be appropriate for adult patients who have failed initial therapy; in addition, ceftidoren, telithromycin, gatifloxacin, gemifloxacin, levofloxacin, and moxifloxacin could also be used. In time, fluoroquinolone antibiotics approved for use in adults may also be approved by the United States Food and Drug Administration for use in children; until then, however, use in pediatric patients should be restricted to unusual and special circumstances.

Patients who failed initial antimicrobial therapy and who have an inadequate response to an extended-spectrum antimicrobial may be managed either medically or surgically. Medical management would be by use of an antibiotic regimen that would incorporate those agents with the greatest activity in vitro against antibiotic-resistant respiratory bacteria. Ceftriaxone, parenterally administered daily or on alternative days until clinical resolution of illness, would be one anti-infective option. The second option would be a combination of two orally administered antibiotics chosen to maximize activity against gram-positive and -negative bacteria. Clindamycin, in combination with either cefixime or ceftibuten, would be an appropriate regimen. A third option for pediatric patients could be the use of a fluoroquinolone antimicrobial; with appropriate informed consent and parent approval, the failure of two successive antibacterial regimens may be a special circumstance justifying use of an agent otherwise currently unapproved for use in children.

The duration of antimicrobial treatment of acute bacterial sinusitis should be for 10 days under most circumstances, as predicated on appreciable clinical improvement by the third treatment day. This recommendation could be modified as the continuation of treatment for seven days beyond

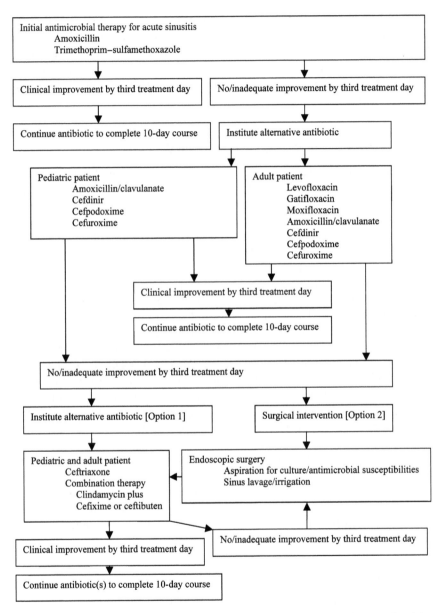

Figure 2 Algorithm for antimicrobial and surgical management of acute sinusitis.

that time where substantial improvement in symptoms following therapy initiation first occurred. One antibiotic, azithromycin, has been approved as a three-day regimen for treatment of acute bacterial sinusitis. However, due to a spectrum of antibacterial activity against the major pathogens causing acute bacterial sinusitis that is reduced when compared to β-lactam antibiotics and fluoroquinolones, and despite the apparently more favorable "short-course" treatment duration, use of azithromycin should be restricted to those patients having a history of significant allergy to penicillin and cephalosporin antibiotics and for whom use of a fluoroquinolone would be inappropriate.

Use of Surgery in the Management of Acute Bacterial Sinusitis

Endoscopic sinus surgery for aspiration of sinus contents for culture and susceptibility testing to guide anti-infective therapy could also be an option for patients who failed initial antimicrobial therapy and who had an inadequate response to an extended-spectrum antibiotic. A secondary benefit may be achieved by endoscopically directed sinus irrigation. Although no evidence would suggest that this intervention is necessary to achieve successful outcome, many patients will perceive an immediate improvement in the severity of the symptoms of sinusitis following irrigation.

Endoscopic sinus surgery generally has no place in the management of uncomplicated acute bacterial sinusitis and should be reserved for patients who have had a complicated course, such as the failure of medical management that was elucidated previously. As well, two additional circumstances may also justify endoscopic sinus surgery in the management of acute bacterial sinusitis. If a person with an episode of acute bacterial sinusitis has a history of frequent episodes of recurring sinusitis, endoscopic sinus surgery performed to identify a mechanical obstruction prohibiting appropriate sinus drainage may allow surgical correction to prevent subsequent recurrences. As well, when acute sinusitis occurs in an immunoincompetent host, knowledge of the infecting pathogen best obtained by fiberoptic sinus endoscopy and aspiration/ lavage can assist in selecting the appropriate anti-infective regimen. However, even for immunoincompetent hosts, "common things happen commonly;" a reasonable alternative would be to restrict endoscopic sinus surgery to those immunoincompetent hosts with acute sinusitis who failed initial empiric medical management.

REFERENCES

1. Conrad DA, Jenson HB. Management of acute bacterial rhinosinusitis. Curr Opin Pediatr 2002; 14:86–90.
2. O'Brien KL, Dowell SF, Schwartz B, Marcy SM, Phillips WR, Gerber MA. Acute sinusitis—principles of judicious use of antimicrobial agents. Pediatrics 1998; 101:174–177.
3. Spector SL, Berstein IL, Li JT, Berger WE, Kaliner MA, Schuller DE, Blessing-Moore J, Dykewicz MS, Fineman S, Lee RE, Nicklas RA. Sinusitis practice parameters. J Allergy Clin Immunol 1998; 102(suppl 6, Part 2):S107–S144.

4. Agency for Health Care Policy and Research: Diagnosis and Treatment of Acute Bacterial Rhinosinusitis. AHCPR Evidence Report/Technology Assessment, Number 9, March 1999 (Rockville, MD).

5. Ioannidis JPA, Lau J. Technical Report: Evidence for the Diagnosis and Treatment of Acute Uncomplicated Sinusitis in Children: A Systemic Overview. Pediatrics 2001; 108(3). URL:http://www.pediatrics.org/cgi/content/full/108/3/e57.

6. American Academy of Pediatrics Subcommittee on Management of Sinusitis and Committee on Quality Improvement. Clinical Practice Guideline: Management of Sinusitis. Pediatrics 2001; 108:798–808.

7. Clement PAR, Bluestone CD, Gordts F, Lusk RP, Otten FWA, Goossens H, Scadding GK, Takahashi H, van Buchem L, van Cauwenberge P, Wald ER. Management of rhinosinusitis in children. Int J Pediatr Otorhinolaryngol 1999; 49(suppl 1):S95–S100.

8. Expert Panel on Pediatric Imaging. Sinusitis in the pediatric population. ACR Appropriateness Criteria, Reston, VA: American College of Radiology, 1999.

9. Sinus and Allergy Health Partnership: Antimicrobial treatment guidelines for acute bacterial rhinosinusitis. Otolaryngol Head Neck Surg 2000; 123(suppl 1, Part 2):S1–S32.

10. Brook I, Gooch WM, Jenkins, SG, Pichichero ME, Reiner SA, Sher L, Yamauchi T. Medical management of acute bacterial sinusitis: recommendations of a clinical advisory committee on pediatric and adult sinusitis. Ann Otol Rhinol Laryngol 2000; 109:2–20.

11. Snow V, Mottur-Pilson C, Hickner JM. Principles of appropriate antibiotic use for acute sinusitis in adults. Ann Intern Med 2001; 134:495–497.

12. Hickner JM, Bartlett JG, Besser RE, Gonzales R, Hoffman JR, Sande MA. Principles of appropriate antibiotic use for acute rhinosinusitis in adults: background. Ann Intern Med 2001; 134:498–505.

13. Sinus and Allergy Health Partnership: Antimicrobial treatment guidelines for acute bacterial rhinosinusitis. Otolaryngol Head Neck Surg 2004; 130(suppl 1): 1S–45S.

14. Poole MD. A mathematical therapeutic outcomes model for sinusitis. Otolaryngol Head Neck Surg 2004; 130(suppl 1):45S–46S.

11

Medical Management of Chronic Rhinosinusitis

Alexander G. Chiu

Division of Rhinology, Department of Otorhinolaryngology—Head and Neck Surgery, University of Pennsylvania, Philadelphia, Pennsylvania, U.S.A.

Daniel G. Becker

Department of Otorhinolaryngology—Head and Neck Surgery, University of Pennsylvania, Philadelphia, Pennsylvania, U.S.A.

Sinusitis is one of the most common health problems in the United States, and accounts for health expenditures in billions of dollars per year. Although acute sinusitis accounts for the majority of these cases, it is estimated that chronic rhinosinusitis (CRS) results in 18 to 22 million U.S. physician office visits annually (1) and causes significant physical, emotional, and functional impairments (2).

The exact etiology of CRS is still unknown, and therefore a clear definition and uniform treatment guidelines have not always been agreed upon. What has come to be known is that CRS represents a cycle of infection and inflammation. Therapy that fails to address both of these aspects may lead to inadequate results. There are currently multiple medications and delivery methods that are used in the medical management of CRS, and a combination of these therapies is needed in order to manage the multiple factors involved in the disease state. Before describing the current medical therapy, we will review the current working definition of CRS and its known inciting factors.

DEFINITION OF CRS

The Sinus and Allergy Health Partnership convened a multidisciplinary task force to develop definitions for CRS that would allow clinicians and researchers to accurately diagnose this condition. Their first publication was in 1997 and the definitions were later revised in 2003 (3). The task force defined CRS as the duration of symptoms for greater 12 consecutive weeks or greater 12 weeks of physical findings. Symptoms include nasal drainage, fatigue, post-nasal drainage, nasal obstruction, and facial pressure. Physical findings are erythema and/or edema of the middle meatus by nasal endoscopy, discolored nasal drainage or polyps, and/or abnormal findings on CT or plain sinus radiographs (3). The criteria not only rely on the duration of symptoms, but also on the objective evidence of inflammation within the sinonasal passages. Inflammation can be brought on by a variety of inciting factors.

INCITING FACTORS IN SINUSITIS

The most common causes of acute rhinosinusitis are preceding viral upper respiratory tract infections and inhalant allergies (4). Both of these inciting factors result in nasal mucosal edema and resultant blockage of the ostiomeatal complex, a functional area in which the anterior ethmoid, frontal, and maxillary sinuses drain. This physical obstruction may lead to hypo-oxygenation of the sinuses and impairment of the mucosal ciliary function. This results in a stasis of secretions that serves as an ideal environment for bacterial invasion.

The distinction between acute and chronic sinusitis is made on the length of symptoms and signs of inflammation. The exact etiology behind CRS is yet unknown, but potential theories have ranged from inadequately treated acute bacterial infections to native fungus (5) and/or superantigens of colonizing bacteria (6). Regardless of cause, the final common pathway is impaired clearance of secretions, damage to the mucosal lining with resultant fibrosis and thickening of the lamina propria (7), and marked tissue eosinophilia (8). Eosinophilic inflammation results in activation of damaging cytokines and factors to the mucosa, and may result in an end pathway of nasal polyps and hypertrophic mucosa. A cycle then develops, as greater mucosal edema and obstruction lead to stasis of secretions and a greater growth of bacteria, which in turn can perpetuate the inflammatory response.

To break this cycle of infection and inflammation, the ideal medical management is made by a combination of therapies aimed at reducing mucosal inflammation, promoting drainage of the sinuses and the release of secretions, and eradicating the inciting bacterial and/or fungal organisms.

ANTIMICROBIAL THERAPY

The organisms recovered from chronically inflamed sinuses are different from those of acute infections. While *Streptococcus pneumoniae* and

Haemophilus influenzae are the most common isolates in acute sinusitis (9,10), polymicrobial flora are present in CRS, which includes both aerobic and anaerobic bacteria. The predominant aerobic isolates include *Staphylococcuys aureus*, coagulase-negative staphylococci, and aerobic gram-negative bacteria such as *Pseudomonas aeruginosa* and *Stenotrophomonas maltophilia*.

Anaerobic bacteria also play a prominent role in CRS. The recovery of these organisms depends on utilization of appropriate methods for their isolation. Although anaerobes are generally isolated from only 10% of patients with acute sinusitis, they can be isolated from up to 67% of patients with chronic infection (11). The predominant species include anaerobic gram-negative bacilli (e.g., *Bacteroides*, *Prevotella*, and *Porpyromonas* spp.) anaerobic gram-positive cocci (*Peptostreptococcus* spp.), and *Fusobacterium* spp. (4).

Many of these aerobic and anaerobic isolates can produce the enzyme β-lactamase (12), which makes the choice of antimicrobial therapy more difficult.

The choice of antibiotics should be made based, whenever possible, on the results of appropriate cultures that led to the recovery of isolates. Susceptibility testing of these organisms should guide the clinician in the choice of antibiotics.

Sample collection sites include the middle meatus and the sphenoethmoidal recess. The maxillary antral tap and lavage are the recognized gold standards for obtaining cultures. However, this is an invasive procedure. Recent studies have shown that endoscopically directed culture swabs and suction aspirators can lead to comparable results (13,14).

However, it is not always possible to obtain a culture using this method, as patients may not present with visible purulence. In these cases, an empirical therapy is chosen.

Empirical antibiotics used for CRS should cover the most common aerobic and anaerobic bacterial organisms found in this condition. Treatment against both aerobic and anaerobic bacteria was shown to be superior to treatment against aerobes alone (14). Examples of proper empiric antibiotics include the combination of a penicillin- and a β-lactamase inhibitor (e.g., clavulanic acid), clindamycin, the combination of metronidazole and a macrolide, or a quinolone also effective against anaerobic bacteria (e.g., moxifloxacin) (see Chap. 9 by Brook) (15).

ANTIMICROBIAL AGENTS

The common β-*lactams* currently available are the penicillins and the cephalosporins. They are time-dependent, and obtaining a concentration above the MIC into the site of infection for greater than 40% to 50% of the time ensures the highest degree of bacterial death (16). These antibiotics are commonly used in the treatment of acute sinusitis, where they have excellent activity against penicillin-susceptible *S. pneumoniae*. In CRS, however, there is a high incidence of multiple drug-resistant *S. pneumoniae* and β-lactamase–producing aerobes and anaerobes. For this reason, amoxicillin in combination with a β-lactamase inhibitor (clavulanate) enhances the activity of amoxicillin against these organisms.

Second-generation cephalosporins have moderate efficacy against intermediate-level penicillin-resistant pneumococci as well as *H. influenzae.* Their use in CRS is limited given their relative lack of activity against aerobic and anaerobic gram-negative organisms.

Among the fluoroquinolones, ciprofloxacin is used in CRS to treat aerobic gram-negative organisms including *Pseudomonas* spp. Newer agents, such as gatifloxacin, moxifloxacin, and gemifloxacin, have activity against gram-positive and -negative aerobic bacteria as well as some oral anaerobes. The activity of these antibiotics is concentration-dependent, and they are also used in for topical preparations.

An effective combination in patients with CRS and osteitic sinonasal bone, effective against the polymicrobial flora, is clindamycin plus trimethoprim–sulfamethoxazole or a third-generation cephalosporin (i.e., cefixime). Clindamycin has good bone penetration, and is effective against resistant strains of *S. pneumoniae* and β-lactam–resistant anaerobes; trimethoprim–sulfamethoxazole cefixime are active against aerobic gram-negative organisms.

Macrolides (i.e., erythromycin, clarithromycin, and azithromycin) and ketolides (e.g., telithromycin) have limited antibacterial use in CRS. There is increasing resistance to the macrolides by *S. pneumoniae* and *S. aureus,* and both classes have little activity against gram-negative enteric aerobes and anaerobes. Despite their limited antimicrobial activity, the macrolides may have a role in the treatment of the inflammatory aspects in CRS.

In vitro studies have shown that macrolides decrease the levels of inflammatory cytokines IL-5, IL-8, and G-CSF and have compared their in vitro effects with that of prednisolone (17). Clinical studies of long-term, low-dose macrolide therapy following endoscopic sinus surgery, which is typically one-half of the doses used for antibacterial effect, have shown subjective and objective improvement as compared to controls (18). More clinical studies are needed, but long-term macrolide therapy may be a well-tolerated anti-inflammatory therapy that can be used to limit the use of steroids in the treatment of CRS. One concern regarding the use of long-term macrolide therapy is the possible selection of antimicrobial resistance to this, as well as other classes of antibiotics.

ANTI-INFLAMMATORY AGENTS

Long-term, low-dose macrolide therapy represents one attempt at controlling the inflammation associated with CRS. Agents that possess anti-inflammatory properties that are well-tolerated are sought to help ease the reliance on systemic corticosteroids.

Corticosteroids are powerful anti-inflammatory agents that affect both the number and function of inflammatory cells. When given systemically, they reduce circulation of basophil, eosinophil, and monocyte counts to 20% of normal (19). They have multiple effects on the inflammatory response in CRS. They inhibit the secretion of growth factors and mediators of inflammatory cell proliferation, the release of arachidonic acid metabolites, the accumulation of neutrophils in the affected tissues, decrease vascular permeability, and thin mucus by inhibiting glycoprotein secretion from submucosal glands (20).

When used in a topical form, nasal steroid sprays have been shown to be safe and effective in alleviating the symptoms of allergic rhinitis (21). Their use in patients with CRS is important in decreasing the size of nasal polyps and diminishing sinomucosal edema (22). There are no set guidelines for the duration of their use, and side effects from long-term use are unknown. Anecdotally, patients with allergic rhinitis and nasal polyps use steroid sprays for many years with little side effects.

Studies involving the use of oral steroids in the treatment of CRS were not done frequently. These agents represent some of our most effective medications, as they have been shown to decrease the size of nasal polyps, diminish mucosal edema, and promote drainage of obstructed sinus ostia (23,24). Some patients with significant and recurrent polyps are maintained on a daily dose of systemic steroids. This can be deleterious to the patients' overall health because of significant side effects. Prolonged oral steroid use may result in muscle wasting and osteoporosis. Bone density scans should be considered in patients on long-term therapy. Extended use may also result in hypertension, redistribution of body fat stores, and may even induce long-lasting suppression of ACTH production, which can result in anterior pituitary and adrenal cortical atrophy. Because of these harmful side effects, steroids are tapered and given in short courses that may span three to four weeks.

Short-term side effects include water retention, mood shifts, and an increase in energy, which may result in sleep deprivation. When treating a bout of CRS, patients are often given a tapering dose of prednisone over a three-week period. It is imperative that the treating physician warn the patient of the potential short- and long-term side effects, and some have even resorted to having patients sign an informed consent form prior to the medical therapy.

ADJUNCTIVE THERAPY

As stated previously, the medical management of CRS rarely depends on a single medication. In many cases, multiple agents with different mechanisms of action are given in hopes of ultimately promoting drainage of secretions and improved oxygenation to obstructed sinus ostia.

One such medication is a decongestant. *Decongestants* are α-adrenergic agonists that act to constrict capacitance vessels and decrease mucosal edema. Topical therapy such as oxymetazoline or neosynephrine may be used in an acute setting, but overuse will result in a rebound effect and rhinitis medicamentosa. Systemic decongestants can be used for longer periods of time, but may cause side effects of insomnia and may exacerbate underlying systemic hypertension (25).

Antihistamines are used in common therapy for patients with underlying allergic rhinitis, but their use in patients without atopy may cause more harm than good. They effectively relieve symptoms of itching, rhinorrhea, and sneezing in allergic patients, but in nonallergic patients may result in thickening of secretions, which may prevent the needed drainage of the sinus ostia.

A well-tolerated medication that thins secretions to facilitate drainage is a high-dose *guaifenesin* (glyceryl guaicolate). Given a daily dose of 2400 mg, patients may experience less nasal congestion and thinner postnasal drainage (26).

Nasal saline irrigations are also helpful in thinning secretions and may provide a mild benefit in nasal congestion. Although poorly studied, hypertonic saline irrigations have been found to improve patient comfort and quality of life, decrease medication use, and diminish the need for surgical therapy (27,28). This can be done with a 60 cc syringe that is cleaned once a week with rubbing alcohol and replaced every month to help limit the chances of contamination and reinfection. There are a number of commercially available delivery methods, including the water pik device and the netty pot. Nasal irrigations can be used for the duration of symptoms and also as a daily prophylactic measure in those who suffer from recurrent sinus infections and allergic symptoms.

Leukotriene inhibitors are systemic medications that block the receptor and/or production of leukotrienes, potent lipid mediators that increase eosinophil recruitment, goblet cell production, mucosal edema, and airway remodeling. Their use in asthma has been well-documented (29), and the class of medications has been recently approved for the use in allergic rhinitis. Their role in CRS and nasal polyposis is much less clear. One case series documents improved subjective and objective results in patients with nasal polyposis on anti-leukotrienes (30), but these studies must be better controlled before a judgment can be made on their utility in the management of CRS and nasal polyposis.

MAXIMAL MEDICAL THERAPY FOR CRS

The definition of maximal medical therapy is not universal. The various medications used, timing, and doses may vary between practitioners and across the various specialties that treat this illness. The aim of maximal medical therapy is, however, uniform to promote drainage of obstructed sinus ostia and stagnant secretions, decrease mucosal edema, and eliminate inciting bacteria and/or fungus.

Table 1 Maximal Medical Therapy for Chronic Sinusitis

Broad-spectrum antibiotic—preferably based on a culture of the middle meatus
Oral prednisone—starting at 60 mg/day and tapered down over three weeks
Nasal hypertonic saline irrigations
Nasal steroid spray
Oral or nasal antihistamine spray if patient has preceding allergic rhinitis
Mucolytic, i.e., guaifenesin

When treating CRS, a CT scan and nasal endoscopy are extremely useful in the initial patient encounter. Pretreatment objective findings of mucosal edema radiographically and/or purulent secretions, and mucosal edema can be used as a baseline to gauge improvement. Quality of life questionnaires, such as the RSOM-31 form or SNOT-20, are also helpful in documenting subjective improvement through the course of therapy.

Once the diagnosis of CRS is made, the treatment regimen consists of a prolonged course of a broad-spectrum antibiotic, oral steroid, nasal saline irrigations, and nasal steroids sprays plus/minus nasal antihistamine sprays based on evidence of atopy (Table 1). The choice of antibiotic is best made with the aid of an endoscopically guided culture of the middle meatus. If one is not attainable, a broad-spectrum antibiotic that covers aerobic gram-positive and -negative bacteria and anaerobes should be chosen. The exact duration of therapy varies, but most preferred to treat with an initial three-week course, with an additional three weeks of therapy for sub-optimal patient response.

The course of antibiotics can be accompanied by a three-week tapering course of oral steroids. A healthy patient is started with 60 mg of prednisone a day for four days, followed by 50 mg a day for four days, 40 mg a day for four days, 30 mg a day for three days, 20 mg a day for three days, and then finally 10 mg a day for three days. During this time period, the patients continues to flush out their nose twice a day with hypertonic saline irrigations and nasal steroid sprays. Other adjunctive methods as outlined above may be tailored to each individual.

After the initial three-week therapy, a repeat CT scan and nasal endoscopy is performed. If there is improvement but still significant findings of sinusitis radiographically or endoscopically, an additional three weeks of antibiotics may be prescribed. After this, if the patient still has subjective symptoms and objective findings of sinusitis, the option of endoscopic sinus surgery is considered.

INFECTIONS FOLLOWING FUNCTIONAL ENDOSCOPIC SINUS SURGERY

Episodes of rhinosinusitis following functional endoscopic sinus surgery have a slightly different microbiology profile, but are open to more options

Table 2 Alternatives to Oral Antibiotics in the Treatment
of Sinusitis in Previously Operated Patients

Topical antibiotic irrigations
Nebulized antibiotics
Intravenous antibiotics

for medical treatments. Endoscopic cultures are more easily obtained in open sinus cavities. This is important in the medical management of these patients, since there is a higher incidence of recovery of aerobic gram-negative organisms and *S. aureus* from patients who have had previous surgery compared to non-operated patients (31). Because of the high prevalence of these potentially antimicrobial-resistant organisms, empirical treatment of bacterial infections in these patients is not advised. Endoscopic-directed cultures should be obtained, and antibiotic coverage should be tailored to the corresponding sensitivities. Rigid nasal endoscopy can be used to direct a cultured swab or leukens trap to collect mucus directly from the involved maxillary or ethmoid sinus cavities. Studies have shown equal sensitivity between the different methods of culture collection and near- equivalence to the maxillary antral tap (13,14).

Open sinus cavities are not only easier to culture, but they are also more accessible to topical medications. New alternatives in delivery methods of antibiotics and anti-inflammatory medications have been employed to directly administer powerful medications to diseased mucosa, and at the same time limit the systemic distribution and potential side effects (Table 2). These methods were ineffective in delivering medicine to the non-operated sinuses (32), but hold promise in those patients who have cavities that are widely exposed and easily accessible.

NEBULIZED MEDICATIONS

Nebulized medications have long been known to be an effective delivery mechanism in management of lower respiratory tract infections (33,34). Recently, this delivery method is being used to treat acute exacerbations of CRS in previously operated patients. Intravenous antibiotics are compounded to a nebulized form and delivered to the sinus mucosa through an aerosilezed machine. The choice of the nebulized antibiotic should be based on the results of a culture. Studies have shown an increase in disease-free intervals and greater 75% response over a 12-week follow-up period (35). Other medications, such as betamethasone, have been tried in an attempt to deliver a strong course of steroids topically and spare the patient from the harmful systemic side effects.

TOPICAL ANTIBIOTIC IRRIGATIONS

Topical preparations share a similar principle as the nebulized medications in that they represent an attempt to deliver intravenous preparations of antibiotics in a topical form directly to the diseased mucosa. Although these preparations are in widespread use, their use has not yet been well documented in the medical literature. Many of the commonly used preparations are directed at aerobic gram-negative organisms commonly seen in patients who have undergone previous surgery. Ceftazadime (36), gentamicin, and tobramycin are examples.

Tobramycin preparations have specifically been used in cystic fibrosis patients awaiting lung transplantation. The sinus and respiratory mucosa of these patients are frequently colonized with *Pseudomonas*. Transplant programs have used antibiotic irrigations as a preventive measure against colonization with *Pseudomonas* in patients awaiting a lung transplant (37). Studies examining the use of tobramycin irrigations in children with cystic fibrosis have shown a significant decrease in revision sinus procedures and polyp reformation (38).

Topical irrigations aimed at the treatment of *S. aureus* sinus infections have their foundation in the vascular access literature. Methicillin-resistant *S. aureus* has been increasingly recovered from infected sinuses following sinus surgery. Mupirocin and betadine nasal irrigations are often being utilized in an attempt to treat these patients without using intravenous antibiotics.

In addition to topical antibiotics, there are also other medications that have been used in a topical preparation in the treatment of CRS and nasal polyps. One case series demonstrated a decrease in the incidence of post-surgical recurrences of nasal polyps following the topical use of a diuretic (furosemide) (39). Antifungals are also used in a nasal irrigation. Amphotericin B has been shown in two prospective, non-controlled trials to decrease nasal polyps. These studies have a limited follow-up, but have shown the irrigations to be well tolerated and have demonstrated good subjective and objective results (40,41). Even though many of these studies were not randomized or compared to a control group, they show potential for the management of the difficult-to-treat patients, where the other options are much more invasive (i.e., intravenous antibiotics and/or revision surgery).

INTRAVENOUS ANTIBIOTICS

The use of intravenous antibiotics in the treatment of CRS has been traditionally reserved for orbital and/or intracranial complications of the disease process. Their use has been well-documented in the management of pediatric sinusitis as an alternative to sinus surgery, as well as the treatment of pediatric orbital complications from ethmoid sinusitis (42,43). Antibiotics that cross the blood–brain barrier are used in conjunction with surgical therapy in the management of epidural collections stemming from frontal sinusitis, and in the management of a Pott's puffy tumor or osteomyelitis of the frontal bone following an acute frontal sinus infection. At least a three-week course of a culture-based parenteral antibiotic is given. When indicated, this is followed, by an additional course of oral therapy to complete a total six weeks, of therapy. If a culture is unavailable, broad-spectrum antibiotics such as a combination of clindamycin or metronidazole with a fourth generation cephalosporin (cefepime or ceftazidime) or single therapy with a carbapenem (i.e., imipenem, meropenem) provide coverage for both anaerobes and aerobes. There are some who are advocating the use of intravenous antibiotics in patients with CRS for patients who have either had unsuccessful surgery, or who have refused surgery, and base their rationale on comparing the disease process of this condition to that of osteomyelitis (44).

There is both clinical and experimental evidence to suggest that the bone underlying the diseased sinus mucosa is involved in CRS. In experimentally induced sinusitis with *P. aeruginosa* using an animal model, Bolger et al. (45) demonstrated bone changes as early as four days after infection of a maxillary sinus. These changes included a coordinated osteoclasis and appositional bone formation adjacent to the sinus, as well as subsequent intramembranous bone formation.

Clinical experience with computed tomography and nasal endoscopy has shown bone to undergo resorption followed by subsequent hyperostosis. In addition, studies have shown that ethmoid bone underwent rapid remodeling in CRS that was histologically identical to the remodeling seen in osteomyelitis (46).

Follow-up studies have demonstrated that rabbits inoculated with bacterial organisms develop CRS and have histological evidence of chronic osteomyelitis (47,48). It appears that inflammation spreads through widened Haversian canal system within the bone and can spread to involve the opposite side. This may help to explain the recalcitrance of severe CRS to medical and surgical therapy, and the clinical observation for tendency of disease persistence in localized areas until the underlying bone is removed.

The translation of this research to clinical use where intravenous antimicrobial therapy was given to patients with CRS has not been as persuasive. The studies published so far have largely been uncontrolled, non-randomized case series of a limited number of patients. The majority of indications are for recalcitrant infections resistant to oral antibiotics. The efficacy of the treatment varies among the studies (29–89%), but they are uniform in their relative high rate of complications (14–26%) (49,50) and have resulted in a relapse rate of 89% at a mean follow-up of 11.5 weeks in one study (51). They range from the benign, such as diarrhea, to the serious and life-threatening, such as septic thrombophlebitis and neutropenia (52). Until more studies are performed, intravenous antibiotic use should be reserved for those select cases in which orbital and/or intracranial complications arise, or in a chronic infection in which there are no other oral antibiotic alternatives.

ASPIRIN DESENSITIZATION

The classic Samter's triad consists of nasal polyps, asthma, and sensitivity to aspirin or NSAIDS that exacerbates the above conditions. Recognition of this disease is not always easily made, since there can be a lag time between presentation of the components of the triad. Studies of these patients have shown that an increase in serum leukotrienes with response to aspirin (ASA) provocation that has a direct result in eosinophil recruitment with subsequent polyp formation and airway remodeling. Clinically, these patients are difficult-to-treat, and do relatively poorly following surgery as compared to non-ASA sensitive patients.

ASA desensitization is the slow introduction of aspirin in a controlled, monitored setting. In vitro studies have shown a subsequent decrease in serum leukotrienes to normal levels one year following aspirin desensitization (53). Clinical studies have shown significant reductions in prednisone requirements, polyp reformation, and improvement in pulmonary function in follow-up as long as six years (54). Patients are often asked to take 650 mg twice a day for improved nasal breathing, but only 81 mg is required to maintain a desensitized state.

CONCLUSION

The recognition of CRS as a disease of both inflammation and infection is the first key step in its medical management. There are multiple choices of antibiotics and anti-inflammatory agents, and a combination of both is needed for an extended period of time. Infections following sinus surgery are even more difficult to treat, and antibiotic coverage should be based on an endoscopically guided culture. There are currently more alternatives to conventional therapy in these patients in which medications can be applied topically to the diseased mucosa.

REFERENCES

1. Benninger MS, Holzer SE, Lau J. Diagnosis and treatment of uncomplicated acute bacterial rhinosinusitis: summary of the Agency for Health Care Policy and Research evidence-based report. Otolaryngol Head Neck Surg 2000; 122:1–7.
2. Senior B, Glaze C, Benninger MS. Use of the rhinosinusitis disability index in rhinologic disease. Am J Rhinol 2001; 15:15–20.
3. Benninger MS, Ferguson BJ, Hadley JA, et al. Adult chronic rhinosinusitis: definitions, diagnosis, epidemiology, and pathophysiology. Otolaryngol Head Neck Surg 2003; 129:S1–S32.

4. Taghizadeh F, Hadley JA, Osguthorpe JD. Pharmacological treatments for rhinosinusitis. Expert Opin 2002; 3:305–313.
5. Ponikau JU, Sherris DA, Kern EB, et al. The diagnosis and incidence of allergic fungal sinusitis. Mayo Clin Proc 1999; 74:877–884.
6. Bernstein JM, Ballow M, Schlievert PM, et al. A superantigen hypothesis for the pathogenesis of chronic hyperplastic sinusitis with massive nasal polyposis. Am J Rhinol 2003; 17:321–326.
7. Bolger WE, Leonard D, Dick EJ, et al. Gram negative sinusitis: a bacteriologic and histologic study in rabbits. Am J Rhinol 1997; 11:15–25.
8. Kaliner MA, Osguthorpe JD, Fireman P, et al. Sinusitis: bench to bedside. Current findings, future directions. Otolaryngol Head Neck Surg 1997; 116:S1–S20.
9. Gwaltney JM. Acute community-acquired sinusitis. Clin Infect Dis 1996; 23: 1209–1225.
10. Brook I. Microbiology and management of sinusitis. J Otolaryngol 1996; 25:249–256.
11. Finegold SM, Flynn MJ, Rose FV, et al. Bacteriologic findings associated with chronic maxillary sinusitis in adults. Clin Infect Dis 2002; 35:428–433.
12. Brook I, Yocum P, Frazier EH. Bacteriology and β-lactamase activity in acute and chronic maxillary sinusitis. Arch Otolaryngol Head Neck Surg 1996; 122:418–422.
13. Nadel DM, Lanza DC, Kennedy DW. Endoscopically guided cultures in chronic sinusitis. Am J Rhinol 1998; 12:233–241.
14. Brook I, Frazier EH, Foote PA. Microbiology of chronic maxillary sinusitis: comparison between specimens obtained by sinus endoscopy and by surgical drainage. J Med Microbiol 1997; 46:430–432.
15. Brook I, Thompson DH, Frazier EH. Microbiology and management of chronic maxillary sinusitis. Arch Otolaryngol Head Neck Surg 1994; 120:1317–1320.
16. Brook I. Microbiology and antimicrobial management of sinusitis. Otolaryngol Clin North Am 2004; 37:253–266.
17. Brook I, Yocum P. Antimicrobial management of chronic sinusitis in children. J Laryngol Otol 1995; 109:1159–1162.
18. Wallwork B, Coman W, Feron F, et al. Clarithromycin and prednisolone inhibit cytokine production in chronic rhinosinusitis. Laryngoscope 2002; 112:1827–1830.
19. Moriyama H, Yanagi K, Ohtori N, et al. Evaluation of endoscopic sinus surgery for chronic sinusitis: post-operative erythromycin therapy. Rhinology 1995; 33:166–170.
20. Clerico DM. Medical treatment of chronic sinus disease. In: Diseases of the Sinuses. London: BC Dekker, 2001.
21. Schleimer RP. Glucocorticoids: their mechanism of action and use in allergic diseases. Allergy: Principles and Practice. Mosby 2003; 912–914.
22. Nuutinen J, Ruoppi P, Suonpaa J. One dose beclomethasone dipropionate aerosol in the treatment of seasonal allergic rhinitis. A preliminary report. Rhinology 1987; 25:121–127.
23. Chalton R, Mackay I, Wilson R, Cole P. Double blind placebo controlled trial of betamethasone nasal drops for nasal polyposis. Br Med J Clin Res Educ 1985; 291:788.

24. Mygand N. Effects of corticosteroid therapy in non-allergic rhinosinusitis. Acta Otolaryngol 1996; 116:164–166.
25. Damm M, Jungehulsing M, Eckel HE, et al. Effects of systemic steroid treatment in chronic polypoid rhinosinusitis evaluated with magnetic resonance imaging. Otolaryngol Head Neck Surg 1999; 120:517–523.
26. Radack K, Deck CC. Are oral decongestants safe in hypertension? An evaluation of the evidence and a framework for assessing clinical trials. Ann Allergy 1986; 56:396–401.
27. Wawrose SF, Tami TA, Amoils CP. The role of guaifenesin in the treatment of sinonasal disease in patients infected with the human immunodeficiency virus (HIV). Laryngoscope 1992; 102:1225–1228.
28. Brown SL, Graham SG. Nasal irrigations: good or bad? Curr Opin Otolaryngol Head Neck Surg 2004; 12:9–13.
29. Rabago D, Zgierska A, Mundt M, et al. Efficacy of daily hypertonic saline nasal irrigation among patients with sinusitis: a randomized controlled trial. J Fam Pract 2002; 51:1049–1055.
30. Riccioni G, Santilli F, D'Orazio F. The role of anti-leukotrienes in the treatment of asthma. Int J Immunopathol Pharmacol 2002; 15:171–182.
31. Parnes SM, Chuma AV. Acute effects on anti-leukotrienes on sinonasal polyposis and sinusitis. Ear Nose Throat J 2000; 79:18–20.
32. Nadel DM, Lanza DC, Kennedy DW. Endoscopically guided cultures in chronic sinusitis. Am J Rhinol 1998; 12:233–241.
33. Kobayashi T, Baba S. Topical use of antibiotics for chronic sinusitis. Rhinol Suppl 1992; 14:477–481.
34. Klepser ME. Role of nebulized antibiotics for the treatment of respiratory infections. Curr Opin Infect Dis 2004; 17:109–112.
35. Cole PJ. The role of nebulized antibiotics in treating serious resp infections. J Chemother 2001; 13:354–362.
36. Vaughan WC, Carvalho GC. Use of nebulized antibiotics for acute infections in chronic sinusitis. Otolaryngol Head Neck Surg 2002; 127:558–568.
37. Leonard DW, Bolger WE. Topical antibiotic therapy for recalcitrant sinusitis. Laryngoscope 1999; 109:668–670.
38. Davidson TM, Murphy C, Mitchell M, et al. Management of chronic sinusitis in cystic fibrosis. Laryngoscope 1995; 105:354–358.
39. Moss RB, King VV. Management of sinusitis in cystic fibrosis by endoscopic surgery and serial antimicrobial lavage. Reduction in recurrence requiring surgery. Arch Otolaryngol Head Neck Surg 1995; 121:566–572.
40. Passali D, Mezzedimi C, Passali GC, et al. Efficacy of inhalation form of furosemide to prevent postsurgical relapses of rhinosinusal polyposis. J Otorhinolaryngol Rel Spec 2000; 62:307–310.
41. Ricchetti A, Landis BN, Maffioli A, et al. Effect of anti-fungal nasal lavage with amphotericin B on nasal polyposis. J Laryngol Otol 2002; 116(4):261–263.
42. Ponikau JU, Sherris DA, Kita H, Kern EB. Intranasal antifungal treatment in 51 patients with chronic rhinosinusitis. J Allergy Clin Immunol 2002; 110(6):862–866.
43. Buchaman CA, Yellon RF, Bluestone CD. Alternative to endoscopic sinus surgery in the management of pediatric chronic rhinosinusitis refractory to oral antimicrobial therapy. Otolaryngol Head Neck Surg 1999; 120:219–224.

44. Sobol SE, Marchand J, Tewfik TL. Orbital complications of sinusitis in children. J Otolaryngol 2002; 31:131–136.
45. Anand V, Levine H, Friedman M, et al. Intravenous antibiotics for refractory rhinosinusitis in nonsurgical patients: preliminary findings of a prospective study. Am J Rhinol 2003; 17:363–368.
46. Bolger WE, Leonard D, Dick EJ, et al. Gram negative sinusitis: a bacteriologic and histologic study in rabbits. Am J Rhinol 1997; 11:15–25.
47. Hwang P, Montone KT, Gannon FH, et al. Applications of in situ hybridization techniques in the diagnosis of chronic sinusitis. Am J Rhinol 1999; 13: 335–338.
48. Khalid AN, Hunt J, Perloff JR, Kennedy DW. The role of bone in chronic rhinosinusitis. Laryngoscope 2002; 112(11):1951–1957.
49. Perloff JR, Gannon FH, Bolger WE, et al. Bone involvement in sinusitis: an apparent pathway for the spread of disease. Laryngoscope 2000; 110:2095–2099.
50. Don DM, Yellon FR, Casselbrant ML, et al. Efficacy of a stepwise protocol that includes intravenous antibiotic therapy for the management of chronic sinusitis in children and adolescents. Arch Otolaryngol Head Neck Surg 2001; 127:1093–1098.
51. Gross ND, McInnes RJ, Hwang PH. Outpatient intravenous antibiotics for chronic rhinosinusitis. Laryngoscope 2002; 112:1758–1761.
52. Fowler KC, Duncavage JA, Murray JJ, et al. Chronic sinusitis and intravenous antibiotic therapy: resolution, recurrent and adverse events. J Allergy Clin Immunol 2003; 111:s85.
53. Tanner SB, Fowler KC. Intravenous antibiotics for chronic rhinosinusitis: are they effective? Curr Opin Otolaryngol Head Neck Surg 2004; 12:3–8.
54. Gosepath J, Schaefer D, Amedee RG, et al. Individual monitoring of aspirin desensitization. Arch Otolaryngol Head Neck Surg 2001; 127:316–321.
55. Stevenson DD, Hankammer MA, Mathison DA, et al. Aspirin densensitization treatment of aspirin sensitive patients with rhinosinusitis-asthma: long-term outcomes. J Allergy Clin Immunol 1996; 98:751–758.

12

Surgical Management

David Lewis

*Department of Otolaryngology, Harvard Medical School,
Massachusetts Eye and Ear Infirmary, Boston, Massachusetts, U.S.A.*

Nicolas Y. Busaba

*Department of Otolaryngology, Harvard Medical School, VA Boston Healthcare
System, Massachusetts Eye and Ear Infirmary, Boston, Massachusetts, U.S.A.*

INTRODUCTION

The surgical treatment of sinus disease has changed dramatically over the past 20 years in the United States and nearly 30 years in Europe. In the past, otolaryngologists relied on using the nasal speculum and a headlight to diagnose and treat diseases of the nasal cavity and paranasal sinuses. Such an examination only allowed for viewing of the anterior components of the nose, and the observer was unable to adequately view the paranasal sinuses or their ostia. For improved visualization and more thorough treatment, open approaches were the only option. There has also been a conceptual shift away from attempting to surgically exenterate the disease within the paranasal sinuses to simply opening specific areas in order to improve sinus function and allow better aeration and drainage. The amount of tissue removed during sinus surgery is minimized now, and the surgeon relies on opening key functional areas to restore the normal physiology within the paranasal sinuses, which thereby helps to reverse the disease.

Since the introduction of nasal endoscopes, the diagnosis and the treatment of sinus disease have changed remarkably. One now has the ability to view the anatomy of the nasal cavity, and at times, the paranasal

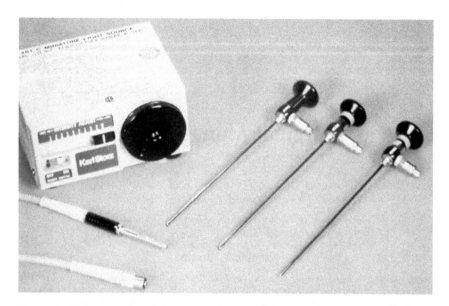

Figure 1 Light source and three 4-mm diameter rigid endoscopes. The endoscopes have a zero, 30-degree, and 70-degree viewing angles.

sinuses themselves, up close and with remarkable detail (Fig. 1). Nasal endoscopes use fiberoptic light cables to transmit light into the nose. Special optical lenses are used for improved viewing. There are both flexible and rigid endoscopes; the latter are available in many different angled optics systems. These scopes allow for excellent visualization of the entire nasal cavity, both in the office and in the operating room, and all of the key paranasal sinus ostia that are involved in sinus disease. The cameras attach to the eyepiece of the endoscope, allow for easy viewing on a television monitor, and also offer the added advantage of using endoscopes for video recording to demonstrate anatomy and pathology to patients in the office, and for teaching purposes.

DIAGNOSTIC WORK-UP

Medical History

When a patient with sinus complaints is referred to the otolaryngologist, the evaluation always begins with a thorough history followed by a careful examination of the nose. (Please refer to the chapter on Clinical Presentation and Diagnosis for a more detailed review on the evaluation of a patient with sinus disease). The patient should be asked about symptoms of facial pain or pressure over individual sinuses, headache, nasal blockage, rhinorrhea, postnasal drip, and hyposmia (Table 1). It is very important to ask

Table 1 Medical History

Symptoms
    Facial pain or pressure
    Headache
    Nasal blockage
    Rhinorrhea
    Post-nasal drip
    Hyposmia and/or hypogeusia
Previous treatment attempts
    Antibiotics
    Steroids
    Antihistamines
    Allergen avoidance
    Previous sinus surgery
Past medical and surgical history
Other medications
Drug allergies
Environmental allergies
Social history including tobacco smoke exposure
Family history
Review of systems

about previous attempts at medical management. What antibiotics have been used to treat the symptoms and for how long were they used? Did they improve the symptoms? Is the patient a smoker or exposed to passive smoke or other irritants? Does the patient have an allergic component to the disease process? If so, have these issues been maximally treated medically with antihistamines, nasal steroids, or other medications? Is the patient a candidate for immunotherapy? Is allergen avoidance a realistic possibility for the patient? What other comorbidities does the patient have? These questions are important to ensure that all patients have been given the most optimal attempt at medical management prior to making any decisions about surgery.

Physical Examination

As part of the head and neck evaluation, a thorough nasal examination should be completed in the office. Anterior rhinoscopy using a headlight or mirror and a nasal speculum should be performed prior to any attempts at nasal decongestion. Any evidence of mucopurulent discharge, nasal polyps, enlarged turbinates, nasal septal deviation, or diseased mucosa should be noted. Using either a rigid or flexible endoscope, one can almost always view the middle meatus and the sphenoethmoid recess. Decongestion and anesthesia with a sprayed mixture of 4% lidocaine with phenylephrine

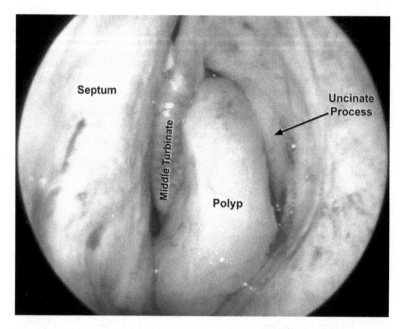

Figure 2 Endoscopic view of an inflammatory polyp in the left middle meatus.

facilitates this part of the examination. The findings noted on anterior rhinoscopy can be confirmed. Additionally, one might see limited areas of inflammation, mucopurulent discharge, and/or polypoid changes that could not be seen during the initial rhinoscopic examination (1) (Fig. 2).

Imaging

Based on the history and examination findings, a decision is made whether or not to obtain a computed tomography (CT) scan. Noncontrast CT scans, particularly in the coronal plane, can be very helpful both for diagnosis and pre-operative planning if surgery is indicated. CT scans can confirm sinusitis, and they can offer the surgeon valuable information about the patient's anatomy that can be used to help avoid complications during surgery. Occasionally, a CT scan can also be useful in ruling out sinus disease in a patient with convincing sinus complaints but no evidence of disease on exam. Additionally, the CT scan has become a valuable tool in image-guided sinus surgery (see following sections).

INDICATIONS FOR PARANASAL SINUS SURGERY

There is currently a wide range of indications for paranasal sinus surgery (Table 2). The most common indication is for chronic rhinosinusitis (CRS).

Table 2 Indications for Paranasal Sinus Surgery

1. Inflammatory or infectious rhinosinusitis
    Chronic rhinosinusitis that failed medical therapy
    Recurrent rhinosinusitis
    Symptomatic nasal polyposis
    Acute or chronic rhinosinusitis with periorbital or intracranial complications
    Invasive fungal sinusitis
    Fungus ball-mycetoma
2. Sinonasal neoplasm (benign and malignant)
3. Repair of skull base defects
    CSF rhinorrhea
    Menigoceles or meningoencephaloceles
4. Approach for excision of intracranial pathology
    Pituitary tumors
    Petrous apex cholesterol granuloma
5. Control of epistaxis
6. Orbital decompression for Graves' ophthalmopathy
7. Removal of sinus foreign bodies
8. Management of nasolacrimal duct obstruction

Patients who continue to have signs and symptoms of rhinosinusitis despite maximal medical therapy are often candidates for sinus surgery. Maximum medical therapy has not been standardized, but typically involves four to six weeks of broad-spectrum oral antibiotics used in conjunction with decongestants and mucolytic agents. Patients with allergies are often also given antihistamines and intranasal steroid sprays. Surgery may also be considered in patients who have repeated episodes of acute rhinosinusitis that clears with antibiotics. Although there is no agreed treatment algorithm for patients with recurrent rhinosinusitis, many rhinologists feel that if the frequency and severity of the patient's symptoms are sufficient to interfere significantly with school or work, then surgery is a reasonable option (2). Prior to surgery, it is important to rule out non-sinus causes of a patient's symptoms, i.e., atypical migraines or other neurologic causes including neuralgia.

Another indication for sinus surgery is to treat patients with symptomatic nasal polyposis. The pathophysiology of polyp formation is poorly understood. However, polyps are commonly associated with asthma and environmental allergies. On the other hand, it is not unusual to diagnose polyps in a patient without atopy or asthma. An antral-choanal polyp is such an example. Unfortunately, medical therapy is rarely sufficient to control nasal polyposis and surgery is often indicated. Patients should be counseled about the high recurrence following surgery. Special attention must be given to those patients with asthma, particularly those with aspirin-sensitivity (Samter's triad). These patients often require preoperative corticosteroids and maximal bronchodilator therapy to optimize their pulmonary status. The corticosteroids may also serve to shrink the polyps and possibly decrease their risk of recurrence. Aspirin-desensitization may also be beneficial in these patients. It is important to note that the differential diagnosis of nasal polyps includes some benign and malignant tumors. Hence, at the time of surgery, tissue specimens should be sent for permanent pathology in all cases. Unilateral disease, a rubbery or fleshy, highly vascular, or ulcerative appearance, or CT evidence of bone destruction should alert one to the possibility of a neoplasm.

In addition to the more common above-mentioned indications, sinus surgery can be performed to treat allergic fungal sinusitis and periorbital and intracranial complications of sinusitis; marsupialize muco(pyo)celes; control epistaxis; remove maxillary sinus foreign bodies; repair anterior skull base cerebrospinal fluid (CSF) leaks or meningo(encephalo)celes; decompress the orbit in patients with Graves' ophthalmopathy; dacrocystorhinostomy; approach and remove pituitary tumors, petrous apex cholesterol granulomas or other skull base lesions; resect benign neoplasms (osteomas, inverting papillomas, or fibrous dysplasia); and decompress the optic nerve (2).

CONTRAINDICATIONS FOR PARANASAL SINUS SURGERY

The only true contraindication to paranasal sinus surgery is the absence of sinus disease. Patients with migraine headaches or other neurological causes of facial pain should not be operated on. Additionally, surgery is not a substitute for medical management; patients with CRS, as mentioned above, should be given maximum medical therapy prior to being offered surgery. A bleeding disorder can place a patient at an increased risk for postoperative hemorrhage, but does not in itself represent a contraindication to surgery.

ENDOSCOPIC (ENDONASAL) SINUS SURGERY

The techniques for performing endoscopic sinus surgery were first described by Messerklinger during the 1970s. These techniques were later introduced into the United States during the mid-1980s by Kennedy, who coined the term "Functional Endoscopic Sinus Surgery" (FESS) to describe a minimally invasive approach to improve drainage of the paranasal sinuses for the treatment of CRS (3–6). Endoscopic endonasal surgery (EES) or endoscopic sinus surgery (ESS) are other terms commonly used to describe the same operation and can be used interchangeably.

FESS involves opening up narrow areas within the nose and paranasal sinuses that are responsible for the pathological changes seen in CRS. Messerklinger studied patterns of mucociliary clearance and noted that in narrow areas of mucosal contact, mucociliary clearance was disrupted (6,7). When this occurs, the mucus becomes either stagnant or recirculated

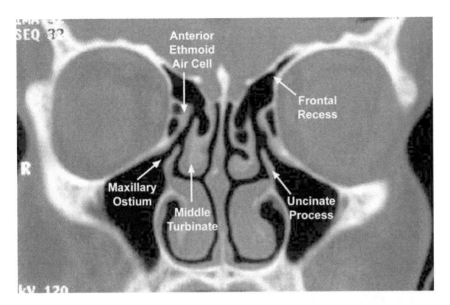

Figure 3 CT image (coronal projection) through the ostiomeatal unit (OMU).

within the affected sinus rather than freely draining into the nasal cavity and nasopharynx. Stagnant or recirculated mucus predisposes the patient to infection, which leads to inflammation that further impedes mucociliary clearance, resulting in increased infection followed by more inflammation, and then a vicious cycle ensues.

The two primary areas of narrowing that can impair mucociliary clearance and lead to problems with CRS are the ethmoidal infundibulum and the frontal recess. These two anatomical points of narrowing are both located in the anterior ethmoid area within the middle meatus. Many rhinologists use the term osteomeatal complex (OMC) or osteomeatal unit (OMU) to describe this functional area where narrowing can occur (Fig. 3). The ethmoidal infundibulum is a three-dimensional space that is a convergence point for mucus flowing from the anterior ethmoid air cells, the maxillary sinus, and the frontal sinus (8). Similarly, the frontal recess is a narrow area in which mucus from the frontal sinus must pass prior to reaching the ethmoidal infundibulum (1,6–8). This area can be further narrowed by projections from the most anterior of the ethmoid air cells, the agger nasi cells (Fig. 4). FESS aims at opening up these two key areas of narrowing to allow adequate drainage of the frontal, anterior ethmoid, and maxillary sinuses. When widespread disease affects all paranasal sinuses, ESS can be tailored to treat all the involved areas.

There are two primary goals of FESS. The first is to open up the narrow areas described above. The second is to perform the surgery in as

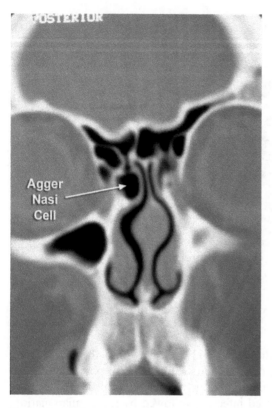

Figure 4 CT image (coronal projection) showing a right agger nasi cell.

atraumatic a manner as possible (1,6–8). Accordingly, sinus surgeons must remove the anatomical areas of obstruction without disturbing the surrounding healthy mucosa. In order to open a narrowed ostiomeatal complex, a thin piece of bone called the uncinate process is carefully removed in its entirety. Additionally, an ethmoid air cell called the ethmoid bulla is typically removed to allow better drainage (Fig. 3). Any further removal of tissue is dependent on the extent of disease. Some believe that an uncinectomy with an ethmoid bullectomy is all that is necessary during FESS and coined the term minimally invasive sinus technique (MIST) (9). The majority of rhinologists recommend a more complete ethmoidectomy in addition to widening of the maxillary ostium and opening of the frontal recess cells. All agree, however, that any diseased mucosa that is not a direct component of the osteomeatal complex should not be removed or manipulated because this surrounding area of disease will eventually revert to normal once there is a wide open area for drainage and aeration (8). In other words, one does not need to strip away all of the diseased mucosa because paranasal sinus

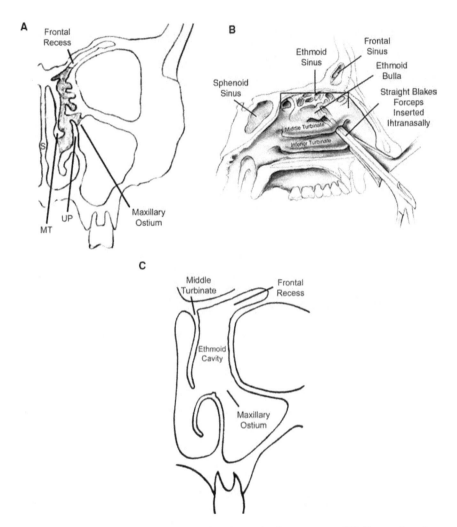

Figure 5 Schematic representation of endoscopic sinus surgery. (**A**) Coronal projection through the OMU. The shaded area represents the ethmoid sinus. (**B**) Schematic drawing of the procedure. (**C**) Ethmoid sinus cavity at the end of surgery with patent maxillary antrostomy and frontal recess. Note that the uncinate process has been removed. *Abbreviations*: UP, uncinate process; MT, middle turbinate; S, septum.

mucosal pathology can be reversed by improving the ventilation and drainage of the involved sinus (Fig. 5).

By minimizing mucosal disruption, one can minimize postoperative scarring. This is very important because some areas of scar tissue formation can be devoid of the respiratory epithelium required for mucociliary clearance. If there are large areas of scar, then mucus will stagnate. Additionally, mucosal

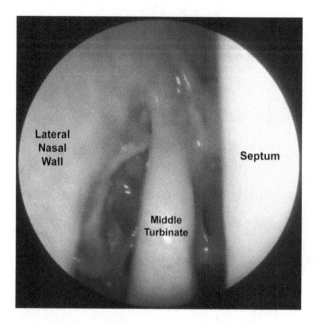

Figure 6 Adhesions in a right ethmoid cavity in a patient with previous endoscopic ethmoidectomy.

disruption with scarring often results in fibrous adhesions that can re-obstruct the drainage of mucus resulting in recurrence of sinus disease (Fig. 6). In these instances, a revision surgery may be required.

The role of several anatomical findings that are noted on CT or nasal endoscopy in the pathophysiology of rhinosinusitis is controversial (10). These include Haller cells, agger nasi cells, concha bullosa, and paradoxical middle turbinate. A Haller cell is an ethmoidal cell that is located along the floor of the orbit and can narrow the maxillary outflow tract (Fig. 7). An agger nasi cell is the anterior-most cell of the ethmoid sinus and may represent pneumatization of the lacrimal bone. Agger nasi cells can narrow the frontal recess (Fig. 4). A concha bullosa is a pneumatized middle turbinate. When large, it can conceivably narrow the OMU (Fig. 8). A paradoxical middle turbinate is convex along its lateral wall instead of the medial wall (Fig. 9). Similar to a concha bullosa, a paradoxical middle turbinate can narrow the OMU. All of the above-mentioned anatomical findings are very prevalent and may be better labeled as anatomical variants, not anomalies. Surgery is not indicated to treat them in the absence of clinical rhinosinusitis. On the other hand, these anatomical findings need to be addressed during ESS that is indicated to treat CRS.

The concept of OMU is valid when the pathophysiology of the CRS is believed to be infectious. More recent theories about the pathogenesis of

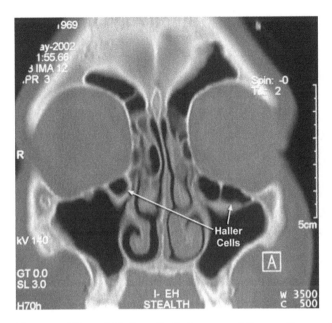

Figure 7 Bilateral Haller cells that narrowed the maxillary outflow tract as seen on a CT scan (coronal projection).

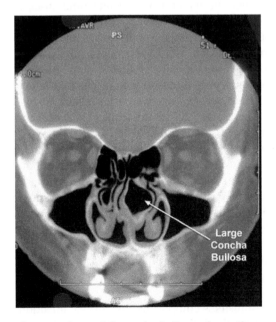

Figure 8 Large left concha bullosa. A smaller concha bullosa can be seen on the right side. (CT scan; coronal projection).

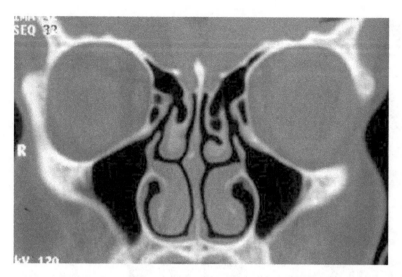

Figure 9 Paradoxical left middle turbinate. Note that the middle turbinate is convex on the lateral surface.

rhinosinusitis stress the role of inflammation as the primary event, i.e., rhinosinusitis is primarily an inflammatory and not an infectious disease. The inflammation is believed to be predominantly caused by the inflammatory mediators that are released by eosinophils, usually in response to the presence of fungi or other superantigens in the nose or sinus mucus (eosinophilic CRS) (11,12). In such a case, the role of ESS is to reduce the offending antigen load by allowing repeated cleaning of inspissated mucus from the sinus cavities in the office by opening their ostia, which in turn can reduce the inflammation. Therefore, ESS in this clinical scenario has a complementary function, and is not a substitute to medical therapy.

The patients who undergo ESS typically are given perioperative antibiotics. Coverage is aimed at preventing acute infection by normal flora that has pathogenic potential, such as *Staphylococcus aureus, Streptococcus pneumoniae, Haemophilus influenzae,* or alpha streptococci. A common choice for an antibiotic would be a first-generation cephalosporin, such as cephalexin. Other choices include clindamycin or azithromycin, the former of which covers anaerobes as well. It should be noted that although there are data to support the use of perioperative antibiotics for other types of surgery, there is no proven benefit to the use of postoperative prophylactic antibiotics after ESS (13,14).

When inflammatory rhinosinusits is complicated by chronic infection, at least 2 weeks of culture driven antibiotics may be used perioperatively in order to decrease intraoperative bleeding.

The majority of ESSs can be done on an outpatient basis. The surgery typically takes between 45 minutes and two hours to perform, depending on the extent of surgery. Although this rarely is a painful surgery, patients are sent home with a prescription for analgesics, which at times contain a narcotic. However, many patients only require regular acetaminophen for analgesia. Like in any other surgery, patients are instructed that they must avoid aspirin and nonsteroidal anti-inflammatory medications for two weeks prior to and at least one week after surgery. Patients can often return to work after a couple of days; however, they are advised to avoid physical exertion for one to two weeks. Additionally, they are instructed to avoid hot liquids and spicy foods to prevent intranasal vasodilation that might result in epistaxis.

Postoperative care is of utmost importance. In order to prevent recurrence of the disease secondary to scarring, patients must return for intranasal debridements on a routine basis for up to six weeks after surgery. If intranasal packing was placed for hemostasis, it can be removed on the first postoperative day. Any material that may have been used to stent open the middle meatus is typically removed at the first or second office visit. If adhesions are found between the middle turbinate and lateral nasal wall or restenosis is noted of the maxillary antrostomy or frontal recess at any point during routine follow up, this can often be successfully treated under local anesthesia in the office. Additionally, irrigation is a very effective method that patients can use at home to remove crusts and clots. Many surgeons have their patients started on saline irrigations immediately after surgery and continue irrigating until the healing process is complete. Using a combination of nasal irrigation and in-office debridements, one can often prevent complications that might otherwise have resulted in recurrence of disease and the need for revision surgery (8,15).

COMPLICATIONS OF ENDOSCOPIC SINUS SURGERY

When sinus surgery is performed by experienced surgeons who have a detailed knowledge of sinus anatomy, complications are extremely rare. However, complications can and do occasionally occur, even with the most seasoned of surgeons (Table 3). A small amount of bleeding is expected postoperatively. Nasal packing, and, at times, hemostasis in the operating room can control major bleeding. Postoperative infection is uncommon. When an infection does occur, office debridement and an oral antibiotic which is determined by culture of the sinus cavity are usually sufficient treatment. As mentioned above, scarring with adhesions and restenosis of ostia can occur. If the office-based treatments fail, then these patients may require a revision surgery.

The paranasal sinuses are surrounded by a number of important structures, which can be potentially injured during sinus surgery. Injury to the anterior skull base can result in a CSF leak. If this is identified during

Table 3 Complications

Bleeding
Infection
Adhesions
Restenosis
CSF leak
Periorbital hematoma
Subcutaneous emphysema
Diplopia
Blindness
Epiphora

---

surgery, then it can be repaired at the time of the incident. If a CSF leak is noted postoperatively, then the patient is placed on bed rest with the head elevated, either with or without placement of a lumbar drain depending on the severity of the leak. These leaks may close spontaneously. Those that do not close can be repaired via either an endoscopic or an open approach, the latter being performed by a neurosurgeon (8,16). Injury to the medial wall of the orbit can result in a retro-orbital hematoma, diplopia, subcutaneous orbital emphysema, or blindness. If the lamina papyracea and periorbita are entered, then blood can accumulate in the orbit. Usually this only results in periorbital ecchymosis; however, patients must be closely monitored for signs of increased intraocular pressure. An ophthalmologist should be consulted immediately because an elevated intraocular pressure for a prolonged interval causes ischemia to the optic nerve, which can result in blindness. Direct injury to the optic nerve along the superior-lateral wall of the sphenoid sinus or posterior aspect of the lamina papyracea (in the region of annulus of Zinn) can similarly cause blindness. The presence of an Onodi cell (a posterior ethmoid air cell that is lateral and at times posterior to the sphenoid sinus) is associated with an increased incidence of optic nerve injury since the nerve may be dehiscent and pass through the cell. Such an anatomic variant can be detected on a preoperative CT (Fig. 10). Blindness can also rarely result from the dissection of local anesthetic containing decongestants (epinephrine) towards the orbital apex, which can cause spasm of the central retinal artery. Diplopia can occur if inadvertent entry into the orbit results in injury to the medial rectus muscle or violation of the periorbita that results in extensive herniation of intraorbital fat. Subcutaneous orbital emphysema occurs if there is injury to the lamina papyracea and the patient inadvertently performs a Valsalva maneuver during vomiting, sneezing, or nose blowing, which usually resolves spontaneously.

Damage to the nasolacrimal duct may occur following sinus surgery, resulting in epiphora and possibly dacrocystitis. The nasolacrimal duct runs

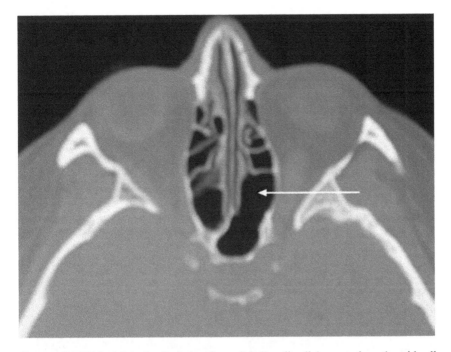

Figure 10 CT (axial projection) showing a left Onodi cell (a posterior ethmoid cell that extends lateral and at times posterior to the sphenoid sinus).

anterior to the anteromedial wall of the maxillary sinus. Hence, an aggressive anterior maxillary antrostomy can accidentally damage this duct as it travels to the inferior meatus (8,16).

Fortunately, these complications are very uncommon. However, patients must be aware of and understand the implications of each of these complications prior to consenting to any form of sinus surgery.

IMAGE GUIDANCE SYSTEMS

The advent of image-guided sinus surgery has had a dramatic impact on ESS. Although it is not a substitute for experience and anatomical knowledge, image-guided surgery has allowed rhinologists to perform challenging and complicated endoscopic procedures with increased confidence and precision. Image guidance systems consist of a computer workstation that displays three-dimensional images of the patient's paranasal sinuses using information obtained from preoperative CT scans. Either an infrared or an electromagnetic signal is used to track the position of a probe or surgical instrument relative to the patient's head (17). Hence, a surgeon can place the tip of an instrument on, for example, the middle turbinate, and see a

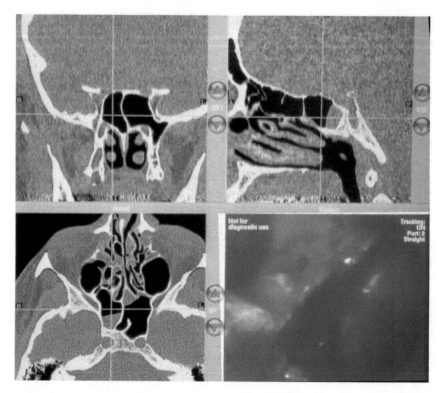

Figure 11   Image guidance system. Right upper, left upper, and left lower images are sagittal, coronal, and axial projections of CT scan with the cross-hairs indicating the position of the probe during surgery. The probe is inside the right sphenoid sinus. The right lower image shows a simultaneous endoscopic view into the sphenoid sinus.

real-time representation of the probe in coronal, axial, and sagittal planes. This can be done to within 2 mm of accuracy (18–20). They can, therefore, be used to confirm certain anatomical locations that are of interest to the surgeon, for example, the lamina papyracea, the skull base, the frontal recess, the sphenoid sinus, or any other area accessible by the probe (Fig. 11). This is particularly helpful in revision cases where the normal anatomical landmarks are obscured. The major limitations to widespread use of this technology are the increased cost and operative time that it requires (18).

MICRODEBRIDERS AND SINUS SURGERY

Mechanical debriders are becoming more and more popular in the field of ESS. These powered instruments precisely shave tissue using an oscillating burr connected to a suction machine (Fig. 12). When used correctly, these mechanical microdebriders can minimize trauma to the tissues and help to

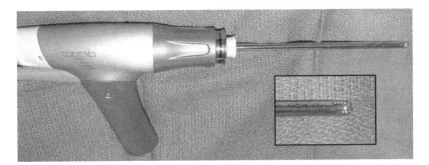

Figure 12 A picture of a microdebrider (Diego Microdebrider; Xomed, USA). The insert is a magnified view of the tip of the microdebrider showing its serrated edges ("aggressive cutter"), which has a 4 mm diameter tip.

preserve normal tissue. In contrast, the use of traditional endoscopic instruments can occasionally tear or strip away healthy mucosa leaving exposed bone, which results in increased crusting and risk of scarring (21,22). The microdebrider can remove diseased tissue quickly and efficiently, which is particularly helpful in cases of nasal polyposis when there can be profuse intraoperative bleeding. The main disadvantages to this technology are the cost, the slightly increased set-up time required, and the repeated clogging of the instrument by the resected tissue. Additionally, aggressive use of a microdebrider through an iatrogenic or disease-related dehiscence of the lamina papyracea or fovea ethmoidalis (roof of the ethmoid sinus) can lead to injury of intraorbital or intracranial structures, respectively.

TYPES OF PARANASAL SINUS SURGERY

The type of surgery performed on a patient depends on the extent and nature of the disease. Now that ESS has become the standard of care for the surgical management of uncomplicated CRS, open approaches to the sinuses are utilized far less often than in the past. Nonetheless, many open procedures are still indicated in select cases. Additionally, there are instances when only a single paranasal sinus needs to be surgically addressed. This section describes the various surgical approaches specific to each individual paranasal sinus.

Maxillary Sinus Surgery

Antral Puncture and Lavage

This procedure takes approximately 10 minutes and can be performed under local anesthesia via two approaches: the canine fossa or the inferior meatus. In the first approach, a small stab incision is made in the upper gingivobuccal sulcus and the anterior bony wall of the maxillary sinus is then entered. In

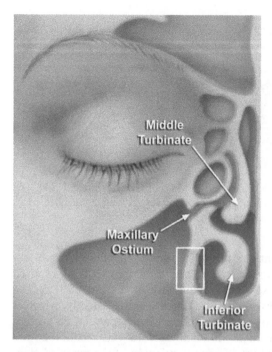

Figure 13 Schematic representation of the right maxillary sinus. The white rectangle represents the area in the inferior meatus where antral puncture or inferior nasoantral window is performed.

the latter approach, the thin bone of the medial maxillary wall is punctured in the inferior meatus (Fig. 13). Either approach can be performed under local anesthesia. The maxillary sinus cavity may then be aspirated and the contents sent for microbiology. The cavity can also be irrigated (lavage) with saline or antibiotic-containing solution. This procedure is indicated for symptomatic relief of acute maxillary sinusitis or for obtaining a culture to guide in the choice of an antimicrobial, usually in the ICU setting or with immunocompromised patients. The main disadvantages are the discomfort and the risk of bleeding.

Inferior Nasoantral Window

The technique is similar to antral puncture through the inferior meatus (Fig. 13). However, in this instance, a wider opening is created in the medial wall of the maxillary sinus to allow for permanent drainage and aeration. The procedure can be performed under local or general anesthesia. This procedure can be particularly helpful in patients with congenital or acquired ciliary dyskinesia since it provides for gravitational drainage of the maxillary sinus secretions. However, there is a high incidence of stenosis or complete closure of the window. In addition, maxillary sinus disease may persist despite a patent inferior nasoantral window since the mucociliary clearance drives the mucus towards the natural ostium and that may still be obstructed.

Endoscopic Middle Meatal Antrostomy

As mentioned earlier in this chapter, ESS has become the mainstay of surgical treatment of both chronic and recurrent maxillary rhinosinusitis. In order to gain endoscopic access to the maxillary sinus, one must surgically remove the uncinate process in order to open up the ethmoidal infundibulum. Once this is done, the natural maxillary sinus ostium can typically be seen. This can be enlarged if necessary through the posterior fontanelle (Fig. 14). Obstructive anatomic abnormalities, such as Haller cells, can also be addressed. This is usually sufficient to treat the maxillary disease without the need for stripping the maxillary sinus mucosa. Establishing adequate aeration and drainage of the maxillary sinus by opening its natural ostium can reverse the disease in the sinus mucosa. This technique is also utilized to remove mycotic "fungus balls" or symptomatic mucus retention cysts, marsupialize muco(pyo)celes of the maxillary sinus, and excise antrochoanal polyps (23,24) (Fig. 15). In the latter cases, a 30-degree or a 70-degree rigid endoscope is used to view the entirety of the maxillary sinus cavity to ensure complete excision, which reduces recurrence. The main advantages in using an endoscopic approach is that it avoids the need for an incision, it is relatively quick, and often can be performed on an outpatient basis. The primary disadvantage is the risk of being unable to fully remove disease in the most lateral recesses of the sinus or along its floor. This is particularly relevant during excision antrochoanal polyp or maxillary sinus retention cyst where recurrences following endoscopic approach can be up to 50% (24). For this reason, many surgeons will often consent select patients for a Caldwell-Luc procedure (see following section) in case an endoscopic approach does not provide adequate exposure to sufficiently treat the disease. Clinical failures of middle meatal antrostomy can be attributed to ciliary dyskinesia or to its occlusion by scar tissue. Optimal postoperative care with office endoscopic debridement in the immediate postoperative period can prevent adhesions in the middle meatus and hence occlusion of the antrostomy.

Caldwell-Luc Procedure

The Caldwell-Luc procedure has been used for over a hundred years to gain access to the maxillary sinus. The Caldwell-Luc procedure involves opening up the anterior wall of the maxillary sinus through the upper gingivobuccal sulcus. A flap of gingiva and periosteum is used to obtain access to the sinus. Unlike the endoscopic approach, the maxillary sinus mucosa is typically stripped and removed during a Caldwell-Luc operation. The procedure

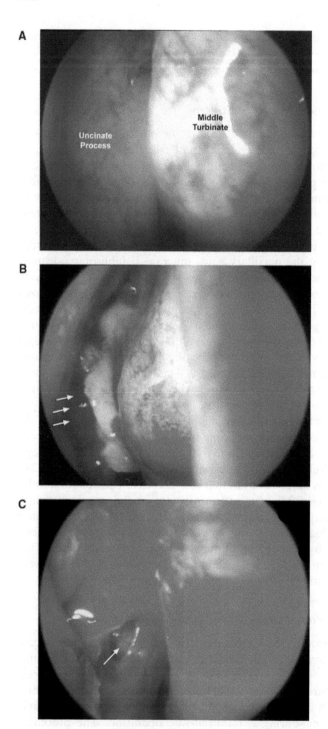

Figure 14 (*Caption on facing page*)

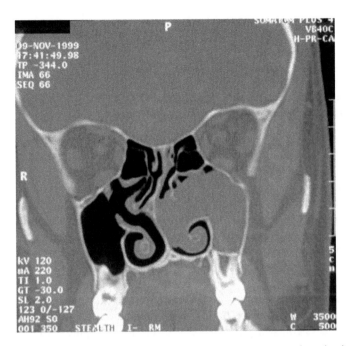

Figure 15 Left antrochoanal polyp. (CT image; coronal projection).

takes approximately one hour. Postoperatively, the patient may or may not have packing in the sinus depending on the amount of bleeding during the case. Some surgeons will apply ice to the upper lip or a pressure dressing to minimize postoperative swelling. Prophylactic antibiotics targeted at normal oral flora are often given perioperatively for five to seven days. Complications are relatively uncommon and include facial swelling, bleeding, and infection. Transient, or rarely permanent, anesthesia of the upper lip and teeth due to a stretch-on or a transection of the infraorbital nerve can occur. This typically subsides within weeks to months in the earlier case but is permanent in the latter (25). An oroantral fistula can develop from nonhealing of the gingivobuccal sulcus incision.

Current indications for the Caldwell-Luc procedure include the removal of mycotic "fungus balls," symptomatic multiseptate mucoceles of the maxillary sinus, antrochoanal polyps that cannot be removed in their

---

Figure 14 (*Facing page*) Endoscopic intraoperative views during right middle meatal antrostomy. (A) View of the middle meatus showing the uncinate process. (B) An incision (*arrows*) is made at the attachment of the uncinate process. (C) The maxillary ostium (*arrow*) is visualized following the uncinectomy.

Table 4 Indications for Caldwell-Luc

Removal of mycotic "fungus balls"
Symptomatic multiseptate mucoceles of the maxillary sinus
Antrochoanal polyps
Biopsy and/or removal of neoplasms or other masses
Exposure to the pterygopalatine fossa (particularly for epistaxis control)
Oroantral fistula repair

---

entirety via ESS, and neoplasms (Table 4). Additionally, this procedure provides excellent exposure to the pterygopalatine fossa and can be used for closure of oroantral fistula and the biopsy of lesions within the maxillary sinus that are suspicious for malignancy (26). A relative contraindication to the procedure involves those pediatric patients with deciduous teeth because entry into the sinus by this approach may damage the permanent dentition. The advantage of this procedure is the increased exposure and access to the maxillary sinus. The disadvantages are the potential risks listed above that are associated with the procedure and the need for an external incision, which increases postoperative pain. In addition, maxillary sinus mucoceles can form several years following the procedure due to entrapment of the sinus mucosa (27).

Ethmoid Sinus Surgery

Endoscopic Endonasal Ethmoidectomy

As previously mentioned, FESS involves opening the anterior ethmoid air cells in order to improve aeration and drainage with the paranasal sinuses (ostiomeatal unit). Depending on the extent of the disease, the amount of surgery can range from opening up a single ethmoid air cell to opening every cell. The least extensive surgery involves opening the ethmoid bulla and removal of the uncinate process. Agger nasi cells, when present, are removed in patients with frontal sinusitis. Penetrating the basal lamella (insertion of the middle turbinate along the lateral nasal wall) is needed to gain access to the posterior ethmoid cells to treat disease in that area. Healthy mucosa in uninvolved ethmoid cells is preserved. Similarly, the middle turbinate is commonly preserved (Fig. 5). At times, a partial anterior–inferior middle turbinectomy is performed to reduce middle meatal adhesions and facilitate viewing of the middle meatal antrostomy in the office.

Indications for endoscopic ethmoidectomy have been already mentioned earlier in this chapter. The advantages are that there is no incision required and the patients recover quickly with minimal postoperative pain. The potential complications of the procedure were detailed earlier in the chapter. In addition, ethmoid mucoceles can form several years following

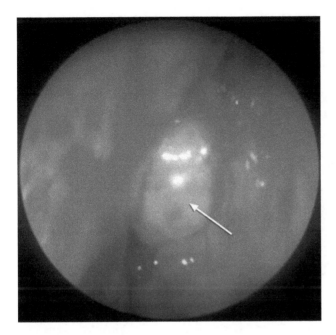

Figure 16 Endoscopic view of an ethmoid mucocele (*arrow*) in a patient with previous endoscopic ethmoidectomy.

the surgery, secondary to entrapment of sinus mucosa (Figs. 16 and 17) (28). Avoiding trauma to healthy mucosa and repeated postoperative cleaning and debridement of the ethmoid cavity can reduce the incidence of mucoceles.

External Ethmoidectomy

An external ethmoidectomy requires that a skin incision be made in order to enter the ethmoid and therefore results in an often barely perceptible scar on the lateral aspect of the nasal dorsum. This procedure takes one to two hours. As with other sinus surgeries, prophylactic perioperative antibiotics are often given. Patients are instructed to place ice over the wound for 24 hours postoperatively and sutures are removed on postoperative day 5. Intranasal postoperative care is similar to the endoscopic procedures, as are the potential complications of the procedure. Additional possible complications include medial canthal scarring and injury to the trochlea or enopthalmos if too much bone is removed (27). The main advantage of this procedure is that it provides excellent visualization and exposure of the medial orbit, ethmoid sinuses, and anterior skull base. Additionally, when the procedure is performed to treat acute ethmoiditis with periorbital abscess, a drain that can be used for irrigation of the ethmoid cavity can be placed. The main disadvantage is that it

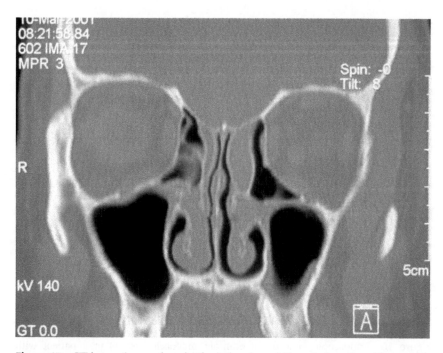

Figure 17 CT image (coronal projection) showing a left posterior ethmoid mucocele that formed five years following an endoscopic ethmoidectomy.

requires an incision, that can result in a cosmetic deformity. Additionally, the incision carries the risk of a sinocutaneous fistula.

External ethmoidectomy continues to have a role in otolaryngology. Although it no longer is used for the treatment of CRS, it is currently indicated for the treatment of acute ethmoiditis complicated by a periorbital or orbital abscess. This approach is also used for the following: for open dacrocystorhinostomy, for complete excision of ethmoid mucocele's with frontal or orbital extension, for orbital decompression or exanteration, for repair of CSF leak or anterior skull base meningo(encephalo)celes, and additionally, as an adjunctive procedure to assist with craniofacial resections and medial maxillectomies (27). Although there are no absolute contraindications to this procedure, one might argue that it is not an acceptable first-line surgical therapy for CRS given the widely available and less morbid endoscopic approaches.

Sphenoid Sinus Surgery

Endoscopic Endonasal Sphenoidotomy

Like the maxillary and ethmoid sinuses, the sphenoid sinus can be similarly opened via an endoscopic approach. The sphenoid sinus can be opened up in conjunction with an endoscopic ethmoidectomy in cases with pansinusitis.

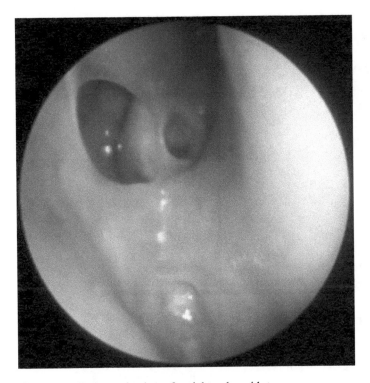

Figure 18 Endoscopic view of a right sphenoidotomy.

On the other hand, isolated sphenoid sinus disease can be successfully treated by an endoscopic sphenoidotomy without the need for an ethmoidectomy (29). In such a case, the sphenoid ostium is accessed between the nasal septum medially, the roof of the posterior choana inferiorly, and the middle and superior turbinates laterally. The sphenoid ostium is above the level of the sinus floor and, therefore, the sphenoidotomy is enlarged in an inferior and medial direction. The posterior septum (vomer bone) and the intersinus septum may be drilled for improved drainage and access, if necessary. As is the case with sinus surgery in general, nondiseased mucosa is preserved (Fig. 18).

Indications for sphenoidotomy include sphenoid sinusitis with or without polyposis, especially in patients with symptoms of retro-orbital headaches or pressure, the removal of or marsupialization of mucoceles or mucopyeloceles, the removal of mycotic "fungus balls," or to assist neurosurgeons in their approach to removing pituitary lesions or other skull base lesions (Fig. 19). The management of these patients is the same as for other endoscopic surgeries; however, it should be noted that the internal carotid artery and the optic nerve run along the lateral and superior

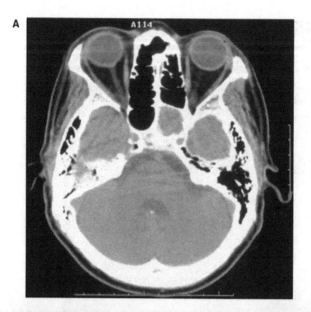

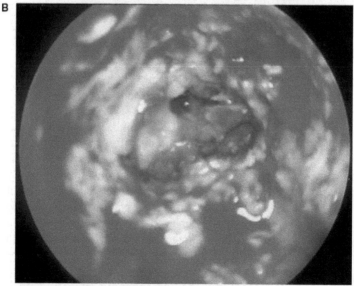

Figure 19 A patient who presented with occipital and vertex headache and was later diagnosed with chronic invasive fungal sinusitis based on the clinical presentation and histopathology. (A) CT scan (axial projection) showing a completely opacified left sphenoid sinus. (B) Intraoperative endoscopic view of the sinus cavity following sphenoidotomy. The sphenoid sinus was filled with fungal debris and hyphae.

walls of the sphenoid sinus, and either can be dehiscent. Hence, surgeons must look carefully for any bony dehiscences on CT scan and be extra cautious when working in this area. Complications of the procedure include bleeding, stenosis/closure of the sphenoidotomy, and injury to the vital structures that are in close proximity to the sinus.

External Spenoethmoidectomy

The majority of sphenoid sinus lesions can be addressed via an endoscopic approach; however, in select cases, an external sphenoethmoidectomy can be used to approach this sinus. This involves performing an external ethmoidectomy and then opening the anterior wall of the sphenoid to gain access to the sinus. This opening is then connected to the natural ostium. A middle turbinectomy is also performed for improved access. The main indication for this approach is for access to skull base tumors or repair of large defects in the skull base. Similar to an external ethmoidectomy, the main advantage of an external sphenoidotomy is that it can provide increased exposure, working room, and if necessary, can be used in conjunction with a microscope for improved visualization. The disadvantage is that it requires an external incision with its potential complications (see external ethmoidectomy).

Frontal Sinus Surgery

Trephination

Frontal sinus trephination involves making an opening in the inferior wall of the frontal sinus through an incision along the inferior aspect of the medial eyebrow. The inferior wall of the frontal sinus is devoid of bone marrow, which averts the risk of developing osteomyelitis in the setting of frontal sinusitis. The sinus cavity is then irrigated with saline or antibiotic-containing solution. The entire procedure takes less than 30 minutes. A drain may be placed for continued irrigation of the sinus. This procedure is indicated in cases of complicated acute frontal sinusitis. Additionally, it can be used in conjunction with endoscopic approaches to the frontal sinus in chronic frontal sinusitis or frontal sinus mucoceles, when the trephination is used to positively identify the frontal duct and pass a catheter through it into the nasal passage to stent it and prevent its stenosis. The main advantage to this approach is that it provides fast and easy access to the frontal sinus. It also affords the surgeon an opportunity to place a drain in the sinus for irrigation. Its main disadvantages are its associated scarring, risk of sinocutaneous fistula formation, and risk of trochlea injury that can cause diplopia.

Lynch Procedure (External Frontoethmoidectomy)

This procedure is performed via an external ethmoidectomy approach. The floor of the frontal sinus is entered. The opening is then widened to include

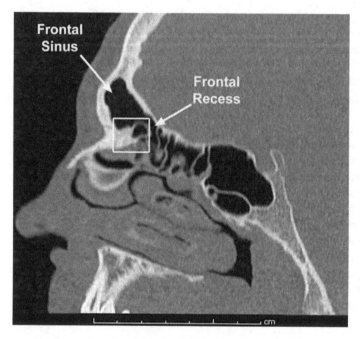

Figure 20 CT image (sagittal projection) through the frontal recess. The "white square" indicates the area that is opened during a Lynch procedure and endoscopic approaches to the frontal sinus.

the frontal duct, which is in turn enlarged to establish what is considered an adequate communication with the anterior ethmoid sinus (Fig. 20). The surgery takes one to two hours to perform and aims at achieving permanent drainage and aeration of the frontal sinus. Accordingly, it is indicated to treat symptomatic frontal sinusitis and frontal sinus muco(pyo)celes. The procedure is currently very rarely performed due to a high failure rate. The frontoethmoid opening occludes in up to 50% of cases, leading to recurrent disease and formation of frontal sinus mucoceles (30). In addition, the surgery entails an external incision with the associated cosmetic issues.

Lothrop Procedure

The Lothrop procedure was originally described as an open approach to treat chronic frontal rhinosinusitis. In this procedure, a common frontal sinus cavity and recess is created by means of removing the bone that divides the left and right sinuses as well as the floor of the frontal sinus. In addition, a portion of the superior nasal septum is resected. The surgery takes one to two hours to perform. Indications for the Lothrop procedure include the treatment of patients with recurrence of frontal sinusitis despite surgery and to remove frontoethmoid mucoceles, osteomas, or inverting papillomas.

This procedure fell out of favor because of a high incidence of restenosis with recurrence of frontal sinus disease.

Endoscopic Frontal Sinusotomy

An endoscopic anterior ethmoidectomy is first performed. The frontal recess air cells of the anterior ethmoid are opened to expose the frontal duct (Fig. 21). This area is anterior to the anterior ethmoid artery as it crosses along the roof of the ethmoid sinus and just posterior to the anterior attachment of the middle turbinate. Openings into supra-orbital ethmoid air cells can at times be confused with the frontal duct, which has a more medial and anterior location. When present, agger nasi cells are opened to widen the frontal recess (Fig. 4). What is to be done once the frontal duct is identified is controversial. Some warn against instrumentation of the duct itself since this can lead to its stenosis. For these surgeons, opening the frontal recess air cells and treating the anterior ethmoid sinus disease is adequate. On the other hand, others recommend widening the duct by either removing part of its inflamed mucosa or by drilling the bony walls anteriorly and along the floor of the frontal sinus with a long handle drill (Fig. 20).

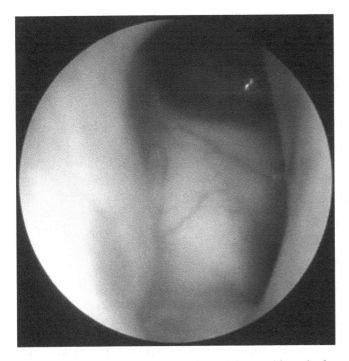

Figure 21 Endoscopic view of the frontal duct and into the frontal sinus following endoscopic frontal sinusotomy.

In recalcitrant cases of frontal sinusitis or those with fibro-osseous stenosis of the frontal duct/recess, the floor of the frontal sinus is drilled in addition to the upper nasal septum, which may then be extended to the floor of the contralateral frontal sinus (modified Lothrop procedure) (31,32). The newly created opening is at times maintained by placing a stent for four to 12 months following the surgery (33). These cases can usually be performed in about two hours. Perioperative antibiotics are typically used, and postoperative care is similar to that of other endoscopic procedures. Indications for endoscopic frontal sinus surgery include the treatment of patients with chronic frontal sinusitis; to remove frontoethmoid mucoceles, osteomas, or inverting papillomas; or to treat recurrent disease as a salvage procedure for osteoplastic flap operation failures (see following sections) (Fig. 22) (32–36).

Most surgeons advocate performing endoscopic frontal sinus procedures with the aid of computer guidance systems (31,34,37). Even so, it should be noted that these procedures involve working extremely close to the anterior cranial fossa, medial orbit, and lacrimal sac; hence, only very experienced surgeons should perform this surgery in order to prevent complications. When they do occur, the complications are typically the same as

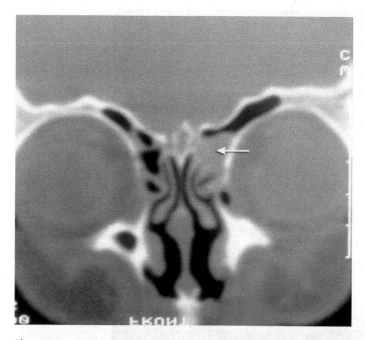

Figure 22 CT image (coronal projection) showing soft tissue opacity in the left frontal recess. This patient suffered from recurrent left frontal sinusitis and was successfully treated by an endoscopic frontal sinusotomy.

those with other endoscopic approaches. Additionally, there appears to be a high incidence of recurrent frontal sinus disease due to restenosis of the frontal recess (31,32,34–37).

Like the other endoscopic approaches, the advantages are that there is no incision required and patients recover quickly with minimal postoperative pain. The main disadvantage of the endoscopic approach is that there appears to be a higher recurrence rate with these procedures when compared to the osteoplastic frontal sinus obliteration (see following sections). The area that is opened via the endoscopic approaches, including drilling of the floor of the frontal sinus, is similar to the one opened by a Lynch or Lothrop procedure (Fig. 20). Hence, there is no reason to expect a higher success rate with the endoscopic approaches compared to the external ones. The success of the endoscopic approach should not be judged until adequate long-term follow-up is conducted, since frontal sinus mucoceles can form more than 10 years following the surgery.

Osteoplastic Frontal Sinus Obliteration

The osteoplastic frontal sinus obliteration procedure is an effective means to eradicate disease in patients who have recurrent or chronic frontal sinusitis despite attempts at improving drainage via the endoscopic route. The procedure takes about two hours. Additional indications are frontal sinus mucoceles, repair of CSF leaks originating from the posterior wall of the frontal sinus, repair of certain frontal sinus fractures, and repair of frontal sinocutaneous fistula (30,38). Its main rationale is the high failure rate of procedures that aim at opening the frontal recess/duct, hence leading to persistent symptoms and, at times, the formation of mucoceles. Therefore, the frontal sinus is obliterated to circumvent the consequences of an occluded frontal recess.

This procedure involves making a skin incision in either the scalp, the mid-forehead, or the eyebrow. The scalp incision that is made above the hairline (bicoronal incision) requires longer operative time and increases intraoperative blood loss but offers superior cosmetics. The supraciliary incision (above the eyebrow) offers more direct access to the frontal sinus and hence reduces operative time and blood loss. However, it is associated with higher incidence of scalp hypesthesia and sometimes long term pain due to transaction of the supratrochlear and supraorbital nerves. The mid-forehead incision offers a compromise. This is made along a skin crease in the forehead and, therefore, has acceptable cosmetics. It also affords direct access to the anterior wall of the sinus with a short operative time and minimal blood loss (38). The bone of the anterior wall of the frontal sinus is then carefully raised in order to open up the sinus. The mucosa of the sinus is completely removed. A large frontal sinus with extensive lateral recesses poses a challenge at removing the entire sinus mucosa. The opening of the frontal duct is then occluded with fascia or other material, such as bone wax. Fat is harvested from the abdomen and used to obliterate the sinus cavity. The anterior bony wall is then reflected into position. Drains are placed under both the scalp and the abdomen incisions for a few days after the surgery. For this reason, patients typically stay in the hospital as inpatients until the drains come out. Perioperative antibiotics are given and there is no intranasal postoperative care. Sutures are removed within one week.

The main advantage to this procedure is that it has a low failure rate (30,38). The disadvantages are that this procedure involves a large incision and is associated with increased length of hospital stay. Permanent frontal scalp hypesthesia may develop, especially following a supraciliary incision since it may transect the supraorbital and supratrochlear nerves. Additional complications include headache, abdominal or scalp wound seroma, hematoma or abscess, headache, dural laceration, and recurrence of disease (33,37). Despite these potential complications, this is a safe and very effective procedure, when done by an experienced surgeon. However, this procedure is not indicated for patients with uncomplicated frontal sinus disease who are undergoing surgery for the first time. These patients are better served by endoscopic procedures.

ANTIBIOTIC COVERAGE IN PARANASAL SINUS SURGERY: PROPHYLACTIC AND POST SURGERY

The role of prophylactic antibiotic coverage in paranasal sinus surgery is controversial (13,14). In addition, there is a lack of consensus regarding antibiotic choice and the duration of such therapy.

It is common practice, however, to put patients on antibiotic coverage following sinus surgery for a duration ranging from 48 hours to two weeks. We recommend a 10- to 14-day course. The choice of the antibiotic is dictated by the surgical approach, nature of the disease process, likely bacteria based on published medical literature, and, when available, preoperative or intraoperative bacteriology culture results.

The chosen antibiotic should have adequate coverage against skin flora such as *Streptococcus* spp. and *S. aureus* and the likely pathogenic bacteria in the involved sinus(es) for surgery via an external approach that require a skin incision. Antibiotic coverage for anaerobic bacteria present in the oral flora is needed for transoral approaches such as Caldwell-Luc procedure. In addition, an antibiotic with demonstrated activity against nasal flora, *S. aureus*, and likely paranasal sinus pathogens is selected for endonasal approaches, both conventional and endoscopic procedures.

The antibiotic of choice should preferably have an easy administration schedule (QD or BID dosing), be well-tolerated, and be available in intravenous as well as equivalent oral formulations. Ability to cross the blood–brain barrier is essential during surgery in patients with periorbital or intracranial complications from sinusitis or iatrogenic CSF rhinorrhea (violation of the base of the skull).

LASERS AND SINUS SURGERY

Presently, lasers have a limited role in sinus surgery. Over the years, various investigators have attempted to use lasers to aid in the eradication of sinus disease. For the most part, these attempts have been somewhat successful; however, the use of lasers is expensive and can be time-consuming. Therefore, the use of lasers has not gained widespread acceptance.

The CO_2 laser has not been found successful in the treatment of sinus disease. It has a wavelength that gets absorbed by water, and its thermal energy is concentrated with very little spread to the surrounding soft tissues. The principle difficulties in applying the CO_2 laser to sinus disease treatment is that it requires a relatively dry field for hemostasis, it results in significant smoke accumulation, and most importantly, its mid-infrared light cannot travel through a fiberoptic cable. Thus, tissues must be visualized directly in order to be treated with the CO_2 laser (39).

In contrast, the Nd:YAG, KTP/532, Argon, and Ho:YAG lasers can be carried through fiberoptic cables. Fiberoptic threads can be passed into instruments, that are designed for intranasal use. Hence, the instruments that transmit the laser energy can be handled manually and placed directly onto tissues with ease and precision. Each of these has advantages and disadvantages related to depth of penetration, scatter of thermal energy, and their ability to coagulate small blood vessels. These lasers have been used to treat inferior turbinate hypertrophy with moderate success (39). They can also be used to remove nasal lesions, such as nasal papillomata, pyogenic granuloma, and other small superficial lesions (40).

A common application of laser technique is the treatment of hereditary hemorrhagic telangiectasias. This is an autosomal-dominant disease characterized by telangiectatic lesions primarily in mucosalized areas, such as the nose, mouth, and gastrointestinal tract. These patients often suffer from severe bouts of epistaxis throughout their lives. The Nd:YAG and KTP/532 lasers have each been used successfully to ablate these lesions (39–43). Patients often require retreatment, however, every four to six months. Ho:YAG laser with its capability to vaporize bone has been used in intranasal endoscopic dacryocystorhinostomy. It did not gain widespread popularity since it does not offer any significant advantage over using cold instruments to justify the added cost and operative time.

CONCLUSION

Paranasal sinus surgery has several indications; the most common is CRS that failed medical therapy. The approach and extent of surgery is dictated by the nature of the disease and the involved sinuses. Endoscopic approaches that are made possible with the technological advances in fiberoptics have gained widespread use. They offer a minimally invasive technique that has a low morbidity and high success rate for treating inflammatory paranasal sinus pathology. The surgery is not risk free, however. Image guidance systems can make the surgery safer. Surgery is often an adjunct to medical therapy. A better understanding of the pathogenesis of rhinosinusitis allows for better delineation of the role of medical therapy and surgery.

REFERENCES

1. Kennedy DW, Zinreich SJ, Rosenbaum AE, Johns ME. Functional endoscopic sinus surgery. Theory and diagnostic evaluation. Arch Otolaryngol 1985; 111:576–582.
2. Rice DH. Indications for endoscopic sinus surgery. Ear Nose Throat J 1994; 73:461–464, 466.
3. Messerklinger W. Background and evolution of endoscopic sinus surgery. Ear Nose Throat J 1994; 73:449–450.
4. Stammberger H. The evolution of functional endoscopic sinus surgery. Ear Nose Throat J 1994; 73:451, 454–455.
5. Vining EM, Kennedy DW. The transmigration of endoscopic sinus surgery from Europe to the United States. Ear Nose Throat J 1994; 73:456–458, 460.
6. Kennedy DW. Functional endoscopic sinus surgery. Technique. Arch Otolaryngol 1985; 111:643–649.
7. Messerklinger W. On the drainage of the normal frontal sinus of man. Acta Otolaryngol 1967; 63:176–181.
8. Stammberger H, Hasler G. Functional Endoscopic Sinus Surgery: The Messerklinger Technique. St Louis, MO: Mosby, 1991.
9. Catalano PJ. Minimally invasive sinus technique: what is it? Should we consider it? Curr Opin Otolaryngol Head Neck Surg 2004; 12:34–37.
10. Kieff DA, Busaba NY. Non-dental related isolated chronic maxillary sinus opacification does not correlate with ipsilateral intranasal structural abnormalities. Ann Otol Rhinol Laryngol 2004; 113:474–476.
11. Taylor MJ, Ponikau JU, Sherris DA, Kern EB, Gaffey TA, Kephart G, Kita H. Detection of fungal organisms in eosinophilic mucin using a fluorescein-labeled chitin-specific binding protein. Otolaryngol Head Neck Surg 2002; 127: 377–383.
12. Ferguson BJ. Categorization of eosinophilic chronic rhinosinusitis. Curr Opin Otolaryngol Head Neck Surg 2004; 12:237–242.
13. Annys E, Jorissen M. Short term effects of antibiotics (Zinnat) after endoscopic sinus surgery. Acta Otorhinolaryngol Belg 2000; 54(1):23–28.
14. Hasselgren PO, Ivarsson L, Risberg B, Seeman T. Effects of prophylactic antibiotics in vascular surgery. A prospective, randomized, double-blind study. Ann Surg 1984 Jul; 200(1):86–92.
15. Gross CW, Gross WE. Post-operative care for functional endoscopic sinus surgery. Ear Nose Throat J 1994; 73:476–479.

16. Stankiewicz JA. Complications of endoscopic sinus surgery. Otolaryngol Clin North Am 1989; 22:749–758.
17. Parikh SR, Fried MP. Navigational systems for sinus surgery: new developments. J Otolaryngol 2002; 31(suppl 1):S24—S27.
18. Metson R. Image-guided sinus surgery: lessons learned from the first 1000 cases. Otolaryngol Head Neck Surg 2003; 128:8–13.
19. Metson R, Gliklich RE, Cosenza M. A comparison of image guidance systems for sinus surgery. Laryngoscope 1998; 108(8 Pt 1):1164–1170.
20. Fried MP, Kleefield J, Gopal H, Reardon E, Ho BT, Kuhn FA. Image-guided endoscopic surgery: results of accuracy and performance in a multicenter clinical study using an electromagnetic tracking system. Laryngoscope 1997; 107:594–601.
21. Selivanova O, Kuehnemund M, Mann WJ, Amedee RG. Comparison of conventional instruments and mechanical debriders for surgery of patients with chronic sinusitis. Am J Rhinol 2003; 17:197–202.
22. Bernstein JM, Lebowitz RA, Jacobs JB. Initial report on postoperative healing after endoscopic sinus surgery with the microdebrider. Otolaryngol Head Neck Surg 1998; 118:800–803.
23. Busaba NY, Salman SD. Maxillary sinus mucoceles: clinical presentation and long-term results of endoscopic surgical treatment. Laryngoscope 1999; 109:1446–1449.
24. Busaba NY, Kieff DA. Endoscopic sinus surgery for inflammatory maxillary sinus pathology. Larynogoscope 2002; 112:1378–1383.
25. Goodman WS. The Caldwell-Luc procedure. Otolaryngol Clin North Am 1976; 9:187–195.
26. Schaefer SD, Gustafson RO, Bansberg SF. Sinus surgery. In: Bailey BJ, Calhoun KH, eds. Head and Neck Surgery—Otolaryngology. 3rd ed. Philadelphia, PA: Lippincott Williams and Wilkins, 2001:359–370.
27. Weber R, Keerl R, Draf W. Endonasal endoscopic surgery of maxillary sinus mucoceles after Caldwell-Luc operation. Laryngorhinootologie 2000; 79: 532–535.
28. Busaba NY, Salman SD. Ethmoid mucocele as a late complication of endoscopic ethmoidectomy. Otolaryngol Head Neck Surg 2003; 128:517–522.
29. Kieff DA, Busaba NY. Treatment of isolated sphenoid sinus inflammatory disease by endoscopic sphenoidotomy without ethmoidectomy. Laryngoscope 2002; 112:2186–2188.
30. Hardy JM, Montgomery WW. Osteoplastic frontal sinusotomy: an analysis of 250 operations. Ann Otol Rhinol Laryngol 1976; 85(4 Pt 1):523–532.
31. Wormald PJ, Ananda A, Nair S. Modified endoscopic Lothrop as a salvage for the failed osteoplastic flap with obliteration. Laryngoscope 2003; 113: 1988–1992.
32. Stankiewicz JA, Wachter B. The endoscopic modified Lothrop procedure for salvage of chronic frontal sinusitis after osteoplastic flap failure. Otolaryngol Head Neck Surg 2003; 129:678–683.
33. Neal DG. External ethmoidectomy. Otolaryngol Clin North Am 1985; 18:55–60.
34. Kountakis SE, Gross CW. Long-term results of the Lothrop operation. Curr Opin Otolaryngol Head Neck Surg 2003; 11:37–40.

35. Gross CW, Harrison SE. The modified Lothrop procedure: indications, results, and complications. Otolaryngol Clin North Am 2001; 34:133–137.
36. Casiano RR, Livingston JA. Endoscopic Lothrop procedure: the University of Miami experience. Am J Rhinol 1998; 12:335–339.
37. Samaha M, Cosenza MJ, Metson R. Endoscopic frontal sinus drillout in 100 patients. Arch Otolaryngol Head Neck Surg 2003; 129:854–858.
38. Montgomery WW. State-of-the-art for osteoplastic frontal sinus operation. Otolaryngol Clin North Am 2001; 34:167–177.
39. Rathfoot CJ, Duncavage J, Shapshay SM. Laser use in the paranasal sinuses. Otolaryngol Clin North Am 1996; 29:943–948.
40. Shah RK, Dhingra JK, Shapshay SM. Hereditary hemorrhagic telangiectasia: a review of 76 cases. Laryngoscope 2002; 112:767–773.
41. Parkin JL, Dixon JA. Laser photocoagulation in hereditary hemorrhagic telangiectasia. Otolaryngol Head Neck Surg 1981; 89:204–208.
42. Levine HL. Lasers in endonasal surgery. Otolaryngol Clin North Am 1997; 30:451–455.
43. Levine HL. Endoscopy and the KTP/532 laser for nasal sinus disease. Ann Otol Rhinol Laryngol 1989; 98(1 Pt 1):46–51.

13

Complications of Acute and Chronic Sinusitis and Their Management

Gary Schwartz and Steve White
Vanderbilt University Medical Center, Nashville, Tennessee, U.S.A.

INTRODUCTION

Sinusitis is a common condition that is usually treated uneventfully on an outpatient basis. Admission to a hospital is rare, as are the complications stemming from sinusitis (Table 1). Although not exactly known, the incidence of complications from sinusitis is thought to be low. One study found a 3% incidence of complications in hospitalized patients (1). In addition,

Table 1 Complications of Sinusitis

Local complications
Mucocele
Osteomyelitis (Pott's puffy tumor)
Orbital complications
Inflammatory edema
Orbital abscess
Subperiosteal abscess
Cavernous sinus thrombosis
Intracranial complications
Meningitis
Subperiosteal abscess

other studies from referral centers looking at complications only report a few patients per year (2). The rarity of this problem can make physicians complacent about looking for complications and therefore could lead to significant morbidity and mortality. Morbidities can include blindness and neurologic deficits.

Complications from sinusitis are caused by the spread of bacteria from the sinus to the surrounding structures. There are two means by which the spread of infection can occur. The most common route is through direct spread to contiguous areas. The spread of infection occurs through either neurovascular foramina, a defect in the sinus wall from a fracture because of trauma, or a congenital abnormality. Spread of infection to the bony wall can also lead to erosions creating an opening through which infection can progress.

PATHOPHYSIOLOGY

Hematogenous route is the other route for an infection to spread. Either bacteria or septic emboli can get into the bloodstream and reach intracranial sites separated by a distance from the sinus. To some extent, all sinus veins drain intracranially and, therefore, have the potential to spread bacteria to the brain. The frontal sinus, whose venous drainage is almost entirely intracranial, is the most common origin for bacterial spread which can cause intracranial complications. Venous drainage from the sinus runs via the diploic veins that penetrate the bony sinus lining. The inner table diploic veins drain directly into the dural venous plexuses and later into the sagital sinus. The outer table of the sinus drains into both the venous plexuses of the face, which then drain through the ophthalmic veins in the orbits, and the dural sinuses. Bacteria from facial skin infections take the same path, which can lead to intracranial infections. Also draining into the dural sinuses are the cortical veins from the brain parenchyma. As these veins are without valves, blood can flow either antegrade or retrograde. Therefore, septic emboli can start in a frontal sinus, drain into a dural sinus, and flow retrograde into the brain, leading to an abscess. Septic emboli can also seed structures along the drainage path, leading to an epidural or subdural empyema.

LOCAL COMPLICATIONS

Osteomyelitis

A sinus infection can spread to the surrounding bony structures leading to osteomyelitis of either the anterior or posterior walls of the sinus. The spread of infection can be either by direct extension or by valveless veins draining into the sinus. Osteomyelitis is most commonly observed in the walls of the frontal sinuses. Once the bone has become infected, it can erode, allowing the infection to spread under the subperiostium leading to subperiosteal abscess formation. The erosion can affect either the anterior or posterior tables of the sinus, leading to either extracranial or intracranial extension. If the subperiosteal abscess is adjacent to the anterior table of the frontal bone, it is called Pott's puffy tumor after Sir Percival Potts, who first described this condition. This is an extremely rare diagnosis with only 20 cases in the literature (3). Patients with Pott's puffy tumor are always older than six years because the frontal sinus is not pneumatized until this age.

Etiology

Osteomyelitis of the bone overlying the sinus is caused by the same organisms that cause sinusitis. The most common are *Staphylococcus*, *Streptococcus*, and anaerobic bacteria (3,4).

Clinical Presentation

Patients who present with osteomyelitis as a complication of sinusitis frequently present with complaints similar to patients with simple sinusitis. These include headache, photophobia, and fever. If Pott's puffy tumor is present, there will also be swelling in the forehead.

Diagnosis

Diagnosis requires radiographic imaging not only to confirm, but also to rule out any associated intracranial complications. Imaging is most easily accomplished with a CT scan. Routine blood tests such as complete blood cell counts are of little value as they are very nonspecific, but an elevated sedimentation rate may be an indication of osteomyelitis.

Treatment

Treatment for osteomyelitis is by administering intravenous antibiotics for a prolonged period of time, six to eight weeks. The antibiotics chosen need to cover both anaerobic and aerobic organisms. An appropriate empiric choice is a combination of a third-generation cephalosporin (i.e., ceftriaxone) and metronidazole or clindamycin, with consideration given to adding vancomycin or linezolid (also available orally), if there is a significant *Streptococcus pneumoniae* antimicrobial resistance or the involvement of *Staphylococcus* spp. Oral therapy with amoxicillin–clavulanate or the combination of cefixime and metronidazole or clindamycin are also appropriate. The choice of therapy should be adjusted according to adequate cultures. If an abscess is present, surgical drainage is the treatment of choice.

Mucocele

A mucocele is a chronic, cystic lesion of the paranasal sinuses. It grows slowly, taking years to become symptomatic, and the symptoms are typically related to the increasing size of the mucocele. As it enlarges, it can exert pressure on the sinus wall which leads to bony erosion. After eroding through the sinus wall, the mucocele can extend into surrounding structures. Mucoceles most frequently involve the frontal sinus, followed by the ethmoid and maxillary sinuses (5). Symptomatic frontal or ethmoid sinus mucoceles can cause headaches, diplopia, and proptosis. The proptotic globe is typically displaced downward and outward. Maxillary sinus mucoceles are usually an incidental finding on radiographs of the sinus. Mucoceles in this location rarely cause symptoms because the maxillary sinuses are large and the mucoceles rarely become large enough to cause bony abnormalities. Maxillary sinus mucoceles can become symptomatic, if they obstruct the ostium of the maxillary sinus. Mucoceles can also become symptomatic in any sinus when they become infected, forming mucopyocele. Diagnosis is usually made by CT of the sinuses. Symptomatic mucoceles are treated with surgical removal and possible sinus obliteration.

ORBITAL INFECTIONS

Orbital infections can be caused by penetration of the orbit during either surgery or trauma; most frequently the result of a bacterial spread is from an infected sinus. As the orbit is bordered by several sinuses—the frontal, ethmoid, and maxillary—infection from any of these sinuses can potentially spread to the orbit. The ethmoid sinus is almost exclusively implicated in the spread of infection to the orbit. This is related to the thickness of the sinus wall lining the orbit. The thinner the wall, the easier is for infection to spread through it. The ethmoid sinus has the thinnest wall, the lamina papyracea, which lines the lateral wall of the sinus and the medial wall of the orbit. Most orbital infections are, therefore, on the medial side of the orbit. Although much less common, the thicker wall sinuses can also be the source of an orbital infection. Once infection has spread past the sinus wall, the periosteal lining of the sinus wall serves as an additional barrier to protect the orbit from the spread of the infection. If an abscess forms between the wall and periosteum, it is called a subperiosteal abscess. If the periosteum is violated, then an orbital abscess may form.

Etiology

Many organisms can be isolated in patients with orbital infections (Table 2). These may be single or multiple organisms, anaerobic or aerobic organisms, or mixture of both. Frequently, the isolates are the same as those found in the infected sinus. To best determine the type of organism, patients should be divided into two groups. The first group consists children of under 9 years old. These patients typically have single aerobic organisms, which include *alpha* and *beta* hemolytic *Streptococcus* spp., *Staphylococcus* spp., non-*Haemophillus influenzae*, and *Moroxalla catarrhalis* (6). The second group

Table 2   Common Organisms Isolated from Patients with Orbital Infections

Aerobic bacteria
   Streptococcus spp.: *Streptococcoccus pneumoniae, Streptococcus viridans,* and
      Streptococcus viridans
   Staphylococcus spp.: *Staphylococcus aureus,* and *Staphylococcus epidermidis*
   Haemophilus influenzae
   Moraxella catarrhalis
Anaerobic bacteria
   Gram-negative bacilli (*Prevotella, Porphyromonas,* and *Bacteroides* spp.)
   Veillonella parvula
   Peptostreptococcus spp.
   Fusobacterium spp.
   Proprionibacterium spp.
Immunocompromised hosts
   Pseudomonas aeruginosa
   Fungal species: *aspergillosis,* and *mucormycosis*

of patients is over nine years old, and typically have complex infections with mixed aerobic and anaerobic organisms. This is especially true for patients in their teens or older. Although aerobic organisms are frequently the same as those found in younger children, the anaerobic organisms are usually oral flora such as anaerobic gram-negative bacilli, *Peptostreptococus* spp., *Fusobacterium* spp., and *Veillonella parvule.* These rules are not absolute, as there are reports of anaerobic bacteria isolated in young children (7,8). There are several theories that explain the causes of this transition; they include the increased incidence of chronic infections in older children and adults and the relative size of the osteo meatal opening. The relative size of the osteo meatal opening to the sinus cavity is larger in younger individuals compared to that of older ones and therefore less likely to become occluded. Occlusion of the opening blocks the sinus cavity, which becomes anaerobic and promotes the growth of anaerobic organisms.

Diagnosis

In an article, Chandler described a classification system for orbital infection that still in use today (9) (Table 3, Fig. 1). The spectrum of orbital infections is classified into five groups; each represents a progressively more serious infection. Group 1 is preseptal cellulitis, a simple cellulitis of the eyelids which manifests as swelling of the eyelids. Infection is limited to the skin in front of the orbital septum. Group 2 is orbital cellulitis, seen as diffuse edema of the lining of the orbits. It manifests as eyelid swelling and pain with extraocular muscle movement. Group 3, subperiosteal abscess, is characterized by edema of the orbital lining with a collection of fluid below the

Table 3 Chandler Classification

Group 1: Periorbital cellulitis
Group 2: Orbital cellulitis
Group 3: Subperiosteal abscess
Group 4: Orbital abscess
Group 5: Cavernous sinus thrombosis.

Source: From Ref. 9.

periosteum usually involving the medical wall of the orbit. Clinically patients with this condition are similar to Group 2 but proptosis may also be noted. Group 4, orbital abscess, is characterized as a true abscess in the orbital space. This may manifest with proptosis, impaired eye movement, and in the worse case, blindness. Group 5 is cavernous sinus thrombosis with rapidly progressive bilateral chemosis, ophthalmoplegia, retinal engorgement, and loss of visual acuity, along with possible meningeal signs and high fever.

The most important decision in dealing with a patient with a swollen eye is determining whether a preseptal or orbital process exists. Obtaining a thorough history, physical examination, and potentially imaging studies can very often assist in this. Preseptal cellulitis is most often caused by local trauma. The history may reveal an insect bite or other trauma to the skin around the eye, which becomes secondarily infected. This infection is usually insidious in onset. *H. influenzae* type B infection causes rapid eyelid swelling and eyelid closure within hours. With the advent of the *H. influenzae* type B

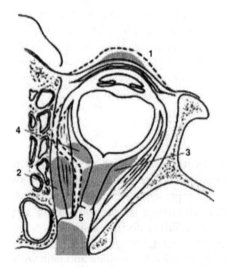

Figure 1 (1) Preseptal cellulitis, (2) Orbital cellulitis, (3) Subperiosteal abscess, (4) Orbital abscess, and (5) Cavernous sinus thrombosis. *Source*: From Ref. 49.

vaccine, a hematogenous source of infection very rarely is identified as the cause of preseptal cellulitis (10). Patients with H. influenzae infection typically develop rapid eyelid swelling with eyelid closure within hours.

As preseptal cellulitis is an inflammatory process, evidence of local eye inflammation is present. Findings include warmth, redness, induration, and pain with palpation. In patients with red swollen eyelids which are boggy, painless to palpation, and not indurated, an allergic reaction or venous congestion because of an underlying sinusitis should be considered. Regardless of the cause of preseptal cellulitis, there should be no visual problem, no proptosis, or no significant pain with eye movement.

Orbital infections (group 2–4) are harder to identify and are typically more insidious in onset. Patients frequently show a history of nasal drainage, headache or pressure, and fever. If infection is in the orbit, visual loss may be present.

Orbital infections may present in a similar way to preseptal infections. These patients present with evidence of orbital inflammation. The presence of eyelid swelling is not indicative of inflammation. As space is limited in the orbit, any inflammatory mass could impact the surrounding structures. A simple orbital infection exerts pressure on the ocular muscles and causes pain with eye movement. If a subperiosteal abscess or abscess forms, there may be pressure placed on the orbit causing proptosis. If the inflammatory process pushes on the optic nerve, blindness may result. Early on, the findings of orbital infection may be minimal, but become more apparent if the infection is allowed to progress.

Imaging

As there can be an overlap in the symptoms of orbital infection, preseptal cellulitis, and other causes of eyelid swelling, some clinicians recommend imaging in all patients with a swollen eye. However, a more common approach would be to reserve imaging studies for those with nonclassic presentations of preseptal cellulitis and those with presumed preseptal cellulitis, who do not improve following one to two days of treatment. All patients with evidence of orbital cellulitis need an imaging study.

The most frequently used imaging study is a CT scan, with or without contrast, using thin slices through the orbit with coronal and axial images. A CT scan is highly sensitive in documenting these infections. Patients with preseptal cellulitis show evidence of eyelid swelling without orbital involvement. The CT scan images of patients with Chandler group 2 (orbital cellulites) frequently show an opacified ethmoid sinus with an ill-defined mass on the orbital side of the lamina papyracea (Fig. 2). In addition, there may also be inflammation of the rectus muscle.

This is the mildest and most common type of orbital infection (Fig. 3). Group 3 (subperiosteal abscess) shows evidence of inflammation with periosteum elevation and rim enhancement, rectus muscle displacement,

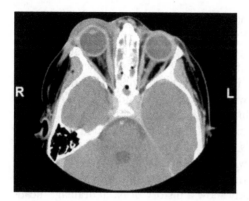

Figure 2 Ethmoid sinusitis with inflammation of the medial wall of the right orbit.

and if large enough, some degree of proptosis of the eye (Fig. 3). Findings for group 4 (orbital abscess) show inflammatory material in the orbital space with proptosis.

An MRI is possibly a better type of imaging study, but can be problematic since most orbital infections are in young children who will need sedating for the procedure. An MRI is best reserved for the complicated infection with intracranial extension, such as cavernous sinus thrombosis (group 5) or epidural abscess. There is no value in obtaining plain radiographs of the sinuses to diagnose an orbital infection.

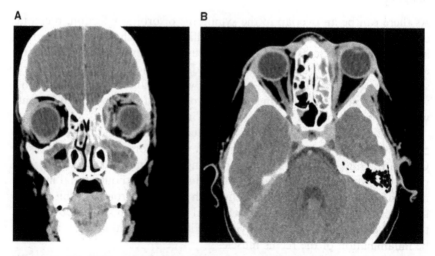

Figure 3 Ethmoid sinusitis with subperiosteal abscess in an adolescent who presented to an emergency department with eyelid swelling and pain with eye movement.

Treatment

Until the past few years, there has been much disagreement on how to treat orbital infections. Until recently, surgical drainage was thought to be necessary in the majority of patients. Now medical management is the treatment of choice in the majority of patients with this type of infection. To successfully treat patients with orbital infections, the patients are to be stratified into low and high risk groups based on likelihood of complications. Low risk patients have over 90% cure rate with antibiotic therapy alone (11). Low risk patients are those under 9 years old, who most likely have single aerobic organisms causing the infection. In addition to young age, low risk patients must also have no visual compromise, at most a modest-sized subperiosteal abscess on the medial side of the orbit, and no evidence of intracranial infection (Table 4). They also must be able to cooperate with frequent ophthalmologic examinations. How frequently an exam must be repeated is not known. Published studies recommend ophthalmic examinations from once a day to multiple times a day (11,12).

The antibiotics selected should be able to cover aerobic gram-positive cocci. Adequate choices include a third-generation cephalosporin (ceftriaxone or cefotaxime) unless there is a high likelihood of recovery of resistant *S. pneumoniae*. In these cases, vancomycin should be given. As anaerobic organisms are rarely seen in young patients, administering antibiotics that cover these organisms is probably unnecessary. Generally, treatment includes less than a week of parenteral antibiotics and is followed by a prolonged period of two to three weeks of oral antibiotic such as high dose of ampicillin/clavulanic acid (90 mg/kg/day in children and 4 g/day in adults) (13,14). In addition to antibiotics, all patients should be started on a nasal decongestant, such as oxymetazoline. Most patients who fit into this low risk category respond appropriately with only antibiotic treatment. However, if the patient's condition deteriorates, it may be necessary to have the abscess and sinus drained. Indications for surgery in this low risk group include visual loss, afferent papillary defect, fever after 36 hours of antibiotic treatment, or absence of clinical improvement after 72 hours. There is no indication for repeating the CT scan when deciding whether to perform surgery or not. Findings on the CT scan

Table 4 Low Risk Group for Complications

Age under 9 years old
No visual compromise
At most, modest-size abscess on medial side of orbit
No evidence of intracranial complication
Ability to cooperate with serial ophthalmologic exams
Not immunocompromised

may worsen before they improve, even in patients who are responding appropriately to antibiotics.

Young children who are not likely to be cured by antibiotics alone include those with subperiosteal abscess not on the medial side of the orbit and those with over 2 mm of proptosis (14).

A more aggressive approach is needed to treat older children and adults, as they have more complex infections that are not as reliably treated with antibiotics alone. Recommended antibiotics for complex infections are a second-generation cephalosporin that covers anaerobic and anaerobic organisms (i.e., cefoxitin or cefotetan), clindamycin, or ampicillin/sulbactam. Other combinations of antibiotics, such as penicillin and metronidazole, can also be used as long as they cover both aerobic and anaerobes. If there is a high likelihood of recovering resistant *S. pneumoniae* vancomycin can be added. Even with the administration of appropriate antibiotics, cultures from an infected sinus or orbital abscess frequently can still grow organisms after several days of therapy. Until the abscess or infected sinus is sterile, there is a risk of the infection spreading. For these patients, a trial of antibiotic therapy alone can be given, but it will likely not cure the infection and place the patient at a continued risk for complications. Some clinicians will wait for 24 hours to see how these patients with complex infections respond, whereas others will proceed to urgent surgery to drain the abscess along with administering parenteral antibiotics. Surgery can be done either endoscopically or through an open approach, depending on the location of the subperiosteal abscesses and the physician's preference.

INTRACRANIAL COMPLICATIONS OF SINUSITIS

Introduction

Intracranial complications of sinusitis are rare, occurring one to three times per year in major referral centers (15–23). Undoubtedly, the advent of antibiotic therapy has decreased the incidence of intracranial infectious complications of sinusitis. Over the three decades spanning 1950–1980, Bradley et al. (24) noted a four-fold decrease in intracranial abscess arising from sinus infection, despite improvements in diagnostic modalities which would otherwise have increased the number of diagnosed cases. Yet, because these intracranial infections represent the most lethal consequences of diagnostic or treatment failure of sinusitis, it is imperative for clinicians to understand the clinical presentation, diagnostic options, and therapeutic approach to treat each of these entities.

Intracranial complications of sinusitis include: (1) meningitis, (2) epidural abscess, (3) subdural abscess, (4) brain abscess, and (5) dural sinus thrombosis. In contrast to intraorbital infections, sinusitis underlies only 3% to 9% of suppurative intracranial infections (15–17,20) and is responsible for less than 1% of cases of meningitis (17).

However, extra-axial abscesses (subdural and epidural) as discrete entities are most commonly of sinogenic origin, and epidural abscess is the most common intracranial complication from sinusitis in some series (15,16,21), although meningitis is more common in other series (23). Meningitis may be under-represented as lumbar puncture is to be avoided in the setting of intracranial space-occupying lesions and would likely only be performed when a CT or MRI scan fails to demonstrate an intracranial abscess or when an intracranial abscess is not considered. Conversely, concomitant sinusitis may fail to be diagnosed in patients diagnosed with meningitis if a neuro-imaging study is not performed, a likelihood in the management of many patients diagnosed with meningitis.

Dural venous sinus thrombosis/thrombophlebitis (sagittal, transverse, and cavernous) is the least common complication, absent in some case series (16,19), and accounting for 3% to 9% of intracranial complications in others (15,18,23). In most cases, venous sinus thrombosis is not an isolated complication, but occurs in concert with subdural suppuration.

Patients commonly have more than one intracranial complication, such as epidural/subdural abscess in association with cerebral abscess and/or meningitis. Table 5 summarizes the relative frequency of each intracranial complication from data pooled from several recent studies that used similar inclusion criteria and selection methods.

Most studies have demonstrated a large male predominance (greater than 3:1, male/female) for intracranial suppuration from sinusitis (16–20,22). This male predominance remains unexplained, but prevails at all age groups and may suggest sex-related anatomical differences in sinus structure/sinus venous drainage.

Pathogenesis

The pathogenesis for intracranial suppuration mirrors that of intraorbital infection. Intracranial infection can develop following direct extension through sinus wall invasion to contiguous bone, and then to intracranial

Table 5 Relative Frequency of Intracranial Complications[a]

Intracranial complication	Relative frequency (%, range)
Meningitis	34% (14–54)
Brain abscess	27% (0–50)
Epidural abscess	23% (0–44)
Subdural abscess	24% (9–86)
Dural sinus thrombosis	8% (0–27)
Percent of patients with >1 intracranial complication	28%

Note: Study reference 30 excluded meningitis cases as a complications.
[a]Pooled data from 131 patients in eight studies (15–17,19,20,23,30,48).

structures through either osteitis or congenital or traumatic defects. In contrast to orbital infections, the more common method of intracranial suppurative spread is by the propagation of septic emboli via calvarial diploic veins and the valveless venous system responsible for drainage of the midface and paranasal sinuses (15,16,20,23).

Although many of these complications arise in the setting of pansinusitis, some intracranial infections are more strongly associated with specific sinus involvement. Meningitis often arises from ethmoid or sphenoid sinus involvement (23). Cavernous sinus thrombosis is also associated with sphenoiditis and ethmoiditis (25,26), although it was more commonly associated with frontal sinusitis prior to use of current antibiotic regimens (25). The frontal sinuses are most frequently implicated in the development of extra-axial and intracerebral abscesses as well as infection of the remaining dural sinuses (15,16,21,23).

Clinical Presentation

Because of the shared pathogenic origin, it common for a patient to have more than one intracranial complication. Therefore, it is difficult to attribute a presenting symptom to an isolated intracranial cause. Similarly, the signs and symptoms of rhinosinusitis also overlap to some degree with the presentation of intracranial infection. Common presenting features will be discussed in this section, and specific presentations more common or unique to a particular intracranial pathological entity will subsequently be discussed. Table 6 summarizes presenting symptoms and signs, collated from recent studies with similar inclusion criteria.

Headache, commonly frontal or retro-orbital, is the overwhelmingly prominent symptom, occurring in approximately 70% of patients with intracranial infection arising from sinusitis. Most patients have fever (>38.5°C) as well. As would be expected, many patients have symptoms of sinonasal disease with purulent rhinorrhea and sinus pressure/pain. Compared to adults,

Table 6 Presenting Symptoms/Signs of Intracranial Infection Arising from Sinusitis[a]

Headache (%)	69
Fever (%)	60
Altered mental status (ranging from confusion to obtundation; %)	41
Nausea/vomiting (%)	30
Cranial nerve palsy (%)	18
Seizure (%)	14
Other focal neurologic signs (hemiparesis/hemiplegia, aphasia, ataxia, motor/sensory deficits; %)	14
Nuchal rigidity (%)	10

[a]Pooled data from 91 patients in seven studies (15–17,19,20,30,48).

children rarely have prominent rhinorrhea or upper respiratory symptoms, and complications often arise during a more acute course of sinusitis.

Patients also commonly have symptoms of increased intracranial pressure, including alterations in mental function, vomiting, and photophobia. Arachnoid irritation may be indicated by nuchal rigidity (15–17,19,20).

Later neurological symptoms and signs for intracranial infections include seizures, focal paresis, and cranial nerve palsies.

Diagnosis

Prior to the advent of computerized cross-sectional neuro-imaging (CT and MRI), diagnosis of space-occupying intracranial infections was primarily based on clinical evaluation and judgment (22).

CT and MRI scans are complementary techniques, each of which can yield diagnostic information helpful in the definitive management of intracranial complications. CT scan is readily available, can demonstrate most cases of intracranial suppuration, and is a technique of choice to evaluate bony involvement. CT scanning is the imaging modality of choice for initial evaluation of complications from sinusitis and for planning sinus surgery because of its superior ability to delineate air–bone and air–soft tissue interfaces. MRI, on the other hand, has better resolution for intracranial pathology and has higher diagnostic accuracy for intracranial infections. In one study comparing CT and MRI for the diagnosis of suppurative complications from sinusitis, CT scan was diagnostic for 36 of 39 cases (92%) compared to 100% with MRI. MRI was also able to detect meningitis in 14 cases compared to three for CT scan. CT scanning missed one subdural abscess and one intracerebral abscess. Both modalities exceeded diagnoses made on clinical grounds, which had an accuracy of 82% overall (22).

Contrasted CT scan may be contraindicated in patients with renal insufficiency or those with life-threatening contrast allergies. MRI should be employed as the first method of evaluation in such cases. If such patients are unsuitable for MRI because of implanted ferromagnetic devices, pacemakers, implanted defibrillators, or other contraindications, patients with renal insufficiency may gain some nephro-protective effect from the administration of *n*-acetyl cysteine (27) or from hydration with sodium bicarbonate (28) prior to contrast administration.

Meningitis

Clinical Presentation

Meningitis most frequently presents as headache. The majority of patients also have fever (>38.5°C) and more than half have neck stiffness/nuchal rigidity. Other symptoms include vomiting, mental status changes, and less commonly, seizures (15,16,20,29). In one series, a patient presented with facial nerve palsy (30).

Bacteriology

As with other sources for bacterial meningitis, *S. pneumoniae* is the most common organism causing meningitis in the setting of sinusitis. Another causative organism, in order of decreasing incidence, is *S. aureus* (especially in sphenoid sinusitis). Rarely, isolates include *H. influenzae, Neisseria meningitidis*, and gram-negative aerobic bacilli (29). The primary pathogen in patients with AIDS is *Cryptococcus neoformans* (29).

Diagnosis

Although meningitis is routinely diagnosed by lumbar puncture and cerebrospinal fluid analyses, the performance of lumbar puncture in the setting of a space-occupying lesion risks trans-tentorial uncal herniation, particularly when the mass is in the temporal fossa (31). As signs and symptoms of space-occupying infection can be subtle or be obscured by the findings that suggest meningitis, CT scan should be obtained prior to lumbar puncture when sinusitis has been diagnosed or clinically suspected. When suspected or known, space-occupying infection (abscess) or increased intracranial pressure precludes lumbar puncture; diagnosis of meningitis can sometimes be made on the basis of contrast-enhanced magnetic resonance imaging. Younis found MRI diagnostic in 14 of 21 patients with meningitis-complicating sinusitis; CT was diagnostic in 3 of 21 patients (22). Contrast-enhanced MRI typically demonstrates dural enhancement along the falx cerebri, tentorium, and dural convexity. Conversely, CT and unenhanced MRI are usually normal, with the exception of findings of sinusitis (22).

Treatment

Isolated meningitis, confirmed by absence of space-occupying lesions on CT scanning or MRI, is treated exclusively with antibiotics. As meningitis can progress rapidly in a fulminating course, especially with the predominance of pneumococcus as the primary pathogen, antibiotic therapy should be initiated as soon as the diagnosis is suspected and prior to neuro-imaging or lumbar puncture (32). Blood culture, on the other hand, should be obtained prior to the administration of antibiotics, as blood collection will not delay therapy.

S. pneumoniae meningitis has a case fatality rate of 20% with significant morbidity among survivors (33). Dexamethasone, when administered either before or with first antibiotic dose, has been shown to decrease unfavorable outcome and mortality (34,35). On the other hand, because vancomycin will only reach the cerebrospinal fluid (CSF) through inflamed meninges, administration of dexamethasone may decrease CSF antibiotic penetration (36). In areas with high prevalence of antibiotic-resistant *S. pneumoniae*, one must weigh the potential decrease in sequellae with the possibility of decreased antibiotic efficacy. Dexamethasone may also be warranted for treatment of cerebral edema secondary to intracranial infection; however, steroid therapy may also contribute to immunosuppression and its role in intracranial suppuration, exclusive of isolated meningitis, has not been rigorously studied. Choice of initial antibiotic therapy consists of a parenteral third-generation cephalosporin (cefotaxime or ceftriaxone) combined with vancomycin to cover resistant *S. pneumoniae*. Further refinement of antibiotic choice should then be made upon review of CSF gram stain and again after results of CSF culture.

In patients with AIDS and contraindication for lumbar puncture, one would need to initiate intravenous therapy with amphotericin B to cover cryptococcus.

Brain Abscess

Clinical Presentation

Headache and fever are the initial prominent symptoms. Moreover, nausea and vomiting are also frequent. Altered mental status—including confusion, decreased mentation, and/or behavioral changes—is an alarming symptom which should be a tip-off that a serious intracranial process is occurring beyond sinusitis or other causes of fever and headache. Intracerebral abscess, in particular, may be associated with behavioral changes, secondary to associated cerebritis. As the majority of brain abscesses from sinusitis occur in the frontal lobes, relatively neurologically silent, these mental status changes may be subtle and unlikely to be associated with focal neurologic deficits (20). Intracerebral abscess also presents a significant risk for seizure development.

Bacteriology

Intracranial and extra-axial abscesses often yield multiple organisms, both aerobic and anaerobic, including *Fusobacterium* spp., anaerobic gram-negative bacilli (*Prevotella* and *Porphyromonas* spp.), anaerobic and microaerophillic streptococci, *Propionibacterium* spp., *Eikenella corrodens*, and *Staphylococcus* spp. However, intraoperative cultures of intracranial abscess cavities may yield no identifiable organism. In the majority of such cases, patients have received oral and/or parenteral antibiotics for the underlying sinusitis. There is often a correlation between the cultures obtained from the sinuses and from the intracranial abscess cavities (37,38). Nevertheless, in some patients the culture results do not correlate between the two sites (15,17). This is likely because of the different microenvironment of intracranial abscess cavities relative to the paranasal sinuses. Brook also suggests that variability in collection techniques, culturing for strict anaerobes, and improper specimen handling to prevent contamination may account for differences in the final organism identification (39). In some cases, however, the presence of sinusitis may be coincidental and not causative of the intracranial suppuration.

Diagnosis

Computed tomography can demonstrate cerebral abscess on the basis of low density attenuation of involved parenchyma and mass effect as well as the later development of ring-enhancement from collagen encapsulation of the necrosis. However, MRI can also demonstrate the early cerebritis phase of abscess formation. In addition, MRI T-1 weighted images can better demonstrate sulcus effacement and mass effect (22).

Treatment

Intracranial abscesses are usually treated by three complementary tactics: (1) immediate initiation of parenteral broad-spectrum antibiotic therapy (prior to neuro-imaging) with good blood–brain barrier traversal; (2) operative drainage of intracranial abscess; and (3) drainage of infected sinuses.

The most commonly used empirical antibiotic choices include the combination of a third-generation cephalosporin (cefotaxime or ceftreaxone), a penicillinase-resistant penicillin, and metronidazole. Vancomycin may substitute the penicillinase-resistant penicillin to cover resistant *S. pneumoniae*. Subsequent antibiotic administration needs to be adjusted based on results from operative cultures. Intravenous antibiotics should be continued for four to eight weeks to maintain high CSF drug levels. As healing occurs and the blood–brain barrier is repaired, adequate drug levels will be achieved only with parenteral administration (15).

A trial of antibiotic therapy alone may be warranted in a selected subset of patients who are deemed clinically stable (40,41). This group would include those in whom the risk of surgery is felt to be inordinately great, either because of the increased neurosurgical risk inherent in operating on deep, dominant, or multiple dispersed lesions or because of increased surgical risk from other health factors. Those patients with early, small abscesses may fall into this category as well, based on relative risk. Patients forgoing surgical drainage should be imaged at least weekly for the first two weeks and bi-weekly through the eight-week course of antibiotic therapy. Clinical deterioration or lack of clinical improvement would necessitate reconsideration of surgical drainage.

Sinus drainage may be performed by open technique or, more commonly, endoscopic technique and should follow intracranial drainage, but during the same course of anesthesia.

Drainage procedures commence as soon as possible after localization of the purulent collection. Although small cerebral abscesses can be treated with a trial of antibiotic therapy, larger ones must be drained either with an open craniotomy or with CT-localized needle drainage procedures, depending on abscess location. Because of seizure risk attendant with cerebral abscess, prophylactic anticonvulsant therapy is warranted and should be initiated as soon as the diagnosis is established.

Extra-axial Abscess (Subdural and Epidural Abscesses)

Clinical Presentation

Patients with subdural abscess, as with other intracranial infections, usually present with headaches, fever, and meningismus. Deterioration of neurologic status can progress rapidly, however, with decreased consciousness and development of seizures (42).

Epidural abscess develops more insidiously, and symptoms may be nonspecific and overshadowed by the symptoms of the patient's sinusitis (Fig. 4) Patients may not present for several weeks, until neurologic deterioration or seizures prompt CNS imaging (42).

Bacteriology

The bacteriology of subdural and epidural abscesses is similar to that previously described for intracerebral abscess (39).

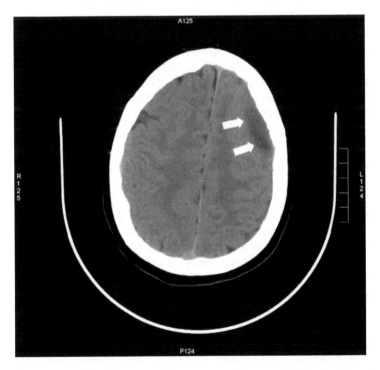

Figure 4 Epidural empyema in a teenager being treated for sinusitis who presented to an emergency department because of new onset seizure.

Diagnosis

MRI is considered as the imaging modality of choice to diagnose both epidural and subdural suppurative collections because of its superior ability to detect abscess not evident on routine CT. In the event that MRI is unavailable or contraindicated, a contrasted CT scan can still reveal the diagnosis in most cases.

Treatment

Subdural pus collections are often loculated and extensive over the cerebral hemisphere and historically have required craniotomy. Multiple burr holes using CT stereotactic localization are now being employed more frequently (15).

Epidural abscesses have also been traditionally treated with neurosurgical drainage. However, a more conservative approach has been suggested for small epidural abscesses, utilizing endoscopic or trephination for sinus drainage and intravenous antibiotics for six weeks. Heran et al. (21) used this approach on a group of four children with epidural abscess with a mean abscess size of 3 cm × 3 cm × 1 cm, without neurologic deficits. Although two patients had transient worsening headache and fever over the first 48 hours, there was no worsening on follow-up imaging, and patients improved over the subsequent two weeks without neurosurgical intervention. Antibiotic therapy was continued for six weeks.

In some cases of epidural abscess with frontal sinusitis and osteomyelitis, exenteration of the frontal sinus (removal of anterior and posterior tables as well as obliteration of the nasofrontal recess) may be warranted (15).

As with intracerebral abscess, drainage of involved sinuses should be coordinated with the neurosurgical procedures and antibiotic therapy should be initiated as soon as possible.

Dural Sinus Thrombosis/Thrombophlebitis

Clinical Presentation

When complicating sinusitis, dural sinus thrombosis rarely occurs in isolation from other intracranial complications. On the other hand, isolated dural sinus thrombosis has myriad causes of which facial/head/neck infections account for only 8%. Patients with major venous sinus thrombosis often appear septic, with high fever, tachycardia, hypotension, and confusion. Headache is almost invariably present. Because of associated cerebral edema and ischemic and/or hemorrhagic infarction, both generalized and focal neurologic symptoms and signs are often present, including decreased or altered consciousness, seizures, paralysis, aphasia, and cranial nerve deficits (26,43–45). In one study, patients who presented with more generalized neurologic impairment, suggesting intracranial hypertension, actually had more diffuse involvement of venous sinuses with thrombosis than did patients with a more focal presentation.

Paradoxically, the patients with the intracranial hypertension presentation had better outcomes than those with focal neurologic impairment (43).

In addition to fever and headache, eye signs will predominate early in the course of septic cavernous sinus thrombosis. As orbital venous congestion progresses, chemosis, periorbital edema, and proptosis can occur. Fundoscopy may reveal papilledema and retinal venous congestion. Ocular movement may become restricted by intraorbital edema and subsequently by oculomotor, trochlear, and abducens nerve palsies. The abducens nerve in particular may be affected early owing to its course within the cavernous sinus, and thus lateral nerve palsy may be noted. Although ocular findings are unilateral initially, progression to bilateral involvement occurs rapidly, usually within 48 hours (25,26).

Bacteriology

For cavernous sinus thrombophlebitis, the most common offending organism is *S. aureus*, accounting for two-thirds of cases (26,46). Other less common organisms include *S. pneumoniae*, gram-negative bacilli, and anaerobes (46).

Diagnosis

Venography can be used for diagnosing venous sinus thrombosis, but its use has largely been supplanted by contrasted MRI with venography (MRV). Contrasted CT scan can demonstrate filling defects within the venous sinus (25), if contraindication for MRI or MRI itself is unavailable. Occasionally the diagnosis is established in the operating room.

Treatment

For septic venous dural sinus thrombosis, management consists of medical therapy in conjunction with drainage of affected pneumatic sinuses and associated areas of intracranial purulence. In addition, anticoagulation has been advocated to facilitate antibiotic penetration, to decrease further propagation of septic thrombus, and to limit a precipitous rise in intracranial pressure. Others have argued that anticoagulation risks increased systemic or intracranial bleeding, including intraorbital bleeding and intracranial bleeding from cortical infarcts or from carotid rupture if the carotid has become infected in it course through the cavernous sinus. Of note, there have been only two cases of intracranial bleeding secondary to anticoagulation and septic cavernous sinus thrombosis (26,47) and no reported cases of intraorbital bleeding. There is also a theoretical risk of further propagation of intracranial infection secondary to a dispersal of septic emboli as the thrombus breaks down.

However, in a small retrospective series of 31 patients with venous sinus thrombosis, Soleau and colleagues demonstrated that observation alone had the poorest results, with clinical improvement in only 2 of 5 patients and hemorrhagic complications in 4 of 5 with one death, whereas systemic

Schwartz and White

anticoagulation resulted in improvement in 75% (8) of patients who were so treated, with no worsening of hemorrhage even in those patients with pretreatment hemorrhage; best results were obtained with a combination of mechanical endovascular clot dissolution and systemic anticoagulation, resulting in clinical improvement in 7 of 8 patients and one death. Chemical thrombolysis (urokinase or tissue plasminogen activator) was successful in restoring venous sinus patency in 6 of 10 patients, but at a significant rate of fatal intracranial hemorrhage (30%) (45). These numbers must be considered in the context of the study limitations inherent with small study size and retrospective data collection.

Options for anticoagulation include intravenous heparin and low-molecular weight heparin, which may have a lower risk of bleeding but is less rapidly reversed. Once the patient becomes stabilized, conversion to oral anticoagulation can be undertaken. Although degree of anticoagulation has also not been definitively established, a general guideline would be essential to maintain an APTT ratio of 1.5 to 2.5 and an INR of 2.0 to 3.0 (26). Duration of anticoagulation should continue until follow-up neuroimaging confirms dissolution of the thrombus, about several weeks; long-term anticoagulation is not required.

REFERENCES

1. Guillen A, Brell E, Cardona E, Claramunt E, Costa J. Pott's puffy tumour: still not an eradicated entity. Child's Nerv Syst 2001; 17:359–362.
2. Verbon A, Husni R, Gordon SM, Lavertu P, Keys TF. Pott's puffy tumor due to *Haemophilus influenzae*: case report and review. Clin Infect Dis 1996; 23: 1305–1307.
3. Laine FJ, Smoker WR. The ostiomeatal unit and endoscopic surgery: anatomy, variation and imaging findings in inflammatory diseases. AJR 1992; 159: 849–857.
4. Clayman GL, Adams GL, Paugh DR, Koopman CF. Intracranial complications of paranasal sinusitis: a combined institutional review. Laryngoscope 1991; 101:234–239.
5. Younis RT, Lazar RH, Bustillo A, Anand VK. Orbital infection as a complication of sinusitis: are diagnostic and treatment trends changing?. Ear Nose Throat J 2002; 81:771–775.
6. Harris GJ. Subperiosteal abscess of the orbit. Age as a factor in the bacteriology and response to treatment. Ophthalmology 1994; 101:585–593.
7. Harris GJ, Bair RL. Anaerobic and aerobic isolates from a subperiosteal orbital abscess in a four year old. Arch Ophthalmol 1996; 114:98–100.
8. Brook I, Friedman EM, Rodriques WJ, Controni G. Complications of sinusitis in children. Pediatrics 1980; 66:568–572.
9. Chandler JR, Langenbrunner DJ, Stevens ER. The pathogenesis of orbital complications in acute sinusitis. Laryngoscope 1970; 80:1414–1428.

10. Schwartz GR, Wright SW. Changing bacteriology of periorbital cellulitis. Ann Emerg Med 1996; 28:617–620.
11. Garcia GH, Harris GJ. Criteria for nonsurgical management of subperiosteal abscess of the orbit. Analysis of outcomes 1988–1998. Ophthalmology 2000; 107:1454–1458.
12. Uzeategui N, Warman R, Smith A, Howard CW. Clinical practice guidelines for the management of orbital cellulitis. J Pediatr Ophtalmol Strabismus 1998; 35:73–79.
13. Sobol SE, Marchand J, Tewfik TL, Manoukian JJ, Schloss MD. Orbital complications of sinusitis in children. J Otolaryngol 2002; 31:131–136.
14. Rahbar R, Robson CD, Petersen RA, DiCanzio J, Rosbe KW, Mcgill TJ. Management of orbital subperiosteal abscess in children. Arch Otolaryngol Head Neck Surg 2001; 127:281–286.
15. Gallagher RM, Gross CW, Phillips CD. Suppurative intracranial complications of sinusitis. Laryngoscope 1998; 108(11 Pt 1):1635–1642.
16. Giannoni CM, Stewart MG, Alford EL. Intracranial complications of sinusitis. Laryngoscope 1997; 107(7):863–867.
17. Giannoni C, Sulek M, Friedman EM. Intracranial complications of sinusitis: a pediatric series. Am J Rhinol 1998; 12(3):173–178.
18. Hytonen M, Atula T, Pitkaranta A. Complications of acute sinusitis in children. Acta Otolaryngol Suppl 2000; 543:154–157.
19. Ong YK, Tan HK. Suppurative intracranial complications of sinusitis in children. Int J Pediatr Otorhinolaryngol 2002; 66(1):49.
20. Albu S, Tomescu E, Bassam S, Merca Z. Intracranial complications of sinusitis. Acta Otorhinolaryngol Belg 2001; 55(4):265–272.
21. Heran NS, Steinbok P, Cochrane DD. Conservative neurosurgical management of intracranial epidural abscesses in children. Neurosurgery 2003; 53(4):893–897 (discussion 7–8).
22. Younis RT, Anand VK, Davidson B. The role of computed tomography and magnetic resonance imaging in patients with sinusitis with complications. Laryngoscope 2002; 112(2):224–229.
23. Younis RT, Lazar RH, Anand VK. Intracranial complications of sinusitis: a 15-year review of 39 cases. Ear Nose Throat J 2002; 81(9):636–638, 40–42, 44.
24. Bradley PJ, Manning KP, Shaw MD. Brain abscess secondary to paranasal sinusitis. J Laryngol Otol 1984; 98(7):719–725.
25. Amran M, Sidek DS, Hamzah M, Abdullah JM, Halim AS, Johari MR, Hitam WH, Ariff AR. Cavernous sinus thrombosis secondary to sinusitis. J Otolaryngol 2002; 31(3):165–169.
26. Bhatia K, Jones NS. Septic cavernous sinus thrombosis secondary to sinusitis: are anticoagulants indicated? A review of the literature. J Laryngol Otol 2002; 116(9):667–676.
27. Birck R, Krzossok S, Markowetz F, Schnulle P, van der Woude FJ, Braun C. Acetylcysteine for prevention of contrast nephropathy: meta-analysis. Lancet 2003; 362(9384):598–603.
28. Merten GJ, Burgess WP, Gray LV, Holleman JH, Roush TS, Kowalchuk GJ, Bersin RM, Van Moore A, Simonton CA, Rittase RA, Norton HJ, Kennedy TP. Prevention of contrast-induced nephropathy with sodium bicarbonate: a randomized controlled trial. JAMA 2004; 291(19):2328–2334.

29. Younis RT, Anand VK, Childress C. Sinusitis complicated by meningitis: current management. Laryngoscope 2001; 111(8):1338–1342.
30. Clayman GL, Adams GL, Paugh DR, Koopmann CF Jr. Intracranial complications of paranasal sinusitis: a combined institutional review. Laryngoscope 1991; 101(3):234–239.
31. Archer BD. Computed tomography before lumbar puncture in acute meningitis: a review of the risks and benefits. CMAJ 1993; 148(6):961–965.
32. Aronin SI, Peduzzi P, Quagliarello VJ. Community-acquired bacterial meningitis: risk stratification for adverse clinical outcome and effect of antibiotic timing. Ann Intern Med 1998; 129(11):862–869.
33. Schuchat A, Robinson K, Wenger JD, Harrison LH, Farley M, Reingold AL, Lefkowitz L, Perkins BA. Bacterial meningitis in the United States in 1995. Active Surveillance Team. N Engl J Med 1997; 337(14):970–976.
34. de Gans J, van de Beek D. Dexamethasone in adults with bacterial meningitis. N Engl J Med 2002; 347(20):1549–1556.
35. van de Beek D, de Gans J, McIntyre P, Prasad K. Steroids in adults with acute bacterial meningitis: a systematic review. Lancet Infect Dis 2004; 4(3):139–143.
36. Quagliarello VJ, Scheld WM. Treatment of bacterial meningitis. N Engl J Med 1997; 336(10):708–716.
37. Brook I, Frazier EH. Microbiology of subperiosteal orbital abscess and associated maxillary sinusitis. Laryngoscope 1996; 106(8):1010–1013.
38. Brook I, Friedman EM, Rodriguez WJ, Controni G. Complications of sinusitis in children. Pediatrics 1980; 66(4):568–572.
39. Brook I. Aerobic and anaerobic bacteriology of intracranial abscesses. Pediatr Neurol 1992; 8(3):210–214.
40. Calfee DP, Wispelwey B. Brain abscess. Semin Neurol 2000; 20(3):353–360.
41. Rosenblum ML, Hoff JT, Norman D, Edwards MS, Berg BO. Nonoperative treatment of brain abscesses in selected high-risk patients. J Neurosurg 1980; 52(2):217–225.
42. Bockova J, Rigamonti D. Intracranial empyema. Pediatr Infect Dis J 2000; 19(8):735–737.
43. Bergui M, Bradac GB. Clinical picture of patients with cerebral venous thrombosis and patterns of dural sinus involvement. Cerebrovasc Dis 2003; 16(3):211–216.
44. Ferro JM, Canhao P, Stam J, Bousser MG, Barinagarrementeria F. Prognosis of cerebral vein and dural sinus thrombosis: results of the International Study on Cerebral Vein and Dural Sinus Thrombosis (ISCVT). Stroke 2004; 35(3): 664–670.
45. Soleau SW, Schmidt R, Stevens S, Osborn A, MacDonald JD. Extensive experience with dural sinus thrombosis. Neurosurgery 2003; 52(3):534–544 (discussion 42–44).
46. Ebright JR, Pace MT, Niazi AF. Septic thrombosis of the cavernous sinuses. Arch Intern Med 2001; 161(22):2671–2676.
47. Southwick FS, Richardson EP Jr, Swartz MN. Septic thrombosis of the dural venous sinuses. Medicine (Baltimore) 1986; 65(2):82–106.
48. Rosenfeld EA, Rowley AH. Infectious intracranial complications of sinusitis, other than meningitis, in children: 12-year review. Clin Infect Dis 1994; 18(5): 750–754.

14

Sinusitis and Asthma

Frank S. Virant

University of Washington, Seattle, Washington, U.S.A.

INTRODUCTION

Sinusitis and asthma are commonly seen simultaneously in clinical practice (1–3). In fact, nearly 50% of asthmatics demonstrate upper airway symptoms and radiographic evidence of rhinosinusitis (4–11). Chronic sinusitis and asthma share several pathophysiological features: chemical mediators, e.g., histamine, cysteinyl leukotrienes, and prostaglandin D_2; cytokines, e.g., interleukin-4 (IL-4), IL-5, IL-9, IL-13, and CCL11 (eotaxin); and cellular mediators, principally eosinophils and T_H2 lymphocytes (12–14). These observations have led to the concept of "one airway ... one disease" rather than the idea of isolated upper and lower airway disorders. At the same time, numerous clinical studies have demonstrated that aggressive medical or surgical treatment of sinusitis improves asthma, suggesting that upper airway inflammation may actually have a causative role in lower airway disease.

This chapter will explore the historical association of sinusitis and asthma, the common inflammatory basis of these disorders, and evidence that sinus therapy can improve concomitant asthma. A brief discussion of possible mechanisms by which sinusitis could exacerbate asthma is followed by implications for patient management.

HISTORICAL ASSOCIATION OF SINUSITIS AND ASTHMA

About two millennia ago, it was Galen's belief that sinusitis caused asthma; this assertion was based on the notion that abnormal secretions dripped from the skull into the lungs, inducing irritation and wheezing. This idea was generally embraced, leading to nasal irrigation and purging to help treat asthma. Ironically, this notion was abandoned in the mid-1600s when early anatomists demonstrated that no direct connection between the skull and lungs existed (15).

Interest in the association between sinusitis and asthma was revived in 1870 when Kratchmer showed that chemical irritation of animal upper airways with ether, cigarette smoke, or sulfur dioxide caused bronchoconstriction (16). At the beginning of the twentieth century, Dixon and Brodie also demonstrated that nasal mechanical or electrical stimuli could induce reflex lower airway obstruction (17).

Clinical observations early in the twentieth century reaffirmed that upper and lower airway diseases were frequently coexistent. Gottlieb observed that 31 of 117 adult asthmatics also had clinical evidence of sinusitis (4). Chobot and Weille (5,6) reported that sinus symptoms were present in as many as 72% of children and adults with asthma. Bullen's review of 400 sinusitis patients revealed a 12% incidence of asthma with many noting that sinus symptoms preceded the appearance of their asthma (18).

Over the last three decades, several studies in adults and children demonstrated that 21 to 31% of asthmatics have significantly abnormal sinus radiographs (mucosal thickening >5 mm, air–fluid levels, or opacification) (7–9,19). In contrast, only 5 to 6% of asymptomatic adults and children showed such radiographic sinus changes (20,21). Collectively, these reports suggest that asthmatics are four to six times more likely to display sinus pathology than healthy non-asthmatics—strong evidence of an association between these diseases.

CHEMICAL, CYTOKINE, AND CELLULAR MEDIATORS OF AIRWAY DISEASE

Further evidence of a relationship between sinusitis and asthma is apparent after comparing chemical, cytokine, and cellular mediators in these diseases (Table 1).

Chemical Mediators

Levels of histamine, prostaglandin D_2, and the cysteinyl leukotrienes (LTC_4, LTD_4, and LTE_4) are all elevated in the maxillary sinuses of patients with chronic eosinophilic sinusitis and in the bronchoalveolar lavage fluid of patients with asthma (12–14,22).

Cytokine Mediators

Both chronic sinusitis and asthma may demonstrate a variety of common cytokine mediators, including IL-4, IL-5, IL-9, IL-13, CCL11 (eotaxin),

Table 1 Chemical, Cytokine, and Cellular Mediators of Airway Disease

Type	Mediator	Effector functions
Chemical	Histamine	Vasodilation, hypersecretion, bronchoconstriction
	Prostaglandin D_2	Smooth muscle constriction
	Leukotriene C_4, D_4, E_4	Vasodilation, hypersecretion, bronchoconstriction
Cytokine	Interleukin 4	Directs B cell to produce specific IgE
	Interleukin 5	Clonal growth factor for eosinophils
	Interleukin 9	T cell, mast cell growth factor
	Interleukin 13	Augments specific IgE secretion
	CCL 11 (eotaxin)	Chemoattractant for eosinophils
	Tumor necrosis factor α	Augments inflammation (fever, pain)
Cellular	Eosinophils	Inflammation, airway hyperresponsiveness
	T_H2 lymphocytes[a]	Produce/release IL-4, IL-5, IL-9, IL-13

[a]T_H2 lymphocytes are a major mediator in *allergic* rhinosinusitis and *allergic* asthma; these cells are a less significant component in *non-allergic* airway inflammation.

and TNF-α. In patients with underlying allergic disease, all of these mediators are present throughout the airway; in non-allergic eosinophilic airway disease, IL-5, eotaxin, and TNF-α are predominating features (23–26).

Cellular Mediators

Almost 80 years ago, Hansel (27) remarked on the histological similarities between chronic sinusitis and persistent asthma: marked eosinophilia, glandular hyperplasia, and stromal edema. More recently, Harlin and coworkers examined the role of the eosinophil in the induction of chronic sinusitis. They examined sinus tissue for the presence of eosinophils and/or major basic protein (MBP—a significant eosinophil-derived granule protein) in 26 adolescent and adult patients with chronic sinusitis. All 13 sinus samples from asthmatics and six of seven samples from allergic rhinitis patients showed significant eosinophils and MBP while none of the six patients with chronic sinusitis without asthma or allergic rhinitis showed significant tissue eosinophils (one had MBP) (28).

Hisamatsu and colleagues (29) showed that MBP at physiologic concentrations in vitro could cause epithelial damage and ciliary dysmotility in sinus mucosal tissue. They concluded that eosinophils could play an important role in increasing the risk for bacterial sinusitis and in the induction of nasal hyperresponsiveness through cholinergic pathways. Potentially, this effect of upper airway eosinophils could also affect bronchial hyperresponsiveness through the same neural pathways (30).

IMPACT OF MEDICAL SINUS THERAPY ON ASTHMA

Over the last two decades, several groups have studied the effect of medical treatment for sinusitis in children with asthma (31). Businco et al. (32) studied 55 asthmatic children with mild to severe maxillary sinus thickening. After 30 days therapy with either nasal corticosteroid plus antihistamine/decongestant or ampicillin plus antihistamine/decongestant, all children showed decreased asthma severity and sinus radiographic improvement. In 1983, Cummings and coworkers compared antibiotics plus nasal corticosteroids and decongestants versus placebo in the treatment of asthmatic children with opacified or markedly thickened maxillary sinuses. Although pulmonary function and bronchial hyperresponsiveness were not significantly changed in either group, the children on active treatment had reduced asthma symptoms and less need for bronchodilators and oral corticosteroids (33). The next year, Rachelefsky et al. (34) treated 48 children who had at least a three-month history of sinusitis and asthma; treatment included prolonged antibiotics and, in select cases, antral lavage. Nearly 80% of the subjects were able to discontinue bronchodilators and more than 50% returned to normal lung function. Independently in 1984, Friedman and colleagues followed the effect of antibiotic treatment in eight children with acute sinusitis and asthma exacerbation; seven of the children showed significant improvement in asthma symptoms. Although pulmonary function did not statistically improve, response to bronchodilator doubled compared with pre-study levels (35).

More recently, Oliveira studied 46 allergic and 20 non-allergic children with sinusitis and asthma. Therapy included 21 days of antibiotics, antihistamines, decongestants, nasal saline irrigation, and five days of oral corticosteroids. By the end of the study, only the children who demonstrated radiographic resolution of their sinusitis had improved pulmonary function and bronchial hyperresponsiveness (36). Additional evidence that upper airway inflammation can affect lower airway disease comes from Corren's research on patients with seasonal allergic rhinitis/bronchial hyperresponsiveness; seasonal nasal corticosteroid treatment alone could prevent increased bronchial hyperresponsiveness (37,38).

IMPACT OF SURGICAL SINUS THERAPY ON ASTHMA

In contrast to medical treatment, the impact of sinus surgical intervention on asthma is variable (39). In 1920, Van der Veer published his clinical observations that asthma was worsened by sinonasal surgery (40). Nearly a decade later, Francis published a series of 13 patients with surgical intervention for chronic sinusitis; nine demonstrated worsening of their lung symptoms after operation (41).

In contrast, Weille's 1936 study of 500 asthmatics revealed a 72% incidence of sinusitis. Ultimately, over half of the 100 subjects who had sinus surgery experienced an improvement in asthma. Ten became totally asymptomatic. At the same time, over 40% of the sinusitis patients who did not have surgery also had asthma improvement (6). Davison's study in 1969 observed that all but one of his 24 patients had at least a 75% improvement in asthma symptoms after sinus drainage (42). In the early 1980s, Slavin and coworkers described similar results in 33 adult sinus surgical patients: 85% had significantly better asthma control and were able to markedly reduce their requirement for oral corticosteroids (43). Over a period of months, though, 40% of those who initially experienced improvement following surgery demonstrated asthma exacerbations. Werth reported on 22 children with chronic sinusitis and asthma in 1984; asthma markedly improved in 20 after sinus surgery (44). The same year, Juntunen et al. described 15 children with persistent chronic sinusitis despite inferior meatal antrostomy and adenoidectomy; even this degree of surgical intervention appeared to improve asthma symptoms and lung function (45).

The last decade has spawned numerous additional studies, primarily, though not exclusively, in adults with nasal/sinus polyps; uniformly, endoscopic sinus surgical intervention improved asthma (46–52).

SINUSITIS AS A TRIGGER FOR ASTHMA—MECHANISMS

Nearly 80 years ago, Gottlieb suggested several ways in which sinusitis might excerbate asthma (Table 2): neural reflexes pathways, nasal obstruction, sinus inflammatory secretions draining into the lower airway, and indirect delivery of inflammatory "signals" through the systemic circulation (4). Recently other researchers have suggested decreased β-adrenergic responsiveness as an additional possible mechanism (30,35). Although controversies remain, the actual process in individual patients is probably a combination of one or more mechanisms (53).

Neural Reflex Pathways

In the early twentieth century, Sluder proposed that asthma was caused by reflexes intiated in the nose and sinuses (54). Subsequent animal research

Table 2 Sinusitis as a Trigger for Asthma—Mechanisms

Neural reflex pathways: trigeminal afferents → CNS → vagal efferents
Nasal obstruction: decreased air filtration, humidification, heating
Sinus inflammatory secretions draining to lower airway: direct effect
Sinus inflammatory mediators exerts systemic effect on lungs: indirect effect
Sinusitis reduces β-adrenergic responsiveness: unknown pathway

after upper airway "irritation" yielded controversial results, including no change in lower airway resistance, bronchodilation, and bronchoconstriction.

In 1969, Kaufman et al. (55) studied non-asthmatics with tic doloreux, inducing increased lower airway resistance by delivering silica into the upper airway. After surgical treatment of tic doloreux with trigeminal nerve resection, this response was blocked, leading the authors to postulate a "nasal-bronchial reflex" mediated through trigeminal afferents and vagal efferents. Other groups demonstrated that nasal provocation with cold air, sulfur dioxide, or petrolatum could also induce pulmonary resistance changes after exposure (56–58).

Salome demonstrated that histamine nasal challenge in symptomatic perennial allergic rhinitis patients could induce at least a 10% decrease in forced expiratory volume in one second (FEV_1) (59). Three other studies on asymptomatic seasonal allergic patients failed to show such a change, suggesting that baseline nasal inflammation was important for this response (60–62).

Corren and coworkers evaluated 10 patients with a previous history of asthma exacerbation during periods of seasonal allergic rhinitis (37). Although spirometry was stable, lower airway methacholine responsiveness increased 30 minutes after nasal radionuclide-labeled nasal antigen challenge—an effect which lasted for 4 hours. A neural mechanism is suggested by the rapidity of this change and verification that antigen did not reach the lower airway.

A decade ago, Brugman et al. (63) studied this issue in rabbits. After the induction of sterile sinus inflammation, they also found no change in lung function but did note increased bronchial responsiveness to histamine. It appeared that these changes could be blocked by preventing inflammatory exudate from progressing beyond the larynx, suggesting that direct deposition of mediators into the lungs was an important mechanism for this effect. Bronchial lavage in "positive reactor" rabbits failed to show histologic signs of inflammation, however, again raising the possibility of a neural pathway.

Nasal Obstruction

Nasal/sinus edema and increased purulent secretions lead to nasal obstruction in patients with rhinosinusitis. This is probably an important mechanism for asthma exacerbation in these patients since several important nasal functions may be bypassed: filtration, humidification, and warming of inspired air (64). When this occurs, the patient is at risk for increased lower airway exposure to allergen, irritants, dry air, and cold air—all known triggers for asthma.

Sinus Inflammatory Secretions Draining to Lower Airway

Based on studies nearly a century ago, clinicians speculated that inflammatory material from the upper airway could directly drain into the lower airway and cause symptoms (4–6,18). In recent years, Huxley (65) showed that nearly 50% of subjects would aspirate upper airway material (radiolabeled) into the lung during sleep or depressed consciousness. This conclusion was criticized because most aspirators had artificially induced subconsciousness and perhaps simply could not clear their pharynx normally. A similar subsequent study by Winfield failed to show significant aspiration episodes (66). Bardin et al. (67) examined the pathway of radiolabeled particles placed in the maxillary sinuses of 13 chronic sinusitis patients (nine with asthma). Although radioactive particles were observed in the nose, sinuses, pharynx, and esophagus, no material could be seen in the lower airway. Collectively, these studies suggest that direct aspiration of inflammatory drainage into the lungs is a minor mechanism for asthma at best.

Sinus Inflammatory Mediators Exerting Systemic Effect on Lungs

Bronchial provocation in asthmatics causes an increase in systemic chemotactic factors and it is known that lower airway disease is more common in patients with systemic inflammatory disorders (68,69). Together, these studies suggest the possibility that sinus inflammatory mediators could induce asthma through systemic pathways. Results from the Brugman study, however, seem to suggest this is unlikely (63). When the rabbits were placed so that inflammatory drainage could not progress past the larynx, lower airway hyperresponsiveness was not observed. Since the degree of sinus inflammation was similar in all test rabbits (despite positioning), it would be anticipated that any systemic mediator effects should also be consistent (and all rabbits would show an effect). Results suggest that if present, a systemic pathway alone is not adequate to enhance bronchial responsiveness.

Sinusitis Reduces β-Adrenergic Responsiveness

Friedman et al. (35) observed that asthmatics demonstrated increased response to β-adrenergic medication after their sinusitis was successfully treated. The authors speculated that sinusitis might somehow reduce overall airway β-adrenergic responsiveness, possibly down-regulating receptors. This could be a spurious effect and simply due to an increased use of β-adrenergic medication in active asthma (a known down-regulator of β-receptors). This postulated mechanism remains a conjecture until further appropriate β-adrenergic receptor studies can be performed.

CLINICAL IMPLICATIONS

Given the association between sinusitis and asthma, it is important to consider both diseases, even when the patient history and complaints focus only on a single entity (Fig. 1).

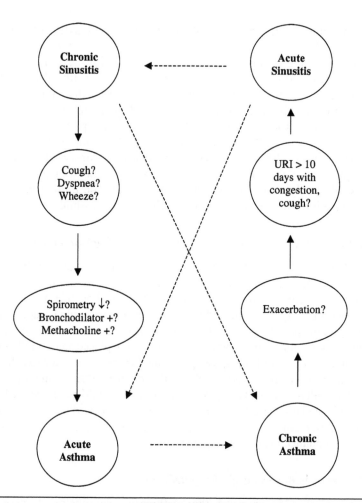

Clinical Implications

- Acute or chronic sinusitis may serve as a trigger for asthma: consider *sinusitis* with prolonged URI symptoms during asthma exacerbation
- Treatment leading to resolution of sinusitis will improve asthma
- Persistent cough/dyspnea during sinusitis exacerbation may reflect *asthma*: check spirometry, response to bronchodilator, methacholine responsiveness
- Prevention of sinusitis reduces the need for antibiotics *and* increased asthma treatment

Figure 1   Association between sinusitis and asthma.

Evaluation of Chronic Sinusitis

When the clinical diagnosis of sinusitis is made, careful attention should be directed to the history of cough, dyspnea, or overt wheezing. If any of these symptoms is present, lung function should be measured (peak expiratory flow rate or spirometry). The importance of even subtle lung function abnormalities can be confirmed by measuring the response to a bronchdilator—significant improvement reflects bronchial hyperresponsiveness. Some patients with refractory chronic sinusitis demonstrate persistent cough and normal lung function. In this setting, a bronchial methacholine challenge can assess whether a component of the patient's cough is due to bronchial hyperresponsiveness (and thus would respond to appropriate medications).

Evaluation of Chronic Asthma

Sinusitis should always be considered as an important trigger for asthma exacerbation. The history is examined for a recent prolonged upper respiratory tract infection (URTI) (beyond 10 to 14 days), particularly with nasal congestion and cough. In this setting, nocturnal cough, especially to the point of vomiting, is suggestive of sinusitis in a child. Supportive evidence for sinusitis includes nasal cytology with predominance of neutrophils and radiographic evidence for significant sinus inflammation (opacification, air–fluid level, or mucosal thickening of greater than 50% of the sinus volume); these findings are only specific in the context of a clinical history of prolonged URTI. In children, a Waters' view radiograph is often a useful screen because it can be easily obtained, is inexpensive, and nearly all new cases of sinusitis will have a maxillary component. In older patients or when isolated ethmoid disease is suspected, a coronal sinus CT is more sensitive (70).

Aggressive treatment of suspected bacterial sinusitis includes appropriate antibiotics (based on likely causative microorganisms) and adjunctive therapy to enhance ostial drainage, e.g., nasal saline, decongestants, and corticosteroids. Saline lavage and decongestants can be useful, particularly early in the course of treatment, to aid in symptom relief and promote mucociliary clearance. Nasal and, in severe cases, oral corticosteroids are a crucial part of treatment in the setting of associated underlying eosinophilic rhinitis (allergic or non-allergic) and asthma. In addition to reducing upper airway edema and purulent rhinorrhea, corticosteroids reduce nasal and associated bronchial hyperresponsiveness.

Prevention of Disease in Patients with Sinusitis and Asthma

When presented with acute sinusitis and asthma, the clinician's first goal is to normalize the sinuses because this alone will improve the lower airway disease. Once stable, prevention starts with exploring the possibility of underlying rhinitis. A baseline evaluation should include nasal cytology to quantify the degree of inflammation when stable, and appropriate skin testing to determine allergic triggers. A long-term approach to prevention begins with environmental control for relevant indoor allergens, e.g., dust mites, animal danders, or molds. If the underlying rhinitis is mild, addition of nasal corticosteroids and possibly leukotriene receptor antagonists during URTIs can often provide a critical reduction in sinus ostial obstruction so that secretion stasis is avoided. When baseline rhinitis is more moderate to severe or when the sinus ostia are known to be compromised, the routine use of nasal corticosteroids and leukotriene receptor antagonists is justified.

CONCLUSIONS

Sinusitis and asthma are frequently encountered simultaneously in patients. In fact, both diseases share many chemical, cytokine, and cellular mediators, suggesting a common pathophysiology. Worsening sinusitis can adversely affect the lower airway. This relationship is apparent from nasal/sinus challenge studies and aggressive medical or surgical treatment of chronic sinusitis often results in improvement in concomitant asthma. Although many ideas have been postulated, the most likely mechanisms for this effect are neural reflex pathways and nasal obstruction.

The close association of upper and lower airway disease has implications for clinical management. Spirometry, and in select cases, methacholine challenge may uncover asthma or bronchial hyperresponsiveness associated with sinusitis. Unexplained exacerbations of asthma should be scrutinized for the possibility of sinusitis. Although sinusitis is a clinical diagnosis, nasal cytology and radiographs may provide supportive evidence.

Ultimately, the key to successful patient management is adequate attention to the upper airway. The initial step is aggressive medical or even surgical therapy to normalize the sinuses. Subsequently, based on the degree of underlying rhinitis, avoidance of environmental triggers and the use of nasal corticosteroids and leukotriene receptor antagonists is crucial for prevention of recurrent rhinosinusitis. Success with this approach is the best way to help the patients control major triggers for their asthma.

REFERENCES

1. Fox RW, Lockey RF. The impact of rhinosinusitis on asthma. Curr Allergy Asthma Rep 2003; 3:513–518.
2. Borish L. Sinusitis and asthma: entering the realm of evidence-based medicine. J Allergy Clin Immunol 2002; 109:606–608.
3. Vinuya RZ. Upper airway disorders and asthma: a syndrome of airway inflammation. Ann Allergy Asthma Immunol 2002; 88:8–15.
4. Gottlieb MJ. Relation of intranasal disease in the production of bronchial asthma. JAMA 1925; 95:105–109.

5. Chobot R. The incidence of sinusitis in asthmatic children. Am J Dis Child 1930; 39:257–264.
6. Weille FL. Studies in asthma: nose and throat in 500 cases of asthma. N Engl J Med 1936; 215:235.
7. Berman SZ, Mathison DA, Stevenson DD, Usselman JA, Shore S, Tan EM. Maxillary sinusitis and bronchial asthma: correlation of roentgenograms, cultures, and thermograms. J Allergy Clin Immunol 1974; 53:311–317.
8. Rachelefsky GS, Goldberg M, Katz RM, Boris G, Gyepes MT, Shapiro MJ, Mickey MR, Finegold SM, Siegel SC. Sinus disease in children with respiratory allergy. J Allergy Clin Immunol 1978; 61:310.
9. Schwartz HJ, Thompson JS, Sher TH, Ross RJ. Occult sinus abnormalities in the asthmatic patient. Arch Intern Med 1987; 147:2194.
10. Bresciani M, Paradis L, Des Roches A, Vernhet H, Vachier I, Godard P, Bousquet J, Chanez P. Rhinosinusitis in severe asthma. J Allergy Clin Immunol 2001; 107:73–80.
11. Pfister R, Lutolf M, Schapowal A, Glatte B, Schmitz M, Menz G. Screening for sinus disease in patients with asthma: a computed tomography-controlled comparision of A-mode ultra sonography and standard radiography. J Allergy Clin Immunol 1994; 94:804–809.
12. Georgitis JW, Matthews BL, Stone B. Chronic sinusitis: characterization of cellular influx and inflammatory mediators in sinus lavage fluid. Int Arch Allergy Immunol 1995; 106:416–421.
13. Steinke JW, Bradley D, Arango P, Crouse CD, Frierson H, Kountakis SE, Kraft M, Borish L. Cysteinyl leukotriene expression in chronic hyperplastic sinusitis-nasal polyposis: importance to eosinophilia and asthma. J Allergy Clin Immunol 2003; 111:342–349.
14. Creticos PS, Peters SP, Adkinson NF Jr, Naclerio RM, Hayes EC, Norman PS, Lichtenstein LM. Peptide leukotriene release after antigen challenge in patients sensitive to ragweed. N Engl J Med 1984; 310:1626–1630.
15. McFadden ER. Nasal-sinus-pulmonary reflexes and bronchial asthma. J Allergy Clin Immunol 1986; 78:1–3.
16. Kratchmer I [cited by Allen W]. Effect on respiration, blood pressure, and carotid pulse of various inhaled and insufflated vapors when stimulating one cranial nerve and various combinations of cranial nerves. Am J Physiol 1928; 87:319–325.
17. Dixon WE, Brodie TG. The bronchial muscles, their innervation and the action of drugs upon them. J Physiol 1903; 29:97–173.
18. Bullen SS. Incidence of asthma in 400 cases of chronic sinusitis. J Allergy 1932; 4:402–407.
19. Zimmerman B, Stringer D, Feanny S. Prevalence of abnormalities found by sinus x-rays in childhood asthma: lack of relation to severity of asthma. J Allergy Clin Immunol 1987; 88:268–273.
20. Kovatch AL, Wald ER, Ledesma-Medina J, Chiponis DM, Bedingfield B. Maxillary sinus radiographs in children with nonrespiratory complaints. Pediatrics 1984; 73:306.
21. Fascenalli FW. Maxillary sinus abnormalities: radiographic evidence in an asymptomatic population. Arch Otolaryngol 1969; 95:190–193.

22. Borish L. The role of leukotrienes in upper and lower airway inflammation and the implications for treatment. Ann Allergy Asthma Immunol 2002; 88: S16–S22.

23. Hamilos DL, Leung DY, Wood R, Bean DK, Song YL, Schotman E, Hamid Q. Eosinophilic infiltration in nonallergic chronic hyperplastic sinusitis with nasal polyps is associated with endothelial VCAM-1 upregulation and expression of TNF-α. 1996; 15:443–450.

24. Bachert C, Wagenmann M, Hauser U, Rudack C. IL-5 synthesis is upregulated in human nasal polyp tissue. J Allergy Clin Immunol 1997; 99:837–842.

25. Minshall EM, Cameron L, Lavigne F, Leung DY, Hamilos D, Garcia-Zepada EA, Rothenberg M, Luster AD, Hamid Q. Eotaxin mRNA and protein expression in chronic sinusitis and allergen-induced nasal responses in seasonal allergic rhinitis. Am J Respir Cell Mol Biol 1997; 17:683–690.

26. Hamilos DL, Leung DYM, Wood R, Cunningham L, Bean DK, Yasruel Z, Schotman E, Hamid Q. Evidence for distinct cytokine expression in allergic versus nonallergic chronic sinusitis. 1995; 96:537–544.

27. Hansel FK. Clinical and histopathologic studies of the nose and sinuses in allergy. L Allergy 1929; 1:43–70.

28. Harlin SL, Ansel DG, Lane SR, Myers J, Kephart GM, Gleich GJ. A clinical and pathologic study of chronic sinusitis: the role of the eosinophil. J Allergy Clin Immunol 1988; 81:867–875.

29. Hisamatsu K, Ganbo T, Nakazawa T, Murakami Y, Gleich GJ, Makiyama K, Koyama H. Cytotoxicity of human eosinophil granule major basic protein to human nasal sinus mucosa in vitro. J Allergy Clin Immunol 1990; 86:52.

30. Slavin RG. Nasal polyps and sinusitis. In: Middleton E, Reed CE, Ellis EF, et al. eds. Allergy, Principles and Practice. 4th ed. St Louis: Mosby, 1992:1455.

31. Scadding G. The effect of medical treatment of sinusitis upon concomitant asthma. Allergy 1999; 54:S136–S140.

32. Businco L, Fiore L, Frediani T, Artuso A, Di Fazio A, Bellioni P. Clinical and therapeutic aspects of sinusitis in children with bronchial asthma. Int J Pediatr Otorhinolaryngol 1981; 3:287–294.

33. Cummings NP, Wood RW, Lere JL, Adinoff AD. Effect of treatment of rhinitis/sinusitis on asthma: results of a double-blind study. Pediatr Res 1983; 17:373.

34. Rachelsfsky GS, Katz RM, Siegel SC. Chronic sinus disease with associated reactive airway disease in children. Pediatrics 1984; 73:525–529.

35. Friedman R, Ackerman M, Wald E, Casselbrant M, Friday G, Fireman P. Asthma and bacterial sinusitis in children. J Allergy Clin Immunol 1984; 74: 185–189.

36. Oliveira CAA, Sole D, Naspitz CK, Rachelefsky GS. Improvement of bronchial hyperresponsiveness in asthmatic children treated for concomitant sinusitis. Ann Allergy Asthma Immunol 1997; 79:70–74.

37. Corren J, Adinoff AD, Irwin CG. Changes in bronchial responsiveness to methacholine following nasal provocation with allergen. J Allergy Clin Immunol 1992; 89:611–618.

38. Corren J, Adinoff AD, Buchmeier AD, Irwin CG. Nasal beclomethasone prevents the seasonal increase in bronchial responsiveness in patients with allergic rhinitis and asthma. J Allergy Clin Immunol 1992; 90:250.

39. Lund VJ. The effect of sinonasal surgery on asthma. Allergy 1999; 54:S141–S145.
40. Van der Veer A Jr. The asthma problem. NY Med J 1920; 112:392–399.
41. Francis C. Prognosis of operations for removal of nasal polyps in asthma. Practitioner 1929; 123:272–278.
42. Davison FW. Chronic sinusitis and infectious asthma. Arch Otolaryngol 1969; 90:110.
43. Slavin RG. Relationship of nasal disease and sinusitis to bronchial asthma. Ann Allergy 1982; 49:76–80.
44. Werth G. The role of sinusitis in severe asthma. Immunol Allergy Proc 1984; 7:45.
45. Juntunen K, Tarkkanen J, Mäkinen J. Caldwell-Luc operation in the treatment of childhood bronchial asthma. Laryngoscope 1984; 94:249–251.
46. Stammberger H. Functional endoscopic sinus surgery. 46. Philadelphia: BC Decker, 1841991:453–457.
47. Wigand ME, Hosemann WG. Results of endoscopic sinus surgery of the paranasal sinuses and anterior skull base. J Otolaryngol 1991; 20:385–390.
48. Jankowski R, Moneret-Vautrin DA, Goetz R, Wayoff M. Incidence of medicosurgical treatment for nasal polyps on the development of associated asthma. Rhinology 1992; 30:249–258.
49. Nishioka GJ, Cook PR, Davis WE, McKinsey JP. Functional endoscopic sinus surgery in patients with chronic sinusitis and asthma. Otolaryngol Head Neck Surg 1994; 110:494–500.
50. Manning SC, Wasserman RL, Silver R, Phillips DL. Results of endoscopic sinus surgery in pediatric patients with chronic sinusitis and asthma. Arch Otolaryngol Head Neck Surg 1994; 120:1142–1145.
51. Senior BA, Kennedy DW. Management of sinusitis in the asthmatic patient. Ann Allergy Asthma Immunol 1996; 77:6–15.
52. Dunlop G, Scadding GK, Lund VJ. Effect of endoscopic sinus surgery on asthma: management in patients with chronic rhinosinusitis, nasal polyposis and asthma. Am J Rhinol 1999; 13(4):261–265.
53. Campanella SG, Asher MI. Current controversies: sinus disease and the lower airways. Pediatr Pulmon 2001; 31:165–172.
54. Sluder G. Asthma as a nasal reflex. JAMA 1919; 73:589–591.
55. Kaufman J, Chen J, Wright GW. The effect of trigeminal resection on reflex bronchoconstriction after nasal and nasopharyngeal irritation in man. Am Rev Respir Dis 1970; 101:768.
56. Nolte D, Berger D. On vagal bronchoconstriction in asthmatic patients by nasal irritation. Eur J Respir Dis 1983; 64(S):110–114.
57. Speizer FE, Frank NR. A comparison of changes in pulmonary flow resistance in healthy volunteers acutely exposed to SO_2 by mouth and by nose. Br J Industr Med 1966; 23:75.
58. Wyllie JW, Kern EB, O'Brien PC, Hyatt RE. Alteration of pulmonary function associated with artificial nasal obstruction. Surg Forum 1976; 27:535.
59. Yan K, Salome C. The response of the airways to nasal stimulation in asthmatics with rhinitis. Eur J Respir Dis 1983; 64:105–108.
60. Hoehne JH, Reed CE. Where is the allergic reaction in ragweed asthma? J Allergy Clin Immunol 1971; 48:36.

61. Rosenberg GL, Rosenthal RR, Norman PS. Inhalation challenge with ragweed pollen in ragweed-sensitive asthmatics. J Allergy Clin Immunol 1983; 71:302.
62. Schumacher MJ, Cota KA, Taussig LM. Pulmonary response to nasal-challenge testing of atopic subjects with stable asthma. J Allergy Clin Immunol 1986; 78:30–35.
63. Brugman SM, Larsen GL, Henson PM, Honor J, Irvin CG. Increased lower airways responsiveness associated with sinusitis in a rabbit model. Am Rev Respir Dis 1993; 147:314.
64. Griffin MP, McFadden ER, Ingram RH. Airway cooling in asthmatic and non-asthmatic subjects during nasal and oral breathing. J Allergy Clin Immunol 1982; 69:354.
65. Huxley EJ, Viroslav J, Gray WR, Pierce AK. Pharyngeal aspiration in normal adults and patients with depressed consciousness. 1978; 64:564.
66. Winfield JB, Sande MA, Gwaltney JM. Aspiration during sleep. JAMA 1973; 233:1288.
67. Bardin PG, Van Heerden BB, Joubert JR. Absence of pulmonary aspiration of sinus contents in patients with asthma and sinusitis. J Allergy Clin Immunol 1990; 86:82–88.
68. Lee TH, Toshikazu N, Papageorgiou N, Iikura Y, Kay AB. Exercise-induced late asthmatic reactions. N Engl J Med 1983; 308:1502.
69. Geddes DM, Corrin B, Brewerton DA, Davies RJ, Turner-Warwick M. Progressive airway obliteration in adults and its association with rheumatoid disease. Q J Med 1977; 46(184):427.
70. McAlister WH, Lusk R, Muntz HR. Comparison of plain radiographs and coronal CT scans in infants and children with recurrent sinusitis. Am J Roentgenol 1989; 153:1259.

15

Rhinosinusitis and Allergy

Desiderio Passàli, Valerio Damiani, Giulio Cesare Passàli,
Francesco Maria Passàli, and Luisa Bellussi
*Ear, Nose, and Throat Department–University of Siena Medical School,
Viale Bracci, Siena, Italy*

EPIDEMIOLOGY

The relationship between rhinosinusitis and allergy has been extensively investigated. In 1978, Rachelefsky et al. showed that 53% of children with atopy had abnormal sinus radiographs (1); and in 1988, Shapiro found sinusal radiological alterations in about 70% of children with allergic rhinitis (2).

In 1992, Benninger reported that 54% of outpatients with chronic rhinosinusitis (CRS) had positive skin-prick tests (3), while Grove et al. found that 50% of patients listed for sinus surgery had positive skin-prick tests (4).

In a 2000 study on 200 patients undergoing endoscopic sinus surgery for CRS, Emanuel and Shah reported that allergy was a contributing factor in 84% of patients; moreover, sensitisation to perennial allergens (house dust) clearly prevailed in patients with both rhinosinusitis and allergic rhinitis (60% of patients) (5). However, the type and severity of the allergy did not correlate with the degree of changes on computed tomography (CT) scans.

In 2001, in a non-peer reviewed publication, Osguthorpe reported a higher incidence of rhinosinusitis in the spring and autumn in the Northeast and South of the United States, which coincides with the pollination of trees, grasses, and weeds during the spring time (6).

More recently (2003), Yariktas et al. showed that 71.2% of patients affected by allergic rhinitis (both seasonal and perennial) in their sample had CT findings suggestive of rhinosinusitis, according to the Lund–Mackay CT-scan staging system. These CT scores were significantly higher among patients with perennial allergic rhinitis, compared to the seasonal allergic rhinitis group ($p < 0.05$) (7).

These and other epidemiological studies lead to the hypothesis that the mucosa of individuals with allergic rhinitis might be expected to be swollen and more liable to obstruct the sinusal ostia, thus reducing ventilation and leading to mucusal retention. These changes produce an intrasinus environment that might be more prone to becoming infected, with subsequent development of an infective rhinosinusitis.

In contrast to the above findings, other studies failed to illustrate an association between infective rhinosinusitis and allergy (8–11). Karlsson and Holmberg did not find an increase in the incidence of infective rhinosinusitis in the pollen season, although they found that 80% of patients affected by bilateral maxillary rhinosinusitis were allergic (8). Hinriksdottir et al. reported that the prevalence of purulent rhinosinusitis was the same in patients with and without allergic rhinitis (9).

Moreover, Iwens and Clement found that the prevalence and extent of sinus mucosal involvement as detemined by CT did not correlate with the patients' atopy (10), and Orobello et al. could not correlate the presence of a positive bacterial culture obtained by sinusal aspiration with atopy in children (11).

These reports highlight the controversy that currently exists regarding the presence of an association between rhinosinusitis and allergy.

PATHOPHYSIOLOGY

The pathophysiology of allergic rhinitis is characterized by an inflammatory response at the nasal level. Nasal allergy is believed to be a result of a three-step process, the first of which is represented by atopy.

Atopy has been defined by the the European Academy of Allergology and Clinical Immunology (EAACI) Nomenclature Task Force as "... a personal or familial tendency to produce IgE antibodies in response to low doses of allergens, usually proteins...." In other words, it represents the genetic predisposition, transmitted as a dominant factor, to become allergic to a definite number of specific allergens (12).

The second step is the sensitization, which begins when the patient is exposed to a specific allergen; this molecule is processed at the nasal mucosal level by the antigen-presenting cells (APCs) and presented, after the migration of APCs to the lamina propria, to CD4 T-Helper and B cells. Activated B cells begin to produce IgEs that in turn will bind to high-affinity IgE receptors of mast cells and basophils and to low-affinity IgE receptors of macrophages, monocytes, platelets, and eosinophils (13). It is still an enigma why, in this phase, innocuous molecules are recognized by the host as foreign ones and why the above interactions incite the production of IgE instead of IgA, IgM, or IgG.

When an allergen to which an individual has already been sensitized comes in contact with the nasal mucosa for a second time, it interacts with specific IgEs that coat the surface of mast cells. This incites cellular degranulation and the release of a number of inflammation mediators (i.e., histamine, leukotrienes, tryptase) (14), leading to the so-called, "early phase response" of the allergic reaction.

Histamine is the most important mediator of the early phase response: it stimulates the H1 receptors, the sensory nerve endings determining itching, and it acts on blood vessels leading to plasma extravasation and congestion that generates the sensation of nasal obstruction.

Leukotrienes also strongly affect the blood vessels of rhinosinusal mucosa, but their effects on nerve endings or glands are less evident. Tryptase breaks down kininogen from blood, leading to the generation of kininis, which in turn causes vasodilatation, edema, and plasma exudation (15).

Moreover, mast cells appear to release some cytokines, namely TNF-α, IL-4, IL-5, and IL-13 in this phase. TNF-α and IL-4 induce the expression of adhesion molecules on the surface of nasal endothelium; moreover, they seem to have a direct chemical-attractant effect for inflammatory cells. IL-5 and IL-13 are strong promoters of activation and survival of eosinophils.

Through the actions of these four molecules (and possibly others that are not yet well defined), another phase ensues in some patients, 4 to 24'hours after the beginning of the inflammatory process. This phase is called the, "late phase response" and is characterized by infiltration of cells and activation at the rhinosinusal mucosal level. Specifically, once inflammatory cells, such as eosinophils, basophils, neutrophils, and mononuclear cells, reach the nasal submucosal tissue, they (by interacting with matrix proteins) release their own mediators. They reach the nasal submucosal tissue thanks to the cytokine-induced expression of adhesion molecules on the endothelium. The inflammatory response is, in this way, perpetuated and enhanced. Whereas pruritus, sneezing, and itching are the major symptoms of the early phase response, the actions of mediators are centered upon nasal hypersecretion and congestion, in the late phase response (16).

This inflammatory process, if stimulated by repeated exposures to allergens, significantly lowers the threshold of patients to other stimuli. After chronic allergenic stimulation, allergic patients typically react strongly to low doses of the causative allergen or to allergens to which they are only mildly sensitised or to non-specific triggers (cold air, smoke, chemicals, etc.). This phenomenon was previously called "priming effect" (17). Nowadays, it has been replaced by the new concept of the "minimal persistent inflammation" (18).

The key element, however, in the development of rhinosinusitis from an allergic inflammation of the nose is the functional obstruction of the ostiomeatal complex, which leads to an alteration in the air and secretion flows to and from the sinuses. In the case of a nasal allergenic challenge allergic rhinitis contributes to this process by causing, mucosal swelling and, if the stimulation persists, thickening of the rhinosinusal mucosa.

Nasal hyperreactivity also plays a role in the pathogenesis of rhinosinusitis. This is mediated by the classical post-gangliar sympathetic and parasympathetic transmitter, as well as other neurotransmitters such as vasoactive intestinal peptide (VIP), somatostatin, and neuropeptide Y (19,20).

These substances are released principally by the sensory nervous endings and represent the effectors of the so-called "neurogenic inflammatory reaction." Independent of the specific cause, the accumulation of undrainable secretions that are unable to pass through narrowed ostia leads to further obstruction and to the development of an anaerobic environment that permits bacterial growth.

Bacterial infection affects mucociliary functionality, which in turn induces further increase in the thickening of the mucosa and ostial obstruction. If this vicious circle is not interrupted, the pathology evolves toward rhinosinusitis, which is the result of continuous rhinosinusal inflammation.

DIAGNOSIS

The process of diagnosing the pathology in the sinus and pharynx in both adults and children involves three diagnostic steps (Table 1).

The key element of the first phase (step I) is the collection of an accurate clinical history. The information that is gathered includes the documentation of nasal and auricular symptoms, the nature of the major triggers, and the timing of symptoms. These symptoms include itching, sneezing, rhinorrea, and nasal congestion. They can be the manifestations of all the pathologies

Table 1 Three-Steps Diagnostic Approach

Step I	Clinical history
	Objective examination
	Active anterior rhinomanometry (AAR)
	Acoustic rhinometry (AR)
	Mucociliary transport time (MCTt)
	Allergy tests (PRICK, intradermal)
Step II	PRIST
	RAST
	Eosinophils count
	Mastocytes degranulation test
Step III	Nasal provocation test (NPT)
	CT

that involve the rhinosinusal area. The differentiation between an acute attack of allergic rhinitis from acute rhinosinusitis, or from the coexistence of both, can be made by comparing the clinical data with the definitions of each condition.

The next phase involves an objective evaluation of the rhinosinusal region, which is performed by using rigid or preferably flexible endoscope.

The careful evaluation of rhinosinusal mucosa already may allow for the differentiation between an allergic and a nonallergic condition. A reddened mucosa is generally found in an infection or in inflammation of the rhinosinusal region, whereas a pale and swollen mucosa is typically present in rhinosinusitis induced by nasal allergy. Crusting of the inflamed mucosa may suggest atrophic rhinitis. The type, quantity, and location of secretions should be recorded.

The nasal cavities should be carefully evaluated for the presence of any anatomical abnormalities (i.e., septal deviation, hypertrophy of turbinates), polyps, foreign bodies, and tumors.

The objective examination of the rhinosinusal region is complemented by an instrumental evaluation of the nasal functions, including active anterior rhinomanometry, acoustic rhinometry, and mucociliary transport time.

Anterior active rhinomanometry is performed in accordance with the instructions of the Committee on Standardization of Rhinomanometry (21). This is an instrumental test that enables an objective evaluation of the patency of the nasal fossae by calculating nasal flows (expressed in cc per second) and pressures (expressed in Pascal). A specific software calculates the nasal resistance values that are essential for the assessment of the pathophysiology of the rhinosinusal region.

Acoustic rhinometry analyzes the sound pulses that are reflected from the interior of nasal fossa and calculate, in this way, the cross-sectional areas and volumes of the nasal cavities (22).

However, this relatively new technique requires further standardization, especially regarding the method of connecting the nosepiece to nostrils and the positioning of the patient's head.

When done in conjunction with a nasal decongestion test, these techniques allow for an accurate and sequential quantification of the abnormalities that were induced by the mucosal congestion and their modification after pharmacological decongestion. The nasal mucociliary function, which is one of the most important and fundamental defense mechanisms of the airways against environmental pollutants, can be evaluated in a specific patient by determining the nasal mucociliary transport time. This is achieved by measuring the time in which a colored substance, placed on the head of the inferior turbinate, reaches the pharynx.

One of the testing substances is a mixture of charcoal powder and 3% saccharine. Charcoal powder is an insoluble tracer, and its use can provide information about the efficiency of the removal of particles entrapped in the outer gel layer of nasal mucus. The saccharine, a soluble marker, enables the determination of times of clearance of the inner sol layer (23). The first diagnostic level is completed by allergological tests.

The skin-prick test is the most widely used allergy test, and represents the primary diagnostic tool for allergy (24). It is simple, inexpensive, and reliable in most patients, and, if properly done (with positive and negative controls) and correctly interpreted, allows for the identification of the causative allergens in most cases.

The second diagnostic level (step II) is aimed at achieving a more thorough evaluation of the allergic problem in the patient. It involves obtaining laboratory tests that include the total IgE dosages (PRIST), specific IgE dosages (RAST), the eosinophil count, and the mastocyte degranulation test.

Among second level tests, PRIST lacks specificity, since other conditions can also raise the total serum IgE levels and more than half of the patients affected by seasonal allergic rhinitis have total IgEs in the physiological range. RAST, determined in both serum and nasal secretion, is more precise and correlates well with the prick test and the nasal challenge results.

The high cost and low sensitivity, compared to those of in vivo tests, are the main limitations of the step II studies.

The third level test (step III), specifically the nasal specific provocation test (NPT), is based upon the pathophysiological mechanisms of allergic sensitization. The symptoms and signs of allergic rhinitis depend mainly on the prevalent or exclusive localization of previously primed mastocytes in the shock organ, the nose.

A properly performed NPT is done in this manner: an active anterior rhinomanometry is done first to exclude any respiratory stenosis (which could invalidate the results of the test), then lactose (the negative control substance) is insufflated into the nasal fossa, followed by a control active anterior rhinomanometry (after 10 min), and thereafter, the administration of a lower concentration (2.5 A.U.) of the lyophilized allergen into the same nasal fossa, and last, an active anterior rhinomanometry (after 10 min).

If nasal resistance is not increased, a higher concentration of the allergen (5, 10, 20, 40, 60, 80 A.U.) is administered and the active anterior rhinomanometry is repeated. The NPT is considered positive when an increase of nasal resistance equal or greater than 100% is registered (25).

The final study is a CT scan. This became the most important diagnostic radiological investigation for the evaluation of both rhinosinusal and intracranial complications and in the preoperative assessment of patients (26).

TREATMENT

According to the International Rhinosinusitis Advisory Board, the major objectives in treating rhinosinusitis are to eradicate the infection, to decrease the duration of the illness, and to prevent the development of complications (27).

Although antibiotics remain the mainstay of therapy for sinusitis (Chap. 9), various general measures, the so-called "adjuvant therapies", are very important, especially in those individuals where allergy is a major contribution to the development of rhinosinusal pathology (Table 2).

In addition to controlling the infection, other important goals are to reduce the mucosal edema, to facilitate the sinusal drainage, to maintain the ostial patency, and to relieve inflammation and allergic response.

All these goals can be achieved by using adjunctive treatments, namely topical decongestants, muco-regulators, corticosteroids, antihistamines, immunotherapy, and nasal irrigation (or douche) with saline solution.

Topical decongestants, administered as nasal drops or sprays, are efficacious only when they are used for a short time (at most, seven days). They act by stimulating the α-adrenergic receptors of the upper airway mucosa, with subsequent vasoconstriction of the mucosal capillaries and shrinking of the edematous mucosa (28). However, after prolonged use these agents lose their efficacy and can induce a rebound rhinitis (also called *rhinitis medicamentosa*). Most topical decongestants are the oximetazoline and tramazoline nasal sprays and are administered two to three times daily.

Mucolytics, or muco-regulating agents, can be safely used in both the prevention and treatment of rhinosinusitis, especially in cases where disorders of mucociliary clearance or of mucus glandular production play a major role in the genesis of the pathology (i.e., cystic fibrosis, immotile cilia syndrome) (29). These agents act by thinning the mucus, with subsequent reduction of mucus stasis and promotion of clearance, and are administrated continuously for four weeks in patients with rhinosinusitis (30).

Oral and parenteral corticosteroids exhibit a strong anti-inflammatory effect and effectively reduce the inflammatory symptoms. However, they have the potential of causing serious systemic side effects and are contraindicated in several conditions, such as heart disease, hypertension, diabetes, obesity, and cataracts, which limits their use to only those with an urgent or severe condition.

Topical nasal steroids act through multiple mechanisms, including vasoconstriction and reduction of edema, suppression of cytokine-production, and inhibition of inflammatory cell migration (31). They work best when

Table 2 Support Therapies for Rhinosinusitis

Topical decongestant
Muco-regulators
Corticosteroids (systemic and topical)
Antihistamines
Immunotherapy
Nasal irrigation

taken regularly on a daily basis in a prophylactic regimen, administered once or twice a day according to the type of steroids administered.

When topical nasal steroids are administered with antibiotic therapy, a decrease in the number of inflammatory cells, a facilitated regression of the radiological alterations, and a significant improvement in patients' symptoms occur (32).

These agents act by reducing the activity of cholinergic receptors, by reducing the number of basophils and eosinophils in the nasal mucosa, and by inhibiting the late phase reaction after exposure to allergens (33). The most commonly used topical nasal steroids administered as nasal sprays are beclomethasone dipropionate, budesonide, flutisolide, and fluticasone dipropionate.

The use of these medications is currently recommended in children older than five years of age. Prospective, randomized, placebo-controlled studies in children from 3 to 12 years of age showed that momentasone has the same rate of side effects as placebo (34,35).

The recommended length of intranasal steroid therapy for acute rhinosinusitis is three to five weeks, followed by a wash-out period and an eventual repetition of the treatment (36). The suggested length of therapy for chronic sinusitis varies from 2 to 16 weeks (37,38).

The untoward effects of these topical drugs include dryness and irritation of nasal mucosa, epistaxis (in about 5% of patients), and rarely, oral candidiasis. These side effects are likely a result of the sterilizing and stabilizing substances that are added to the solutions such as benzalkomium chloride.

H1-antihistamines are also commonly used as adjunct therapy. These agents have mild anti-inflammatory activity (39) and significantly reduce (after four weeks of treatment) sneezing, itching, and rhinorrhea, but their effects on nasal obstruction is less significant (40).

First-generation antihistamines cannot selectively bind to H1-receptors, and therefore they also interact with dopaminergic, serotoninergic, and cholinergic receptors, leading to untoward effects such as dryness of the mouth and constipation. Moreover, these drugs, although very efficacious at the nasal level, easily cross the blood–brain barrier, leading to adverse effects at the central nervous system level (i.e., fatigue, sedation, dizziness) (41).

Second-generation antihistamines are as efficacious as the former generation, but, as they are more lipophobic, they do not cross the blood–brain barrier. Since they selectively bind to H1-histamine receptors (41), they do not cause somnolence, interfere with performance, or possess an anticholinergic effect. However, when combined with drugs metabolized by the P-450 Cytochrome, they can produce torsades de pointes and ventricular arrhythmia (42).

The recently developed third-generation antihistamines have a similar efficacy as the other two classes without their adverse effects (43), and represent a promising tool for the management of allergy-related CRS.

Numerous uncontrolled clinical reports of immunotherapy, both nasal and sublingual, suggest that this mode of therapy may have an important role in the management of allergy-related forms of rhinosinusitis (44).

Although some controversies exist regarding the specific mechanisms of action of immunotherapy, it produces an increase in allergen-specific Ig G-blocking antibodies, is associated with an initial increase and subsequent fall in allergen-specific IgEs levels, and produces a decrease in both the release of histamine from basophils and in the lymphocyte–cytokine response to allergen challenge (45).

More recently, scientific interest has focused on the allergen-specific deviation of the immune response from a Th2 to a Th1 cytokine phenotype and on the induction of CD4+/CD25+ T cells that occurs after administration of immunotherapy (46).

Nishioka observed a significantly better long-term outcome after endoscopic sinus surgery, compared with allergic patients who underwent surgery without having preoperative immunotherapy (47).

Krause recently reported that allergic patients with rhinosinusitis and treated with immunotherapy had a reduced number of infectious episodes after endoscopic sinus surgery (48).

In conclusion, when properly administered, immunotherapy represents a valid therapeutic aid in the management of allergic patients affected by rhinosinusitis. Nasal irrigation (or douche) with saline solution seems to be able to reduce nasal and rhinosinusal dryness, facilitating the clearing of thick mucus and crusts (49). The use of nasal irrigations after surgery in patients operated for CRS has obtained more of a consensus in recent years because of their moisturizing effects and ability to reduce swelling (50). The lack of side effects and low price makes the use of saline solutions more practical.

PREVENTION

The major goal of all the measures taken to prevent rhinosinusitis is to avoid the negative effects of all the risk and predisposing factors that lead to the emergence of the rhinosinusal cycle (Chap. 6).

Preventing allergy-related rhinosinusitis involves reducing the chronic allergic inflammation of rhinosinusal mucosa that can induce a permanent edematous state, blocking the ostiomeatal complex.

A recent Italian epidemiological analysis (51) found that the probability of an allergic patient developing rhinosinusitis is $21.5 \pm 3.4\%$. These results are similar to the 20% risk one noted in the WHO ARIA Document (52).

The concept of "one airway, one disease" in relation to the rhinitis–rhinosinusitis–asthma relationship is strongly endorsed by the data presented above. However, although this relationship is well defined from the theoretical viewpoint, there is paucity of studies that analyze the preventive effects of different treatments of allergic rhinitis on lowering the risk of developing rhinosinusitis.

A recent retrospective study that encompassed 20 years of follow-up found that treatment of nasal allergy can prevent the development of rhinosinusitis and lower airways pathologies (53). However, no differences were noted in the preventive effects of the various treatment modalities (i.e., nasal steroids, antihistamines, immunotherapy).

In conclusion, medical treatment and interference with the early stages of allergic rhinitis are the most important measures that can prevent the development of this condition and its complications.

REFERENCES

1. Rachelefsky GS, Goldberg M, Katz RM, Boris G, Gyepes MT, Shapiro MJ, et al. Sinus disease in children with respiratory allergy. J Allergy Clin Immunol 1978; 61(5):310–314.
2. Shapiro GC. The role of nasal airway obstruction in sinus disease and facial development. J Allergy Clin Immunol 1988; 82:935–940.
3. Benninger M. Rhinitis, sinusitis and their relationship to allergies. Am J Rhinol 1992; 6:37–43.
4. Grove R, Farrior, J. Chronic hyperplastic sinusitis in allergic patients: a bacteriologic study of 200 operative cases. J Allergy Clin Immunol 1990; 11:271.
5. Emanuel IA, Shah SB. Chronic rhinosinusitis: allergy and sinus computed tomography relationships. Otolaryngol Head Neck Surg 2000; 123(6):687–691.
6. Osguthorpe D. Sinusitis: allergy sufferers more susceptible to sinus disorders; interview. Sci Health 2001; April 9.
7. Yariktas M, Doner F, Demirci M. Rhinosinusitis among the patients with perennial or seasonal allergic rhinitis. Asian Pac J Allergy Immunol 2003; 21(2): 75–78.
8. Karlsson G, Holmberg K. Does allergic rhinitis predispose to sinusitis? Acta Otolaryngol Suppl 1994; 515:26–28; discussion 29.
9. Hinriksdottir I, Melen I. Allergic rhinitis and upper respiratory tract infections. Acta Otolaryngol Suppl 1994; 515:30–32.
10. Iwens P, Clement PA. Sinusitis in allergic patients. Rhinology 1994; 32(2): 65–67.
11. Orobello PW Jr, Park RI, Belcher LJ, Eggleston P, Lederman HM, Banks JR, et al. Microbiology of chronic sinusitis in children. Arch Otolaryngol Head Neck Surg 1991; 117(9):980–983.
12. EAACI Nomenclature Task Force. A revised nomenclature for allergy. Allergy 2001; 56:813–824.
13. Van Cauwenberge PB. Nasal sensitisation. Allergy 1997; 52(suppl 33):7–9.
14. Naclerio RM. Allergic rhinitis. N Engl J Med 1991; 325:860–869.
15. Naclerio RM, Proud D, Peters S, Sobotka AK, Lichtenstein L, Norman P. The role of inflammatory mediators in allergic rhinitis. Ear Nose Throat J 1986; 65:206–212.

16. Montefort S, Feather H, Wilson SJ. The expression of leukocyte-endothelial adhesion cells is increased in perennial allergic rhinitis. Am J Respir Cell Mol Biol 1992; 7:393–398.
17. Collen JT. Quantitative intranasal pollen challenges. The priming effect in allergic rhinitis. J Allergy 1969; 43:33–44.
18. Ricca V, Landi M, Ferrero P, Bairo A, Tazzer C, Canonica GW, Ciprandi G. Minimal persistent inflammation is also present in patients with seasonal allergic rhinitis. J Allergy Clin Immunol 2000; 105:54–57.
19. Bousquet J, Chanez P, Vignola AM, Lacoste JY, Michel FB. Eosinopholic inflammation in asthma. Am J Respir Crit Care Med 1994; 150(suppl):S33–S38.
20. Bonini S, Magrini L, Rotiroti G. Basi biologiche dell'infiammazione allergica delle vie aeree. In: Passàli D, Pozzi E, Olivieri D, eds. Allergia e infiammazione delle vie aeree:entità parallele o convergenti? Firenze: Scientific Press,1996: 19–222.
21. Clement PAR. Committee report on standardization of rhinomanometry. Rhinology 1984; 22:151–155.
22. Hilberg O, Jackson AC, Swift DL. Acoustic rhinometry: evaluation of nasal cavity geometry by acoustic reflection. J Appl Physiol 1989; 66:295–303.
23. Passali D, Bellussi L, Bianchini-Ciampoli M, De Seta E. Our experiences in nasal mucociliary transport time determination. Acta Otolaryngol (Stockh) 1984; 97:319–323.
24. Collins-Williams C, Nirami RM, Lamenza C, Chin. Nasal provocative testing with molds in the diagnosis of perennial allergic rhinitis. Ann Allergy 1972; 30:557–561.
25. Passàli D, Anselmi M, Bellussi L, Passàli FM, Passali GC. Storia delle metodiche utilizzate quali test di provocazione nasale aspecifica (TPNA) alla luce di esperienze personali. Riv Orl Aud Fon 1999; 3–4:121–130.
26. Lloyd GAS, Lund VJ, Scadding GK. CT of the paranasal sinuses and bronchial endoscopic surgery: a critical analysis of 100 symptomatic patients. J Laryngol Otol 1991; 105:181–185.
27. International Rhinosinusitis Advisory Board: Infectious Rhinosinusitis in adults: Classification, Etiology and Management. ENT J 1997; 76(suppl 12): 1–22.
28. DelaFuente JC, Davis TA, Davis JA. Pharmacotherapy of allergic rhinitis. Clin Pharmacol Ther 1989; 8:474–485.
29. Davidson TM, Murphy C, Mitchell M, et al. Management of chronic sinusitis in cystic fibrosis. Laryngoscope 1995; 105:354–358.
30. Yuta A, Baraniuk JN. Therapeutic approaches of airway mucus hypersecretion. In: Rogers DF, Lethem MI, eds. Airway Mucus: Basic Mechanisms and Clinical Perspectives. Batel: Birkhauser Verlag, 1997:365–383.
31. Meltzer EP, Orgel HA, Backhaus JW, et al. Intranasal flunisolide spray as an adjunct to oral antibiotic therapy for sinusitis. J Allergy Clin Immunol 1993; 92:812–823.
32. Paurvels R. Mode of action of corticosteroids in asthma and rhinitis. Clin Allergy 1986; 16:281–288.
33. Mabry RL. Interface of allergy and sinus disease. Dallas Med J 1991; 99: 596–599.

34. Brannan MD, Herron JM, Affrime MB. Safety and tolerability of once-daily mometasone furoate aqueous nasal spray in children. Clin Ther 1986; 65: 449–456.

35. Nayak AS, Settipane GA, Pedinoff A, Charous BL, Meltzer EO, Busse WW, et al. Effective dose range of mometasone furoate nasal spray in the treatment of acute rhinosinusitis. Ann Allergy Asthma Immunol 2002; 89(3):271–278.

36. Dolor RJ, Witsell DL, Hellkamp AS, Williams JW Jr, Califf RM, Simel DL. Comparison of cefuroxime with or without intranasal fluticasone for the treatment of rhinosinusitis. The CAFFS trial: a randomized controlled trial. JAMA 2001; 286(24):3097–3105.

37. Parikh A, Scadding GK, Darby Y, Baker RC. Topical corticosteroids in chronic rhinosinusitis: a randomized, double-blind, placebo-controlled trial using fluticasone propionate aqueous nasal spray. Rhinology 2001; 39(2):75–79.

38. Lavigne F, Cameron L, Renzi PM, Planet JF, Christodoulopoulos P, Lamkioued B, et al. Intrasinus administration of topical budesonide to allergic patients with chronic rhinosinusitis following surgery. Laryngoscope 2002; 112(5):858–864.

39. Howarth PH. Assessment of antihistamine efficacy and potency. Clin Exp Allergy 1999; 86:87–97.

40. Braun JJ, Alabert JP, Michel FB, Quiniou M, Rat C, Cougnard J, Czarlewski W, Bousquet J. Adjunct effect of loratadine in the treatment of acute sinusitis in patients with allergic rhinitis. Allergy 1997; 52(6):650–655.

41. Yanai K, Ryu JH, Watanabe T, Iwata R, Ido T, Sawai Y. Histamine H1-receptor occupancy in human brains after single oral doses of histamine H1-antagonists measured by positron emission tomography. Br J Pharmacol 1995; 116:1649–1655.

42. Delpon E, Valenzuela C, Tamargo J. Blockade of cardiac potassium and other channels by antihistamines. Drug Saf 1999; 1:11–18.

43. Casale TB, Andrade C, Qu R. Safety and efficacy of once-daily fexofenadine Hcl in the treatment of autumn seasonal allergic rhinitis. Allergy Asthma Proc 1999; 20:193–198.

44. Benninger M, Anon J, Mabry R. The medical management of rhinosinusitis. Otolaryngol Head Neck Surg 1997; 117:S41–S49.

45. Fireman P. Allergic rhinitis. In: Fireman P, Slavin RG, eds. Atlas of Allergies. 2nd ed. St Louis: Mosby-Wolfe, 1996:141–159.

46. Francis JN, Til SJ, Durham SR. Induction of IL-10+Cd4+Dc25+ T Cells by grass pollen immunotherapy. J Allergy Clin Immunol 2003; 111:1255–1261.

47. Nishioka GJ, Cook PR, McKinsey JP. Immunotherapy in patients undergoing functional endoscopic sinus surgery. Otolaryngol Head Neck Surg 1994; 110:406–412.

48. Krause HF. Allergy and chronic rhinosinusitis. Otolaryngol Head Neck Surg 2003; 128:14–16.

49. Nuutinen J, Holopainen E, Haaletela T, et al. Balanced physiologic saline in the treatment of chronic rhinosinusitis. Rhinology 1986; 24:265–269.

50. Ryan RM, Whittet HB, Norval C, et al. Minimal follow up after functional endoscopic sinus surgery. Does it affect the outcome? Rhinology 1996; 34:44–45.

51. ARIA: Allergic Rhinitis and its Impact on Asthma, Workshop Report, 2001.

52. Passàli D, Bellussi L, Damiani V, Passali GC, Passali FM, Celestino D. Allergic rhinitis in Italy: epidemiology and definition of most commonly used diagnostic and therapeutic modalities. Acta Otorhinolaryngol Ital 2003; 23(4):257–264.
53. Passali D, Damiani V, Mora R, Passali GC, Bellussi L. Natural history of allergic rhinitis: our experience in Italy. Clin Exp All Rev 2003; 3:28–32.

16

Nosocomial Sinusitis

Viveka Westergren and Urban Forsum
Division of Clinical Microbiology, Department of Molecular and Clinical Medicine, Faculty of Health Sciences, Linköping University, Linköping, Sweden

INTRODUCTION

An accurate definition of nosocomial infection identifies "nosocomial" as a disease or symptom initiated during a period of hospital care and under different states of bacterial presence (1). As such, it describes the two dimensions that together are part of the working definition of the concept of nosocomial sinusitis. Of the two particular kinds of sinusitis included in this chapter, however, only one is a "true" nosocomial sinusitis according to the definition above, and this is the sinusitis of critically ill patients in the intensive care unit (ICU) that is related to mechanical ventilation. On the other hand, post–sinus surgery refractory sinusitis, which is considered in the last paragraph of the Introduction section, is not truly a nosocomial sinusitis. Under each subheading, ventilator-associated sinusitis will be dealt with first, followed by post–sinus surgery sinusitis.

In the ICU, critically ill patients commonly have dysfunction of one or more organ systems, including fractures, combined, at least temporarily, with impaired host-defense. They are subjected to multiple invasive diagnostic and therapeutic procedures. Fever is common, either of infectious or noninfectious etiology (2), which may be the sign of a complication when all diagnostic measures are unsuccessful. Devices used for securing the airway are one of those factors (3) that can induce infection associated with fever.

The unique circumstances in the ICU affect the bacterial flora of the patients, the medical staff, and the ward. The presence and the development of bacterial resistance to antimicrobials has become a constant problem. The manner in which antibiotics are utilized regulates the bacterial flora of the ICU both quantitatively and qualitatively, as well as the pattern of bacterial antibiotic sensitivity (4).

The diagnosis of bacterial sinusitis is complicated by the concealed location of the maxillary sinuses, which makes their direct visualization impossible, and by the difficulty in obtaining an uncontaminated sample for culture. An infectious sinusitis in the ICU setting is often over-diagnosed, as most cases of sinus inflammation in this setting are noninfectious reactive inflammatory sinusitis (5), or an infected artificial ventilation-acquired sinopathy. It is quite possible that only a few cases of sinus inflammation in the ICU setting are truly of infectious etiology.

The first publication regarding sinusitis in the ICU setting was in 1974, when four cases were reported (6). During the following decade, similar case reports were published, some of which used purulent nasal discharge or drainage as the means of diagnosis (7–12). In response to the identified problem, retrospective studies were conducted. These studies indicated that infectious sinusitis in the ICU correlated with placement of the nasal tube, and that bacteria grew in 80% to 100% of aspirated samples (13–18). As awareness of the diagnostic obstacles of paranasal sinus disease in the ICU increased, study results have changed over time. In addition to discussing the diagnosis and management of ICU-associated sinusitis, this chapter surveys the results of microbiological and other studies that broadened our understanding of the pathophysiology of this infection.

The post–sinus surgery refractory sinusitis also discussed in this chapter is not a true nosocomial sinusitis by definition. The major indication for sinus surgery is chronic sinusitis. Post–surgery sinusitis is a continuous inflammatory disease of the sinus cavity in which expected healing does not occur and the bacterial floras may persist or change (19).

ETIOLOGY AND PATHOGENESIS

Numerous factors make the critically ill patient susceptible to infections. These include the presence of one or more diseases or injuries, a secondary impaired host-defense, and the need for intensive care in order to survive. Patients who are already immunocompromised (diabetes, chemotherapy, undernourished, etc.) are generally at higher risk for infections, while patients with head injuries and intra paranasal sinus bleeding are at particularly high risk for infectious sinusitis.

In post–sinus surgery sinusitis, the indication for surgery is generally chronic sinusitis with an impaired local (the rhinosinus mucosa) host-defense. Evaluations of short-term endoscopic sinus surgery (ESS) results indicate "first time" failure rates between 5% and 10%. In long-term follow-ups, new surgical procedures are necessary in up to 25% of the patients (20,21). Successful ESS provides improvement in the mucosal ciliary beat (22,23), while scarring with ostial obstruction has repeatedly been identified as a significant surgical complication at revision surgery (20,23–25).

The Nosocomial Bacterial Flora

The patient's indigenous bacterial flora may cause infections, although the bacterial reservoir in the ICU represents an even higher potential risk. Hospitalized patients rapidly become colonized or infected by the ICU flora, which is strongly influenced by the selective pressure caused by antimicrobial agents that are used (26–28). In addition, the therapeutic measures utilized in the patient, such as use of invasive devices and immunomodulating therapy, may enhance the predisposition to infection. Infectious sinusitis in this setting is caused by bacteria and occasionally by fungi. However, the etiology of paranasal sinus during an ICU stay is not only infectious. There are inflammatory conditions, varying from noninfectious sinusitis that does not contain bacteria to noninfectious sinusitis with bacteria, that only represent colonization (29).

Body Position

When lying down, our otherwise upward-directed blood vessels fill better, since their direction has changed. When a healthy individual assumes a recumbent position, the blood vessels in the rhinosinus region become engorged, thus leading to mucosal edema with a significant reduction in the patency of the antral ostiae (30,31). An inflammatory reaction in the mucosa due to allergy or the common cold also increases the nasal airflow resistance up to three times in the horizontal position as compared to the resistance in a healthy individual (32,33). The full significance of the general edema in the rhinosinuses of critically ill patients is not fully understood. Even so, it is common practice in the ICU to position the patient's head at a 30° to 45° elevation to prevent gastrointestinal aspiration (34) and nasal obstruction.

Biofilm

An inert foreign body in the nose, such as a plastic pearl or a tube, can cause a localized purulent secretion (35). In an experimental study in rabbits, it was possible to demonstrate the development of local mucosal reaction with an increasing number of goblet cells, secretion, and accretion surrounding the plastic tube, together with a change of bacterial flora (36). The bacterial accretion of a protective glycocalyx, the formation of biofilm fixed to an endotracheal tube, is a time-dependent event in the mechanically ventilated patient (37). Facultative aerobic bacteria with particularly high adhesive ability and slime production are staphylococci and *Pseudomonas aeruginosa*, which are the most common bacteria of the transmeatal maxillary sinus aspirates in cases of ventilator-associated sinusitis (5). The colonization by staphylococci and *P. aeruginosa* comprises the upper airway and the digestive tract, as well as the lower airway, where they are the two most common bacterial species reported as causative agents of nosocomial pneumonia (1). How interaction and growth of pathogenic organisms in a biofilm further trigger an infection has not yet been determined (38).

A biofilm can be defined as an assemblage of microbial cells that is irreversibly associated (not removed by gentle rinsing) with a surface and enclosed in a matrix of primarily polysaccharide material. (Figure 1 is a drawing of the general biofilm structure, while Figure 2 is a SEM photo of a biofilm.) Biofilms may form on a variety of surfaces including living tissues, indwelling medical devices, industrial or potable water system piping, and natural aquatic systems. The understanding of biofilms has increased during the past decade through the use of the confocal laser scanning microscope to study biofilm ultrastructure and to investigate genes involved in cell (bacteria) adhesion and biofilm formation (38). The course of events from inoculation and sticking to slime/glycocalyx production and formation of biofilm is complex, with probable variations among different strains of bacterial species (39).

Schematically, a biofilm formation by *Staphylococcus epidermidis* can be divided into three steps, where step 1 is the primary adhesion of individual bacteria to a surface, influenced by physical interactions (hydrophobic, electrostatic) that are in turn possibly influenced by cell surface adhesions. Step 2 is cellular aggregation mediated by polysaccharide intercellular adhesins. The polysaccharide intercellular adhesins are products of the icaADBC gene cluster and are virulence factors in the pathogenesis of foreign body infections (40). The generation of a slime exopolysaccharide encasing the

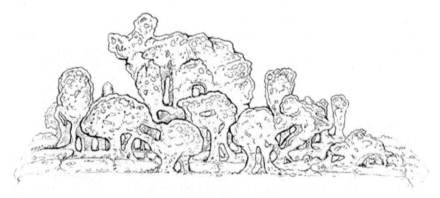

Figure 1 Organization of a mature biofilm, an organized community of bacteria. *Source*: Courtesy of Dr. C. Post, the Center for Genomic Sciences, Allegheny Singer Research Institute.

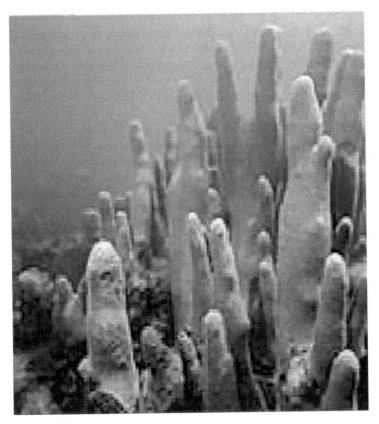

Figure 2 Scanning electron microscope image of a "coral reef" biofilm. *Source*: Courtesy of Dr. C Post, the Center for Genomic Sciences, Allegheny Singer Research Institute.

surface-bound microorganisms in a gelatinous matrix comprises step 3, the final step, although it is not crucial for establishing a biofilm (39).

In a *P. aeruginosa* biofilm formation, step 1 is the primary adhesion of individual bacteria to a targeted surface and it is dependent on functional flagellar motility. The next phase, step 2, requires the synthesis of type IV pili, providing the bacteria with the ability to migrate across the surface and congregate in microcolonies. The development of the biofilm, step 3, is completed with the fabrication of an alginic acid-like exopolysaccharide coded by the algACD gene cluster. Bacteria close to the outer surface may extricate from the biofilm to migrate and colonize new microenvironments (39).

The established biofilm commonly hosts a mixed flora of bacteria in a stationary phase in which the single bacteria has transformed from a planktonic cell to a "town-dweller" where the dense bacterial mass participates in an intercellular signal system. The biofilm coexistence of *Klebsiella pneumoniae* and *P. aeruginosa* can be stable, with *P. aeruginosa* primarily growing as a base biofilm while *K. pneumoniae* forms localized microcolonies in a small part of 10% of the area. The interpretation of this observation is that *P. aeruginosa* is competitive in rapidly colonizing the surface and gains long-term advantage, while *K. pneumoniae* survives due to its ability to attach to the *P. aeruginosa* biofilm, to have a faster growth, and to profit from the surface advantages of the biofilm (41).

The biofilm-associated bacteria attain resistance to several toxic substances, such as chlorine and detergents, as well as antibiotics. Several reports provide reasons and evidence that explain the increased resistance of biofilms to therapeutic interventions. These include the poor penetration of antibiotic into the biofilm, decreased growth rate in a biofilm, capacity of biofilm-specific substances such as exopolysaccharide, formation of persister cells, and quorum-sensing specific effects (42–45). Conjugation (plasmid transfer mechanism) between bacteria included in a biofilm occurs at a greater rate compared to bacteria in the planktonic state (46). The plasmids may carry genes for resistance to multiple antibiotics. Therefore, biofilm-association provides a mechanism for selection and for promoting the spread of antimicrobial resistance.

The formation of biofilms can apply to all biomedical devices used in ICU patients, and not only to nasotracheal and nasogastric tubes. However, these two indwelling devices are mainly used in the rhinosinus area and act as the local source of bacteria, exposing their additive and unprotected surfaces to biofilm formation allowing bacterial density not otherwise possible. The situation is nevertheless hard to avoid, and contamination and infection are difficult to separate (47).

Nitric Oxide

Mechanical ventilation, as applied today, overrides the ventilation of the upper airway and thereby sets aside the outflow of nitric oxide from the maxillary sinuses. The maxillary sinuses were found to be the major endogenous origin of airway nitric oxide in 1995 (48). Measured nasal nitric oxide concentrations are low in newborns with immature sinuses, and thereafter increase and seem to follow the development and pneumatization of the sinuses to the adult higher levels (48). Nasal nitric oxide of various levels, possibly related to animal size and comparable to human values, have been found in several mammals with open paranasal sinuses. In a baboon species that lack sinuses, the measurable nasal nitric oxide is very low (49). Studies that utilized ultrastructural immunolocalization determined that the production sites of nitric oxide are the sinus epithelial cilia and microvilli (50). In Kartagener's syndrome, characterized by the derangement of the cilia and microvilli, an absence of measurable nasally nitric oxide levels has been ascertained (51). As subjects with immotile cilia syndrome and cystic fibrosis also show extremely low nasal nitric oxide levels (51,52), it might be expected that any disorder of the mucosal surface will also have a negative impact on nitric oxide release.

The nitric oxide pulmonary vasodilating effect that enhances pulmonary oxygen uptake (53), as well as the existence of an endogenous source for nitric oxide (54), had already been recognized when it was discovered that the maxillary sinuses are the airway's main endogenous source of nitric oxide.

Nitric oxide has been shown to have an in vivo stimulatory effect on the mucosa ciliary activity that is part of the local innate rhinosinus defense system (55). Patients with chronic airway disease, such as chronic sinusitis or recurrent pneumonia, have low nasal nitric oxide concentrations, as well as significantly impaired mucociliary function as is measured by the ciliary beat frequency and saccharin transport time (52). In addition to this mechanical type of defense, nitric oxide is also involved in other processes that have antibacterial effects. In the in vitro models, immunomodulatory, cytotoxic, and antibacterial effects have been demonstrated to be coupled to inducible nitric oxide synthase (iNOS) released nitric oxide. Experimental results have indicated that the ability of endothelial cells, after phagocytosis, to kill *Escherichia coli* is nitric oxide-dependent, while the effect on *Staphylococcus aureus* remains growth-inhibiting (56). Another possible pathway is quinone compound enhancing of the cytotoxity of phenolic compounds, where nitric oxide promotes their oxidation (57).

The expression of inflammatory leukocytes in attaining increased numbers does not seem to be affected by nitric oxide presence in vivo, but the efficacy does. In mice with induced *K. pneumoniae* pneumonia, the nitric oxide-depleted group had an impairment of phagocytosis and killing function of the bacteria compared to the control group (58). In an experimental animal bacterial challenge of iNOS-deficient mice response compared to a wild-type control, an up-regulated release of polymorphonuclear leukocyte superoxide resulted in a significantly greater percentage of dead polymorphonuclear leukocytes (59).

The nasal concentrations of nitric oxide output show a significant decrease if the maxillary sinus ostiae are obstructed as in nonallergic polyposis (60). In a study of septic ICU patients with radiological sinopathy, the maxillary sinuses were fenestrated as a measure to reduce a possible origin of sepsis, and the maxillary nitric oxide output that was found was significantly lower, together with the iNOS levels, than the levels of the controls (50). However, the decreased nitric oxide output did not correlate with the presence of infection, as only two out of six cultures had bacterial growth. Other inflammatory sinus conditions with decreasing nitric oxide output have been demonstrated by nasal measurements in children with acute sinusitis (61) and in patients with chronic sinusitis, while common cold subjects exhibit values comparable to the controls (62).

Overall, the number of subjects that were so far included in nitric oxide studies is small and more studies are needed before we can proceed beyond hypothetical knowledge and reach the practical level, where the nitric oxide production in the upper airways would be regulated to the advantage of critically ill patients as well as chronic sinusitis patients. Joint research recommendations have been published (63) carefully enumerating how measurements should be carried out in order to be able to compare and combine results of different research groups.

Airway Bypass

Little is known about the local effects on the innate and acquired-host immune defenses of the sinuses by mechanical ventilation airway bypass, which brings about a change in gas-compositions in these cavities. When any nasal medical device is used, it induces traumatic wear and tear of the mucosa. These, as well other factors such as mucosal sinus surgery trauma, may enhance the susceptibility of the mucosa to adhesive bacteria, thereby becoming a receptive surface for biofilm formation. The rapid genetic exchanges by conjugation among the static biofilm bacteria can effect the host–microbe interference. The spread of virulence and pathogenicity determinants can turn a nonpathogenic bacterial strain into a pathogenic strain of the same species (64,65).

Host-Defense

The microbial challenge of the sinus may not be adequately opposed by a deregulated or a perplexed local defense. Primary immunodeficiencies are not entirely rare and are commonly underdiagnosed (66). This is particularly the case among patients with refractory chronic sinusitis who fail to respond to medical and surgical therapy (67). A study that followed individuals after ESS revealed that those with a diagnosis of systemic disease had a significantly higher frequency of poor surgical outcome as validated by their subjective symptomatic score (20,68). Our inadequate recognition of systemic or local human immune defense defects is hampering our understanding of how to improve diagnosis and therapies.

Lactoferrins, avid iron-binding glycoproteins of the transferring family ubiquitously secreted on mucosal surfaces and within specific granules of polymorphonuclear leukocytes, have an antimicrobial effect in their unsaturated form. Initially, this was attributed to their ability to sequester iron that is essential for bacterial growth, but iron-independent antimicrobial activities that rely upon the direct interaction of lactoferrin with its target have also been demonstrated (69,70). Even in lower concentrations, lactoferrin can, by chelating iron, stimulate twitching, a specialized surface motility of bacteria that keeps them wandering, unable to squat to become sessile and form biofilms (71).

Antimicrobial peptides are synthesized in granula of phagocytic cells and are secreted by the epithelia. Once excreted, they avidly bind to many of the potentially pro-inflammatory molecules released by microorganisms, such as lipopolysaccharide. Through this inactivation mechanism, the antimicrobial peptides inhibit the host-cells reactions and restrain undesirable inflammatory responses. They have inducible and constitutive properties, and participate in the innate defense of the sinus and the lungs (72).

Mainly known as components of the gastrointestinal region immune system, β-defensins provide endogenous antimicrobial activities demonstrated in vitro, activities against gram-negative bacteria, protozoa, and fungi. β-defensins are synergistic with lysoszyme and lactoferrin. They also possess immunomodulatory functions with memory T-cells and naïve dendritic cells (73).

Increasing levels of locally acting inflammatory mediators can have unto-ward effects resulting in the production of matrix metalloproteinases (MMPs) and other components of the hosts' extracellular matrix remodeling machinery. MMPs, which comprise of more than 20 calcium and zinc dependent enzymes, can cause persistent pulmonary pathological stromal alterations in asthma, chronic obstructive pulmonary disease, and emphysema. An increase in the levels of MMP-9 that exceeds the regulating tissue inhibitor TIMP-1 has been described in exacerbations of asthma. This is interpreted as an imbalance that allows temporary matrix damage that is followed by abnormal repair (74). An increase in the MMP activity also occurs in rhinosinus disease (75). There is a significant increase within the blood vessel MMP-7-positive epithelial cells in the nasal polyposis patients as compared to the control and the chronic sinusitis patients. MMP-9 has a significant up-regulation effect in epithelial cells of both the nasal polyposis group and the chronic sinusitis group, and some increase in the stroma. The presence of TIMP-1-staining cells shows some increase, but this is not significant in either the nasal polyposis group or the chronic sinusitis group. However, when the staining results where compared to the ELISA immunoas-says, the chronic sinusitis group had significantly higher TIMP-1 levels (75). The difference between the regulations of the MMPs leads to the hypothesis that there are two different tissue-remodeling patterns in sinus diseases, which offer possible new therapies.

Another aberrant course of events in the host inflammatory response seems to occur when the cytokine response increases, possibly becoming un-controllable, resulting in an enhanced intracellular and extracellular bacterial growth, as has been shown in vitro (76). This new approach to host–micro-organism interference is based upon observations in patients with acute respiratory distress syndrome who had a concomitant ventilator-associated pneumonia. The observations revealed that nonsurvivors had a heavier bac-terial, often polymicrobial, load in their bronchoalveolar lavage along with a more intense local inflammatory response of TNF-α, IL-1β, and IL-6, than survivors. This observation reverses the traditional logic that the innate host-defense is influenced by the microbial pressure and suggests that a cytokine boom might make bacterial proliferation more abundant. In vitro growth of the applicable bacterial strains is promoted by adding the cytokines TNF-α, IL-1β, or IL-6 to the growth medium (77). These results provide a new insight into various kinds of difficult rhinosinus diseases, indicating that the presence of bacteria is only an expression of pathology and not the primary agent.

Additional uncontrollable effects on microorganisms occur due to the influence of medications that are commonly used in intensive care units, i.e., the catecholamine inotropes, norepinephrine, and dobutamin. An association between the use of catecholamine injections and an increased rate of infection was observed 70 years ago. This lead to studies which showed that epinephrine promotes in vivo growth and virulence of a number of gram-positive and gram-negative bacteria. An in vitro study of an intravenous catheter milieu used inotrope concentrations at or below the clinical situation and a low bacterial inocula of *S. epidermidis*, attempting to imitate the situation that occurs at the time of an induction of an opportunistic infection. The study showed that the inotropes stimulated the growth of *S. epidermidis* on the intravenous catheters to form biofilm (78). These studies demonstrate the effects of inotropes on the bacterial colonization of a foreign body. Although intravenous catheters are not inserted into the nose for infusion, this could be a reminder that effects might exist that we do not see because we do not expect them, and this is also something to be more aware of, particularly in refractory cases. It could sometimes be worthwhile to stop the use of pharmaceuticals and only use physiologic saline rinse to find the basic level of symptomatology.

EPIDEMIOLOGY

Nosocomial Sinusitis

In general, 5% to 15% of hospitalized patients contract a nosocomial infection. This rate is higher in the ICU, where a one-third of the patients will suffer from a nosocomial infection. Ventilator-associated pneumonia, catheter-related bloodstream infections, surgical site infections, and urinary-catheter related infections account for greater than 80% of these infections (79). Among mechanically ventilated patients, pneumonia has the highest incidence. The complication of an infection prolongs the length of stay, increases the costs of hospitalization, and increases the risk of mortality (1).

Epidemiological studies provided the following conclusions regarding the expected change in the patients' bacterial flora in the ICU setting: (i) In time all patients are colonized by the nosocomial flora; (ii) colonization rate is directly related to the seriousness of the patients condition; and (iii) the same bacterial strains are generally found in the upper as well as the lower airways of individuals (80–82). Johansson et al. (83) demonstrated over 30 years ago that nosocomial colonization in ICU patients predisposes them to pneumonias: pneumonia developed in 23% of nosocomially colonized ICU patients compared to only 3% of noncolonized. Potential pathogenic bacteria are commonly found within 24 hours of admission in mechanically ventilated patients. In samples taken from oropharynx, gastric fluid, sub-glottic space, and trachea, most patients in a study harbor enterococci, *S. epidermidis*, and *Candida* spp. In 59% of the patients, anaerobic bacteria were isolated in the sub-glottic and tracheal samples (84). It has been surmised that colonization starts in the oropharynx, then the stomach, followed by the lower respiratory tract, and that it then spreads upwards, contaminating the tracheal tube (85). Considerable amounts of intraluminal biofilm (density of up to 10^6 CFU/cm^2) made of hospital-acquired bacterial flora was found on tracheal tubes used for 24 hours or less (86). This high microbial load might lead to the development of pneumonia and sinusitis whenever the opportunity arises. The denser the colonization, the harder it becomes to obtain adequate maxillary sinus samples. This practical difficulty explains why recent studies included only a smaller number of positive aspiration cultures (29). A summary of the microbiological findings in specimens obtained by most often the transmeatal route is presented in Table 1. Overall, the results mirror the hospital-acquired flora, and there were significant numbers of anaerobic bacteria when proper methods for their collection and identification were used.

Artificial ventilation-acquired sinopathy is defined as the presence of signs of sinus disease in a mechanically ventilated patient where bacteria, if present, are a predisposing factor but cannot be proved as direct agents that initiate the inflammatory reaction. Indirect imaging pathology is artificial ventilation-acquired sinopathy until further tests confirm a change of diagnosis. In the asymptomatic population, the occurrence rate for sinopathy, such as mucosal thickening, is present in about 40% of individuals, sinus edema of the ethmoids is seen in about 30%, and maxillary sinus edema in about 25% (103).

Fassoulaki et al. (104) showed that in 16 patients who were admitted to the ICU without sinus pathology and were nasotracheally intubated with one side of the nose free, six (38%) developed sinus X-ray pathology (either mucosal thickening, air-fluid levels, or opacification) within 48 to 72 hours. After eight days, 14 (88%) had only a radiological sinopathy ipsilateral to the nasotracheal tube (104). Hansen et al. conducted a similar study and evaluated 12 of 41 patients who underwent CT-scanning because of skull trauma and did not have sinus pathology on admission. These patients were fit with a nasotracheal tube on one side and a nasogastric tube on the other. All had developed sinopathy in less than two days, in seven cases with the initial changes on the nasogastric tube side (105). Other comparative studies report 50% sinus X-ray pathology after five days of mechanical ventilation (106) as compared to only a 10% imaging pathology in tracheotomized patients (107). Strange et al. (108) found that significant risk factors were prolonged intubation time, $p < 0.001$, and use of nasotracheal tube, $p < 0.02$, when they observed eight patients with orotracheal tubes and 12 patients with nasotracheal tubes (108).

All these studies illustrate that radiological sinopathy tends to develop in any mechanically ventilated ICU patient but faster in patients with nasal

Table 1 Prospective ICU Sinusitis Studies Including Maxillary Samples for Culturing with Microbiological Findings

Study	Caplan & Hoyt (13)	Kronberg & Goodwin (15)	Grindlinger et al. (87)	Guérin et al. (88)	Humphrey et al. (89)
Year	1982	1985	1987	1989	1987
Sample route	Transmeatal		Transmeatal	Transmeatal	Transmeatal
Disinfection	Yes	?	Yes	–	Yes
Number of positive cultures	25	4	19	11	24
Current antibiotic therapy	Yes	Yes	Yes	Yes	Yes
Polymicrobial growth	56%	100%	89%	64%	88%
Gram-positive cocci					
Staphylococcus aureus	1	2	6		8
Coagulase-negative staphylococci					
Streptococcaceae	4	1	14	1	8
Enterococci		2			
Streptococcus pyogenes				6	7
Streptococcus pneumonia					
Others		1	2		4
Gram-negative bacilli					
Pseudomonas aeruginosa	12	2	7		8
Acinetobacter species			2	1	3
Klebsiella species	7		3	2	4
Enterobacter species	7	1		1	
Escherichia coli	3		7	3	7
Proteus species	5	2	4	3	
Serratia species					
Haemophilus influenzae					
Others		1	5	1	10
Anaerobes					
Bacteroides species	2	1	3		3
Anaerobic cocci			2		2
Others		3	1		1
Yeasts					
Candida				1	
Others		1			
Total number of isolates	41	17	56	19	65

Study	Aebert et al. (16)	Bell et al. (17)	Linden et al. (18)	Guérin et al. (90)	Fougeront et al. (91)
Year	1988	1988	1988	1989	1990
Sample route	?	Transmeatal	Transmeatal	Transmeatal	?
Disinfection	–	–	Yes	–	–
Number of positive cultures	4	11	21	39	10
Current antibiotic therapy	Yes	Yes[a]	Yes[a]	Yes[a]	?
Polymicrobial growth	50%	46%	42%	54%	30%
Gram-positive cocci					
Staphylococcus aureus	1	3	5	5	6
Coagulase-negative staphylococci					
Streptococcaceae		1	1	4	1
Enterococci					
Streptococcus pyogenes			1	18	6
Streptococcus pneumonia			2	2	
Others		2			
Gram-negative bacilli					
Pseudomonas aeruginosa	4	1	3		
Acinetobacter species	1				1
Klebsiella species		1	2	3	
Enterobacter species			3	5	
Escherichia coli		4		4	
Proteus species		1	1	15	
Serratia species				1	
Haemophilus influenzae		1	1	1	1
Others			3		
Anaerobes					
Bacteroides species			6		
Anaerobic cocci					
Others					
Yeasts					
Candida			1	3	
Others					
Total number of isolates	6	15	28	61	15

Study	Bowers et al. (92)	Michelson et al. (93)	Holzapfel et al. (94)	Rouby et al. (95)	Bert & Lambert-Zechovsky (96)
Year	1991	1992	1993	1994	1995
Sample route	?	?	Transmeatal	Transmeatal	?
Disinfection	–	–	–	Yes	–
Number of positive cultures	4	9	54	44	103
Current antibiotic therapy	Yes[a]	Yes	?	Yes[a]	?
Polymicrobial growth	50%	?	50%	32%	65%
Gram-positive cocci					
Staphylococcus aureus	1	1	10	18	35
Coagulase-negative staphylococci	1				8
Streptococcaceae	1	2	23	13	8
Enterococci			2		5
Streptococcus pyogenes					
Streptococcus pneumonia					
Others			5		4
Gram-negative bacilli					
Pseudomonas aeruginosa	1	4	1	11	26
Acinetobacter species			2	6	20
Klebsiella species			3		20
Enterobacter species	1		3	2	8
Escherichia coli			17	6	13
Proteus species			6	4	11
Serratia species			2	4	3
Haemophilus influenzae	1	1	7		9
Others			4	6	5
Anaerobes					
Bacteroides species			5	2	2
Anaerobic cocci					
Others		3			17
Yeasts					
Candida			4	14	27
Others				1	
Total number of isolates	6	10	92	88	217

Study	Bert & Lambert-Zechovsky (97)	Mevio et al. (98)	George et al. (99)	Westergren et al. (23)	Le Moal et al. (100)
Year	1996	1996	1998	1998	1999
Sample route	Transmeatal	Transmeatal[abc]	Aspirate ?	Canine fossa	Transmeatal
Disinfection	Yes	?	?	Yes[ab]	Yes
Number of positive cultures	271	24	?	7	30
Current antibiotic therapy	?	?	?	Yes[a]	Yes[a]
Polymicrobial growth	58%	50%	82%	57%	73%
Gram-positive cocci					
Staphylococcus aureus	94	10	8		5
Coagulase-negative staphylococci	14		8		2
Streptococcaceae	23	1	10	2	4
Enterococci	14		4	1	3
Streptococcus pyogenes					
Streptococcus pneumonia					1
Others			4	2	
Gram-negative bacilli					
Pseudomonas aeruginosa	64	12	8		7
Acinetobacter species	91	2	2		3
Klebsiella species	35	1	6		1
Enterobacter species	16	2	6		1
Escherichia coli	34	6	5	1	5
Proteus species	32		5		5
Serratia species		1			1
Haemophilus influenzae	16		1		2
Others	30	1	5		3
Anaerobes					
Bacteroides species			1	5	22
Anaerobic cocci			1	1	4
Others			1	5	7
Yeasts					
Candida	62	1	7		1
Others		1			1
Total number of isolates	525	38	84	17	77

Study	Holzapfel et al. (101)	Souweine et al. (102)	Total no.	
Year	1999	2000		
Sample route	Transmeatal	Transmeatal		
Disinfection	Yes	?		
Number of positive cultures	80	24		
Current antibiotic therapy	Yes[a]	Yes		
Polymicrobial growth	42%	62%		
Gram-positive cocci				
Staphylococcus aureus	10	4	233	All gram-positive cocci: 541
Coagulase-negative staphylococci	9	5	46	
Streptococcaceae	30	5	154	
Enterococci		7	39	
Streptococcus pyogenes			38	
Streptococcus pneumonia			10	
Others			21	
Gram-negative bacilli				
Pseudomonas aeruginosa	12	12	195	All gram-negative bacilli: 877
Acinetobacter species	4		138	
Klebsiella species	6		94	
Enterobacter species	6	6	68	
Escherichia coli	12	3	130	
Proteus species	10		103	
Serratia species			11	
Haemophilus influenzae	7		45	

Others	6	1	93	
Anaerobes				All anaerobic bacteria: 115
Bacteroides species	Undefined		50	
Anaerobic cocci	15		10	
Others			40	
Yeasts				All yeasts: 149
Candida	10	5	146	
Others			3	
Total number of isolates	138	48	1682	

Note: ? Information is not included in the publication.

[a] Patients treated with antibiotics at the time of sampling, with some exceptions

[ab] Free bone area

[abc] 22 samples from maxillary exudates and 2 from nasal swabs

devices. Isolated radiological sinopathy is not an infectious disease; however, bacterial sinusitis also has radiological sinopathy.

A prospective study of 1,126 intra-nasotracheally intubated patients in an ICU revealed the presence of bacterial sinusitis in 27 (2%) (98). In another study where 111 patients were randomized to either orotracheal or nasotracheal intubation and the diagnostic requirements were radiographic sinopathy and positive protected-brush culture, a 43% frequency of sinus infection was found in the nasotracheally intubated group (94). Additional data about other clinical studies are discussed in the Diagnosis section.

Post Sinus Surgery Sinusitis

Most operative results represent an improvement (21), but some cases of chronic sinusitis are refractory to surgery. Some types of chronic sinusitis heal better than others after surgery, while others do well without surgery. Facial pain, in particular, is a symptom requiring careful consideration both when planning primary sinus surgery (109) and even more so when it persists post surgery (21,109). Differential diagnoses for facial pain include mid-facial segment pain, tension-type headache, atypical facial pain, migraine, paroxysmal hemicrania, and cluster headache.

One post–sinus surgery follow-up using scintigraphy to assess mucociliary function noted a difference between cases of sinus cysts and cases with hyperplastic mucosal generation; the latter took a longer time to recover normal ciliary function (110). These findings support the hypothesis that there are different types of inflammatory diseases of the paranasal sinuses. Lavigne et al. (112) studied 15 consecutive patients with allergy and chronic sinusitis, all of whom had a rating higher than 12 using the Lund–Mackay staging system (111), but no nasal polyposis or any recognized immunodeficiency. At surgery, mucosa samples were collected and evaluated for lymphocyte subsets (CD3, CD4, CD8), mast cells, eosinophils, and cells expressing IL-4 and IL-5 messenger RNA. At follow-up two years after surgery, there were seven patients who were asymptomatic and eight who did not improve. Those who failed to respond had a significantly increased number of cells expressing IL-5 messenger RNA in the preoperative ethmoid sinus biopsies, $p = 0.007$ (112).

Reports on microbiology findings post–sinus surgery are surprisingly few. Brook and Frazier (113) present a retrospective evaluation of cultures taken from the patients with chronic sinusitis of whom 33 had surgery and 75 did not have surgery. The recovered bacteria presented as a polymicrobial flora with anaerobic bacteria, alone or mixed with aerobic bacteria, in more than 80% of cultures. The post-surgery patients had significantly more often *P. aeruginosa* ($p < 0.001$) and more enteric gram-negative bacilli compared to those who had no surgery. Bhattacharyya et al. (114) presented a retrospective study of the aerobic microbiology of 125 patients who relapsed after ESS. No bacteria grew in cultures from 30% of the patients, which is a frequency similar to the frequency of cultures with only anaerobic bacteria by Brook and Frazier (113).

Similar to that study (113), Bhattacharyya et al. (114) recovered *P. aeruginosa*, as well as enteric gram-negative bacilli and gram-positive cocci (mostly *S. aureus* and *S. epidermidis*).

The culture results of these two studies resemble those of nosocomial sinusitis in the ICU setting (Table 1).

Bhattacharyya et al. (115) prospectively investigated whether infections occurring after ethmoid ESS represent overgrowth of the previous sinonasal flora or represent a new bacterial infection. Cultures from 113 patients were obtained endoscopically and processed only for aerobic bacteria. Baseline postoperative cultures were sterile in 23% of cases, "oral" flora were recovered in 18%, and 60% were colonized showing commonly gram-positive cocci (mainly *Staphylococcus* spp.) in 41%. Twenty acute exacerbations were cultured in 17 patients during the follow-up period of 14.5 months. All these cultures yielded bacteria; they were mostly gram-positive cocci (56% of isolates), half of which were *S. aureus* and 75% of the strains where new compared to baseline cultures. These findings illustrate that most infections arising postoperatively represent a new infection that best requires reculturing to properly select antimicrobial therapy.

Clinical Presentations

It is difficult for critically ill patients to relate symptoms of sinus disease. While many ordinary people present with nonspecific signs and symptoms of sinusitis, these are even more common in the ICU patients as they originate from their critical condition. A decision to search for an infection is made on an individual basis. Fever can arise from a number of non-infectious causes in ICU patients. Fever has a variety of features that need evaluation such as a transient spike, repeated elevations, or persistent fever (116,117). The symptom of nasal suppuration, discussed under the subheading Pathogenesis, is not in itself diagnostic of a sinus infection. The observation of radiographic sinusitis, even accompanied by a positive culture, may not be diagnostic. This was demonstrated by Borman et al. (118) who followed 598 patients; only one of the 26 that required further evaluation developed an infection. Infectious sinusitis mainly presents itself as an alternative cause of a suspected infection in the critically ill patient when other more common causes have been excluded. The series of Figures 3–9 represent photographs obtained during antroscopies of ICU patients who were studied to exclude sinusitis. They illustrate various conditions of normal maxillary sinuses, different kinds of inflammatory or edematous reactions, with and without pus, and the presence of adherent plaques probably representing biofilm.

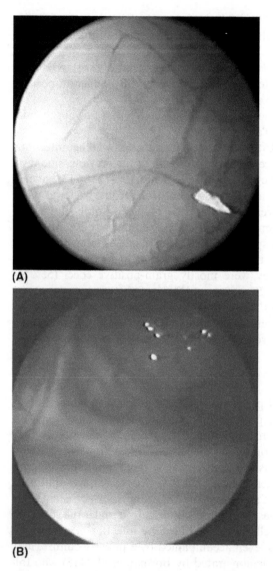

Figure 3 All images are from antroscopies of ICU patients investigated for possible infectious maxillary sinusitis from 1991 to 1994 at the University Hospital, Linköping, Sweden. **(A)** Normal mucosa with visible vessels on the right maxillary sinus. A female patient, 61 years old, had been at the ICU for 21 days with a nasotracheal tube on the left and a nasogastric tube on the right. The left side was unaffected except for the presence of some serous fluid. The patient had secondary to an exchange of cerebroventricular shunts developed meningitis caused by a *Pseudomonas* species and had received antibiotics ceftazidim, piperacillin, and tobramycin. **(B)** Panoramic view of the unaffected right maxillary sinus.

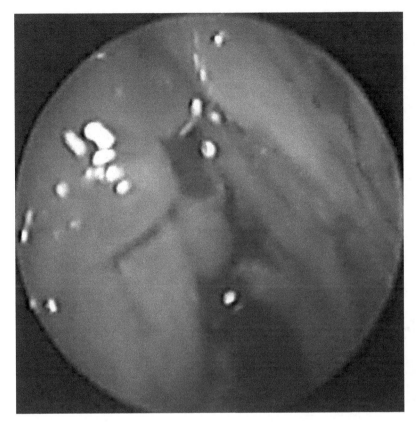

Figure 4 A vitreous edema reaction in the left maxillary sinus without bacterial findings. The patient had had a nasogastric tube for 14 days through the left nasal cavity and received cefuroxim during this period.

DIAGNOSIS OF AN INFECTIOUS SINUSITIS IN THE ICU

The difficulties in obtaining noncontaminated samples from the involved sinus makes it difficult to compare results from different studies (119). Sobin et al. (120) performed a study in healthy people in which they kept the maxillary samples uncontaminated and showed the sinuses to be free from bacteria. Another study showed contradictory results, although the patients were not free from rhinosinus symptoms as sampling was done during septoplasty under general anesthesia, with the occurrence of anaerobic bacteria in all samples, and mixed with aerobes in some (121). There are indications that enclosed cavities such as the nose and paranasal sinuses may harbor different bacterial floras, and that samples of nasal drainage or meatal drainage do not always represent the bacteria that are present within a sinus itself (122–124).

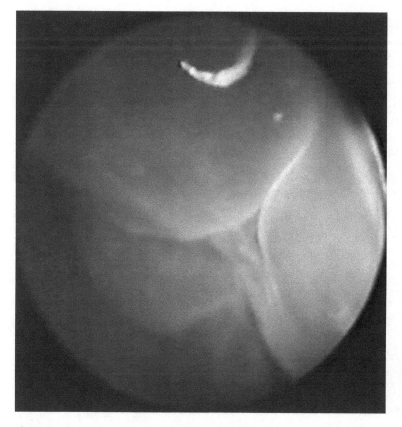

Figure 5   Polypoid mucosa in the right maxillary sinus in a patient with nasotracheal tube in the adjacent nasal cavity for 12 days, without bacteria in cultures from secretion and mucosa.

The formation of a biofilm on medical devices is an immense obstacle to obtaining an uncontaminated maxillary sinus sample via the nose. Some previous publications used nasal discharge cultures to diagnose sinusitis, which should be viewed as documentation of nasal biofilm flora.

Most studies performed in ICU sinusitis cases that employed disinfection prior to transmeatal aspiration failed to document the efficacy of the topical disinfection. Rouby et al. were able to disinfect the septum in only 50% of their control samples (95). The biofilms are resistant to disinfection and the effect of a mechanical surface scrub is temporary (further discussions on biofilms under heading Etiology and Pathogenesis). The site of sinus penetration extends more than an inch into the cavity of the inferior meatus. Even the use of a protected brush combined with a cut off level of $>10^3$ CFU/L for assessing the positivity of a sample may not be sufficient if the bacterial density in

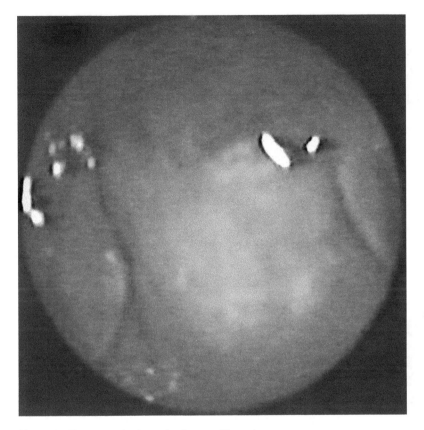

Figure 6 Intense red edema in the maxillary sinus.

the route of penetration is unknown and may be $>10^3$ CFU/L (96). The contact of instruments with the mucosa can result in their contaminations in two-thirds of the samples, and only to refrain from any mucosal contact of the penetrating instrument eliminated contamination (125). It is, therefore, prudent to avoid the nasal routes for obtaining sampling from maxillary sinuses in mechanically ventilated patients. It is, however, important, especially in the ICU setting, to establish the precise diagnosis of sinusitis without delay. The use of endoscopic visualization is the most helpful method in a critically ill patient to diagnose bacterial sinus infection (29,126), preferably, a protected canine fossa route to avoid nasal contamination. This would allow obtaining adequate bacterial cultures, which can assist in recovering the pathogens and selecting the proper antibiotic therapy. The routine study of the bacterial flora at different body sites of the involved patient, and knowledge of the ICU isolates in general, is necessary to know which antibiotics to choose from.

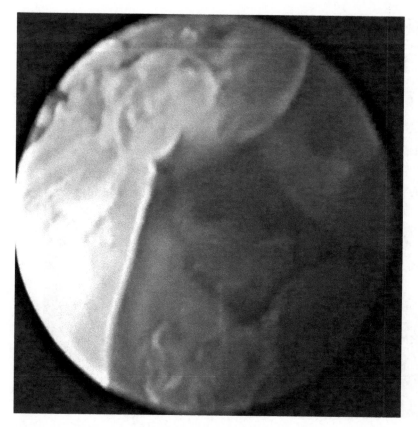

Figure 7 Combination of vitreous edema and intense red edema in the left maxillary sinus. A small amount of serous fluid was removed by suction. The patient had had a nasotracheal tube in the adjacent nasal cavity for 13 days. The antibiotic cefuroxim was given for two days before sinoscopy. Bacterial cultures were negative.

MICROBIOLOGY AND CHOICE OF ANTIMICROBIALS

The choice of proper antimicrobial therapy depends upon identification of the bacteria causing the infection. The validity of the obtained cultures must be carefully considered, and only after such deliberation has been made can an informed choice of antimicrobial therapy be made. The assessments of the bacterial importance of the bacterial isolates in the ICU setting are presented under previous headings in this chapter (Etiology and Pathogenesis/The Nosocomial Bacterial Flora/Biofilm/ Nitric Oxide and Epidemiology in Nosocomial Sinusitis).

Table 1 presents published results from studies of maxillary sinus done in the last 20 years. Since the most common isolate, *S. aureus*, was usually recovered through the transmeatal route, its recovery may be due to

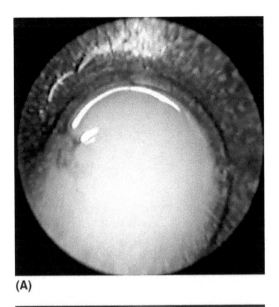

(A)

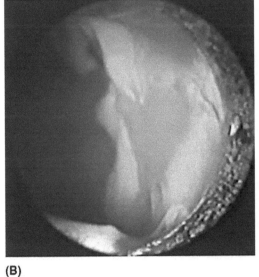

(B)

Figure 8 (A) Pus at primary inspection after removing the trocar, right maxillary sinus. A patient with intracerebral hematoma was nasally intubated for three days, then tracheotomized for eight days before sinoscopy and free of devices in the right nasal cavity. The patient was prescribed intravenous cefuroxim since surgery the first day. Aerobic and anaerobic cultures from the sinuses were negative. (B) At inspection after suction a red, moderate edema with a biofilm in the form of whitish, sticky sheets on a surface that could be considered as biofilm.

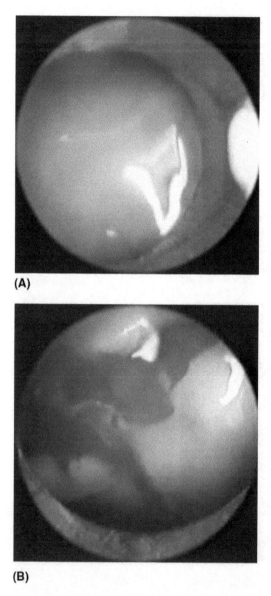

(A)

(B)

Figure 9 (A) Similar finding as in Figure 6(A) seen in another antroscopy of the left maxillary sinus, pus at primary inspection after removing the trocar in a female patient at the ICU for a fortnight and trachetomized after a week. A nasogastric tube in the adjacent nasal cavity was inserted and the patient had had a high dose of cefuroxim for a week. (B) As seen in Figure 7(A) after suction, where a more glassy, red edema of the mucosa can be seen in areas not covered by biofilm, and not removable by suction or rinse. Aerobic and anaerobic cultures from pus and mucosa were negative.

specimens contamination rather than causing an infection, since the vestibulum nasi is a normal site of this bacterium.

Gram-negative bacteria emerged as the major pathogens in the studies that avoided contamination. The isolates most often found are *E. coli, Klebsiella, Acinetobacter, Enterobacter* spp., and *P. aeruginosa*. The combined presence of an *Enterobacteriaceae* species plus *P. aeruginosa* is very common as polymicrobial growth occurs in 59% (Table 1).

Anaerobic bacteria are probably under-represented in most of the studies as proper method for their collection and transportation were not employed, and many studies did not include or even attempt to culture them. However, studies that used proper anaerobic culture illustrated the significance of mixed anaerobic infection in nosocomial sinusitis. In patients, who had been previously treated with antibiotics, the role of yeasts needs to be considered.

The empiric selection of a carbapenem (i.e., imipenem) before cultures are available provides coverage against the aerobic gram-negative species including most *P. aeruginosa* as well as anaerobes. A quinolone such as levofloxacin, providing covering *Enterobacteriaceae*, *P. aeruginosa* and several of the aerobic gram-positive cocci including some resistant strains is an alternative.

Specific therapy can be chosen when culture results become available. The decision should also take into consideration the bacterial strains recovered from patients and the environment in the specific ICU and their antimicrobial susceptibility. The choice should be done in consultation with the hospital infection control unit, and be based upon the need of an individual patient as well as the control of the nosocomial spread of bacterial resistance.

TREATMENT

In addition to antimicrobial therapy, surgical drainage may be also needed to achieve cure of maxillary empyema. Repeated lavages are recommended along with attempts to shrink the patients' bacterial load. If the patient's condition permits, the prefered advice is waiting for the identification of the pathogenic bacteria and their susceptibility to guide the choice or lead to avoidance of antibiotic therapy. Antibiotics are more effective against planktonic bacteria (i.e., in the free-floating microbial phase) in the sinuses (127), as is the case after a lavage, before a new biofilm has a chance to form. However, once a biofilm has formed, antimicrobial agents usually do not have effect and assessing bacterial sensitivity by minimum inhibitory concentration (MIC) may not be applicable. With the help of the Calgary Biofilm Device, it is possible to measure a minimum biofilm eradication concentration (MBEC) (128). Some gram-positive cocci may have identical sensitivity to antibiotics in the planktonic or biofilm state, while *P. aeruginosa* strains that are susceptible in the planktonic state become multi-resistant as a biofilm (129). To use of MBEC to determine antimicrobial susceptibility in the biofilm is highly recommended.

If the sinusitis is adjacent to a nasal cavity with a medical device, it is helpful to remove the device to reduce the microbial load in the nose and its efflux into the sinuses. The utility of re-intubation should be reconsidered, as this constitutes a risk factor for ventilation-associated pneumonia that may be due to aspiration of biofilm material (130). Removal of the nasotracheal tube may be the treatment of choice, however, there are no studies to support this, though normalization of the condition using ultrasound (131) and the resolution of fever (118) have been reported. In the authors' experience, patients generally undergo a decrease in body temperature of 1°C to 2°C one to two days following antral lavage. These of nasotracheal or the nasogastric tube was not a risk factor in the development of a nosocomial sinusitis, and a higher statistical significance correlation was found only with nasal colonization with enteric gram-negative bacteria ($p = 0.0007$) and Glasgow coma score ≤ 7 ($p = 0.0001$) (99).

Weaning the patient off mechanical ventilation so that all medical devices can be removed is the most effective treatment of sinusitis. Improving the patient's psychological status increases the upper airway nitric oxide flow (132) and supports the continuous restoration of normal sinus physiology. There are humanitarian aspects in the care of ICU patients, which might be the key to their improvement.

Some patients with a probable systemic disease may fail both medical therapy and endoscopic surgery. Using Denker's procedure, a radical surgery, as a last resort in such patients brought about symptomatic improvement (20,133). However, the creation of a widely open sinus cavity destroys the ciliary transport system and the patients have to rinse their sinuses daily with saline. The post-Denker sinus cavity is easy to inspect which facilitates removal of polyps and cysts (20).

COMPLICATIONS

Colonization of the sinuses is common in critically ill patients. The development of biofilm could shield the undisturbed bacterial communities that can become the potential origin of the microbial agents of pneumonia which carries about 50% mortality (130) in the ICU, or sepsis. Although radiographic sinopathy along with nosocomial colonization can occur prior to the development of pneumonia (94), the role of sinusitis is still unclear. Pneumonia is also recognized as carrying a high risk of complication that is enhanced by the severity of the patient illness, and in the upper airway and gastric nosocomial colonization (130). Sinusitis is often diagnosed along with other concomitant infections (118,134). In one study of patients who had nasotracheal and nasogastric tubes, the patients were randomized to either receiving extra attention including scheduled sinus CT scans, or to a control group that was treated and followed routinely. In the study group of 199, 80 patients developed infectious sinusitis, diagnosed based on CT findings and positive aspiration culture, and antibiotics were used more frequently in this group ($p = 0.03$). No sinusitis was diagnosed in the control group of 200 patients. The study group developed significantly fewer pneumonias ($p = 0.02$) but not significantly fewer septicemias (101).

The other complications of acute and chronic sinusitis, including nosocomial complications, are presented in Chapter 13.

PREVENTION

Keeping the nasal cavities free of devices is the most effective preventive measure. Nosocomial sinusitis can also occur in orotracheally intubated patients, although the frequency is somewhat lower (95). In intensive care settings, several pros and cons must be considered about the use of nasal or oral routes for devices (135), and a decision must be made on an individual basis. Other preventive strategies involve the use of infection prevention practices that reduce the transfer of nosocomial flora (i.e., careful handwashing by the staff, the implementation of one team per patient) and the proper choice of antibiotics to avoid the development of resistance.

Several new avenues of research show promise for newer means of prevention. Nebulization of gentamicin into tracheal tubes avoids systemic antibiotics and can reach topical concentrations that exceed the MBEC (136). Antimicrobial coatings of polyurethane and silicone are being tested (137). Slow release of nitric oxide coating may have antimicrobial properties that decrease *P. aeruginosa* adhesion (138). Oxygen glow discharge that changes the surface properties of polyvinylchloride endotracheal tubes reduced the adhesive ability of *P. aeruginosa* 70% (139). Ongoing experiments with chemical wet treatments on endotracheal tubes using sodium hydroxide (NaOH) and silver nitrate ($AgNO_3$) have completely inhibited the adhesion of *P. aeruginosa* for a period of 72 hours (140). These results point toward the potential of future adaptation of respiratory devices which may prevent their colonization with potential pathogens.

Selective decontamination of the digestive tract showed significantly decreased mortality in ICU patients (141). This method attempts to preserve the indigenous intestinal flora, as it possesses protective effect against secondary colonization with potentially pathogenic gram-negative bacteria. Nonabsorbed topical antibiotics, e.g., polymyxin E, tobramycin, and amphotericin B, are administered as an oral mixture through the gastric tube. Where oral colonization has already taken place, nebulization is used. A reduction of ventilator-associated pneumonia is difficult to evaluate, and there exists the risk that enhanced bacterial resistance would result if selective digestive decontamination was in general use. The method has not yet been validated in a convincing way, and should be avoided in milieus harboring methicillin-resistant *S. aureus*, vancomycin-resistant enterococci, or multi-resistant *Acinetobacter* spp. (142).

REFERENCES

1. Emori T, Gaynes R. An overview of nosocomial infections, including the role of microbiology laboratory. Clin Microbiol Rev 1993; 6:428–442.
2. Blech M-F. Impact de l'antibioprophylaxie sur l'écologie microbienne. Ann Fr Anesth Réanim 1994; 13:S45–50.
3. Vallandigham JC, Johanson Jr WG. Infections associated with endotracheal intubation and tracheostomy. In: Bisno AL, Waldvogel FA, eds. Infections Associated with Indwelling Devices. American Society for Microbiology, 1989:179–197.
4. Cunha BA, Shea KW. Fever in the intensive care unit. Infect Dis Clin North Am 1996; 10:185–209.
5. Westergren V, Lundblad L, Hellquist HB, Forsum U. Ventilator-associated sinusitis: a review. Clin Infect Dis 1998; 27:851–864.
6. Arens J, LeJeune Jr F, Webre D. Maxillary sinusitis, a complication of nasotracheal intubation. Anesthesiology 1974; 40:415–416.
7. Gallagher TJ, Civetta JM. Acute maxillary sinusitis complicating nasotracheal intubation: a case report. Anesth Analg 1976; 55:885–886.
8. Pope T, Stelling C, Leitner Y. Maxillary sinusitis after nasotracheal intubation. South Med J 1981; 74:610–612.
9. Knodel AR, Beekman JF. Unexplained fevers in patients with nasotracheal intubation. JAMA 1982; 248:868–870.
10. O'Reilly MJ, Reddick EJ, Black W, Carter PL, Erhardt J, Fill W, Maughn D, Sado A, Klatt GR. Sepsis from sinusitis in nasotracheally intubated patients. A diagnostic dilemma. Am J Surg 1984; 147:601–604.
11. Meyer P, Guérin JM, Habib Y, Levy C. Pseudomonas thoracic empyema secondary to nosocomial rhinosinusitis. Eur Respir J 1988; 1:868–869.
12. Wolf M, Zillinsky I, Lieberman P. Acute mycotic sinusitis with bacterial sepsis in orotracheal intubation and nasogastric tubing: a case report and review of the literature. Otolaryngol Head Neck Surg 1988; 98:615–617.
13. Caplan ES, Hoyt NJ. Nosocomial sinusitis. JAMA 1982; 247:639–641.
14. Deutschman CS, Wilton PB, Sinow J, Thienprasit P, Konstatinides FN, Cerra FB. Paranasal sinusitis: a common complication of nasotracheal intubation in neurosurgical patients. Neurosurgery 1985; 17:296–299.
15. Kronberg FG, Goodwin WJ. Sinusitis in intensive care unit patients. Laryngoscope 1985; 95:936–938.
16. Aebert H, Hünefeld G, Regel G. Paranasal sinusitis and sepsis in ICU patients with nasotracheal intubation. Intens Care Med 1988; 15:27–30.
17. Bell R, Page G, Bynoe R, Dunham M, Brill A. Post-traumatic sinusitis. J Trauma 1988; 28:923–930.
18. Linden B, Aguilar E, Allen S. Sinusitis in the nasotracheally intubated patient. Arch Otolaryngol Head Neck Surg 1988; 114:860–861.

19. Lund VJ, Draf W, Gwaltney JM Jr, Hoffman SR, Huizing EH, Jones JG, Jones JK, Kennedy DW, Lusk RP, Mackay IS, Moriyama H, Nacleiro RM, Stankiewics JA, van Cauwenberge P, Vining EM. Quantification for staging sinusitis. Ann Oto Rhino Laryngol 1995; 167 (Suppl):17–21.
20. Wreesman VB, Fokkens WJ, Knegt PP. Refractory chronic sinusitis: evaluation of symptom improvement after Denker's procedure. Otolaryngol Head Neck Surg 2001; 125:495–500.
21. Palmer JN, Kennedy DW. Medical management in functional endoscopic sinus surgery failures. Curr Opin Otolaryngol Head Neck Surg 2003; 11: 6–12.
22. Abdel-Hak B, Gunkel A, Kanonier G, Schrott-Fischer A, Ulmer H, Thumfart W. Ciliary beat frequency, olfaction, and endoscopic sinus surgery. ORL J Otorhinolaryngol Relat Spec 1998; 60:202–205.
23. Chambers DW, Davis WE, Cook PR, Nishioka GJ, Rudman DT. Long-term outcome analysis of functional endoscopic sinus surgery: correlation of symptoms with endoscopic examination findings and potential prognostic variables. Laryngoscope 1997; 107:504–510.
24. Chan KH, Winslow CP, Abzug MJ. Persistent rhinosinusitis in children after endoscopic sinus surgery. Otolaryngol Head Neck Surg 1999; 121:577–580.
25. Richtsmeier WJ. Top 10 reasons for endoscopic maxillary sinus surgery failure. Laryngoscope 2001; 111:1952–1956.
26. Jarvis WR. The epidemiology of colonization. Infect Control Hosp Epidemiol 1996; 17:47–52.
27. Hanberger H, Hoffmann M, Lindgren S, Nilsson LE. High incidence of antibiotic resistance among bacteria in 4 intensive care units at university hospital in Sweden. Scand J Infect Dis 1997; 29:607–614.
28. Hoth JJ, Franklin GA, Stassen NA, Girard SM, Rodriguez RJ, Rodriguez JL. Prophylactic antibiotics adversely affect nosocomial pneumonia in trauma patients. J Trauma 2003; 55:249–255.
29. Westergren V, Lundblad L, Forsum U. Ventilator-associated sinusitis: antroscopy findings and bacteriology when excluding the contaminants. Acta Otolaryngol 1998; 118:574–580.
30. Rundcrantz H. Postural variations of nasal patency. Acta Otolaryngol 1969; 68:435–443.
31. Aust R, Drettner B. The patency of the maxillary sinus ostium in relation to body posture. Acta Otolaryngol 1975; 80:443–448.
32. Rundcrantz H. Posture and congestion of nasal mucosa in allergic rhinitis. Acta Otolaryngol 1964; 58:283–287.
33. Hasegawa M, Saito Y. Postural variations in nasal resistance and symptomatology in allergic rhinitis. Acta Otolaryngol 1979; 88:268–272.
34. Vincent J-L. Nosocomial infections in adult intensive-care units. Lancet 2003; 361:2068–2077.
35. Baker MD. Foreign bodies of the ears and nose in childhood. Pediatr Emerg Care 1987; 3:67–70.
36. Westergren V, Otori N, Stierna P. Experimental nasal intubation: a study of changes in nasoantral mucosa and bacterial flora. Laryngoscope 1999; 109:1068–1073.

37. Sottile FD, Marrie TJ, Prough DS, Hobgood CD, Gower DJ, Webb LX, Costerton JW, Gristina AG. Nosocomial pulmonary infection: possible etiologic significance of bacterial adhesion to endotracheal tubes. Crit Care Med 1996; 14:265–270.

38. Donlan RM. Biofilms: microbial life on surfaces. Emerg Infect Dis 2002; 8:881–890.

39. Dunne WM Jr. Bacterial adhesion: seen any good biofilms lately? Clin Microbiol Rev 2002; 15:155–166.

40. Rupp ME, Ulphani JS, Fey PD, Bartscht K, Mack D. Characterization of the importance of polysaccharide intercellular adhesin/hemagglutinin of *Staphylococcus epidermidis* in the pathogenesis of biomaterial-based infection in a mouse foreign body infection model. Infect Immun 1999; 67: 2627–2632.

41. Stewart PS, Camper AK, Handran SD, Huang C-T, Warnecke M. Spatial distribution and coexistence of *Klebsiella pneumoniae* and *Pseudomonas aeruginosa* in biofilms. Microb Ecol 1997; 33:2–10.

42. Watnick P, Kolter R. Biofilm, city of microbes. J Bacteriol 2000; 182: 2675–2679.

43. Mah TF, O'Toole GA. Mechanisms of biofilm resistance to antimicrobial agents. Trends Microbiol 2001; 9:34–39.

44. Gilbert P, Allison DG, McBain AJ. Biofilms in vitro and in vivo: Do singular mechanisms imply cross-resistance? Symp Ser Soc Appl Microbiol 2002; 31:98S–110S.

45. Stewart PS. Mechanisms of antibiotic resistance on bacterial biofilms. Int J Med Microbiol 2002; 292:107–113.

46. Roberts AP, Pratten J, Wilson M, Mullany P. Transfer of a conjugative transposon, Tn5397, in a model oral biofilm. FEMS Microbiol Lett 1999; 177:636.

47. Bauer TT, Torres A, Ferrer R, Heyer CM, Schultze-Werninghaus G, Rasche K. Biofilm formation in endotracheal tubes. Association between pneumonia and the persistence of pathogens. Monaldi Arch Chest Dis 2002; 57:84–87.

48. Lundberg JON, Farkas-Szallasi T, Weitzberg E, Rinder J, Lidholm J, Änggard A, Hökfelt T, Lundberg JM, Alving K. High nitric oxide production in human paranasal sinuses. Nature Med 1995; 1:370–373.

49. Lewandowski K, Busch T, Lohbrunner H, Rensing S, Keske U, Gerlach H, Falke KJ. Low nitric oxide concentration in exhaled gas and nasal airways of mammals without paranasal sinuses. J Appl Physiol 1998; 85:405–410.

50. Deja M, Busch T, Bachmann S, Riskowski K, Campean V, Wiedmann B, Schwabe M, Hell B, Pfeilschifter J, Falke KJ, Lewandowski K. Reduced nitric oxide in sinus epithelium of patients with radiologic maxillary sinusitis and sepsis. Am J Respir Crit Care Med 2003; 168:265–266.

51. Lundberg JON, Weitzberg E, Nordvall SL, Kuylenstierna R, Lundberg JM, Alving K. Primarily nasal origin of exhaled nitric oxide and absence in Kartagerner's syndrome. Eur Respir J 1994; 7:1501–1504.

52. Lindberg S, Cervin A, Runer T. Low levels of nasal nitric oxide (NO) correlate to impaired mucociliary function in the upper airways. Acta Otolaryngol 1997; 117:728–735.

53. Frostell CG, Blomqvist H, Hedenstierna G, Lundberg J, Zapol WM. Inhaled nitric oxide selectively reverses human hypoxic pulmonary vasoconstriction without causing systemic vasodilation. Anesthesiology 1993; 78:427–435.

54. Gerlach H, Rossaint R, Pappert D, Knorr M, Falke KJ. Autoinhalation of nitric oxide after endogenous synthesis in the nasopharynx. Lancet 1994; 343:518–519.

55. Runer T, Cervin A, Lindberg S, Uddman R. Nitric oxide is a regulator of mucociliary activity in the upper respiratory tract. Otolaryngol Head Neck Surg 1998; 119:278–282.

56. Zhang B, Cao GL, Cross A, Domachowske JB, Rosen GM. Differential antibacterial activity of nitric oxide from the isozyme nitric oxide synthase transduced into endothelial cells. Nitric Oxide 2002; 7:42–49.

57. Urion AM, López-Gresa P, González C, Primo J, Martínez A, Herrera G, Escudero JC, O'Connor J-E, Blanco M. Nitric oxide promotes strong cytotoxicity of phenolic compounds against *Escherichia coli*: the influence of antioxidant defenses. Free Rad Biol Med 2003; 35:1373–1381.

58. Tsai WS, Strieter RM, Zisman DA, Wilkowski JM, Bucknell KA, Chen G-H, Standiford, TJ. Nitric oxide is required for effective innate immunity against *Klebsiella pneumoniae*. Infect Immun 1997; 65:1870–1875.

59. Gyurko R, Boustany G, Huang PL, Kantarci A, Van Dyke TE, Genco CA, Gibson FC III. Mice lacking inducible nitric oxide synthase demonstrate impaired killing of *Porphyromonas gingivalis*. Infect Immun 2003; 71: 4917–4924.

60. Arnal JF, Flores P, Rami J, Murris-Espin M, Pasto I, Aguilla M, Serrano E, Didier A. Nasal nitric oxide concentration in paranasal sinus inflammatory diseases. Eur Respir J 1999; 13:307–312.

61. Baraldi E, Azzolin NM, Biban P, Zacchello F. Effect of antibiotic therapy on nasal nitric oxide concentration in children with acute sinusitis. Am J Respir Crit Care Med 1997; 155:1680–1683.

62. Lindberg S, Cervin A, Runer T. Nitric oxide (NO) production in the upper airways is decreased in chronic sinusitis. Acta Otolaryngol 1997; 117: 113–117.

63. American Thoracic Society. Recommendations for standardized procedures for the online and offline measurement of exhaled lower respiratory nitric oxide and nasal nitric oxide in adults and children. Am J Respir Crit Care Med 1999; 160:2104–2117.

64. Hacker J, Blum-Oehler G, Muhldorfer I, Tschape H. Pathogenicity islands of virulent bacteria: Structure, function and impact on microbial evolution. Mol Micro 1997; 23:1089–1097.

65. Curtis MA. Summary: Microbiological perspective. Mol Immunol 2003; 40: 477–479.

66. Cooper MA, Pommering TL, Koranyi K. Primary immunodeficiences. Am Fam Physician 2003; 68:1919, 1923, 1926.

67. Sethi DS, Winkelstein JA, Lederman H, Loury MC. Immunologic defects in patients with chronic recurrent sinusitis: diagnosis and management. Otolaryngol Head Neck Surg 1995; 112:242–247.

68. Sharp HR, Rowe-Jones JM, Mackay IS. The outcome of endoscopic sinus surgery: correlation with computerized tomography score and systematic disease. Clin Otolaryngol 1999; 24:39–42.
69. Farnaud S, Evans RW. Lactoferrin—a multifunctional protein with antimicrobial properties. Mol Immunol 2003; 40:395–405.
70. Nibbering PH, Ravensbergen E, Welling MM, van Berkel LA, van Berkel PHC, Pauwels EKJ, Nuijens JH. Human lactoferrin and peptides derived from its N terminus are highly effective against infections with antibiotic-resistant bacteria. Infect Immun 2001; 69:1469–1476.
71. Singh PK, Parsek MR, Greenberg EP, Welsh MJ. A component of innate immunity prevents bacterial biofilm development. Nature 2002; 417:552–555.
72. Devine DA. Antimicrobial peptides in defence of the oral and respiratory tracts. Mol Immunol 2003; 40:431–443.
73. O'Neil DA. Regulation of expression of β-defensins: Endogenous enteric peptide antibiotics. Mol Immun 2003; 40:445–450.
74. Cataldo DD, Gueders MM, Rocks N, Sounni NE, Evrard B, Bartsch P, Louis R, Noel A, Foidart JM. Pathogenic role of matrix metalloproteases and their inhibitors in asthma and chronic obstructive pulmonary disease and therapeutic relevance of matrix metalloproteases inhibitors. Cell Mol Biol 2003; 49:875–884.
75. Watelet JB, Bachert C, Claeys C, Van Cauwenberge P. Matrix metalloproteinases MMP-7, MMP-9 and their tissue inhibitor TIMP-1: expression in chronic sinusitis vs. nasal polyposis. Allergy 2004; 59:54–60.
76. Meduri GU. Clinical review: A paradigm shift: the bidirectional effect of inflammation on bacterial growth. Clinical implications for patients with acute respiratory distress syndrome. Critical Care 2002; 6:24–29.
77. Meduri GU, Kanangat S, Stefan J, Tolley E, Schaberg D. Cytokines IL-1β, IL-6, and TNF-α enhance in vitro growth of bacteria. Am J Respir Crit Care Med 1999; 160:961–967.
78. Lyte M, Freestone PPE, Neal CP, Olson BA, Haigh RD, Bayston R, Williams PH. Stimulation of Staphylococcus epidermidis growth and biofilm formation by catecholamine inotropes. Lancet 2003; 361:130–135.
79. Eggiman P, Pittet D. Infection control in the ICU. Chest 2001; 120:2059–2093.
80. Johansson W, Pierce A, Sanford J. Changing pharyngeal flora of hospitalized patients. New Engl J Med 1969; 281:1137–1140.
81. Schwartz S, Dowling J, Benkovic C, DeQuittner-Buchanan M, Prostko T, Yee R. Sources of gram-negative bacilli colonizing the trachea of intubated patients. J Inf Dis 1978; 138:227–231.
82. Donaldsson S, Azizi S, Dal Nogare A. Characteristics of aerobic Gram-negative bacteria colonizing critically ill patients. Am Rev Respir Dis 1991; 144:202–207.
83. Johansson WG Jr, Pierce AK, Sanford JP, Thomas GD. Nosocomial respiratory infections with gram-negative bacilli: the significance of colonization of the respiratory tract. Ann Intern Med 1972; 77:701–706.
84. Agvald-Ohman C, Wernerman J, Nord CE, Edlund C. Anaerobic bacteria commonly colonize the lower airways of intubated patients. Clin Microbiol Infect 2003; 9:397–405.

85. Feldman C, Kassel M, Cantrell J, Kaka S, Morar R, Goolam Mahomed A, Philips JI. The presence and sequence of endotracheal colonization in patients undergoing mechanical ventilation. Eur Respir J 1999; 13:546–551.

86. Inglis TJJ, Millar MR, Jones G, Robinson DA. Tracheal biofilm as a source of bacterial colonization of the lung. J Clin Microbiol 1989; 27:2014–2018.

87. Grindlinger GA, Niehoff J, Hughes SL, Humphrey MA, Simpson G. Acute paranasal sinusitis related to nasotracheal intubation of head-injured patients. Crit Care Med 1987; 15:214–217.

88. Guérin JM, Meyer P, Lévy C, Reizine D, Habib Y, Tran Ba Huy P, Segrestaa JM. Sinusites aiguës sphénoidales consecutive à l'intubation naso-trachéale. Sem Hôp Paris 1987; 63:3671–3674.

89. Humphrey MA, Simpson GT, Grindlinger GA. Clinical characteristics of nosocomial sinusitis. Ann Otol Rhinol Laryn 1987; 96:687–690.

90. Guérin JM, Meyer P, Segrestaa JM, Reizine D, Levy C. Sinusites nosocomiales et intubation nasotrachéale. Ètude prospective à partir de 53 patients. Ann Med Interne 1989; 140:106–107.

91. Fougeront B, Bodin L, Lamas G, Bokowy C, Elbez M. Sinusites de reanima-tion. Ann Oto-Lar Chir C-F 1990; 107:329–332.

92. Bowers B, Purdue G, Hunt J. Paranasal sinusitis in burn patients following nasotracheal intubation. Arch Surg 1991; 126:1411–1412.

93. Michelson A, Schuster B, Kamp H-D. Paranasal sinusitis associated with nasotracheal and orotracheal long-term intubation. Arch Otolarngol Head Neck Surg 1992; 118:937–939.

94. Holzapfel L, Chevret S, Madinier G, Ohen F, Demingeon G, Coupry A, Chaudet M. Influence of long-term oro- or nasotracheal intubation on noso-comial maxillary sinusitis and pneumonia: Results of prospective, randomized, clinical trial. Crit Care Med 1993; 21:1132–1138.

95. Rouby J-J, Laurent P, Gosnach M, Cambau E, Lamas G, Zouaoui A, Leguillou J-L, Bodin L, Do Khac T, Marsault C, Poète P, Nicolas M-H, Jarlier V, Viars P. Risk factors and clinical relevance of nosocomial maxillary sinusitis in the critically ill. Am J Respir Crit Care Med 1994; 150:776–783.

96. Bert F, Lambert-Zechovsky N. Microbiology of nosocomial sinusitis in inten-sive care unit patients. J Infect 1995; 31:5–8.

97. Bert F, Lambert-Zechovsky N. Sinusitis in mechanically ventilated patients and its role in the pathogenesis of nosocomial pneumonia. Eur J Clin Micro-biol Infect Dis 1996; 15:533–544.

98. Mevio E, Benazzo M, Quaglieri S, Mencherini S. Sinus infection in intensive care patients. Rhinology 1996; 34:232–236.

99. George DL, Falk PS, Meduri GU, Leeper KV Jr, Wunderink RG, Steere EL, Nunnally FK, Beckford, Mayhall CG. Nosocomial sinusitis in patients in the medical intensive care unit: a prospective epidemiological study. Clin Infect Dis 1998; 27:463–470.

100. Le Moal G, Lemerre D, Grollier G, Desmont C, Klossek J-M, Robert R. Nosocomial sinusitis with isolation of anaerobic bacteria in ICU patients. Intens Care Med 1999; 25:1066–1071.

101. Holzapfel L, Chastang C, Demingeon G, Bohe J, Piralla B, Coupry A. A randomized study assessing the systematic search for maxillary sinusitis in

nasotracheally mechanically ventilated patients. Am J Respir Crit Care Med 1999; 159:695–701.

102. Souweine B, Mom T, Traore O, Aublet-Cuvelier B, Bret L, Sirot J, Deteix P, Gilain L, Boyer L. Ventilator-associated sinusitis: microbiological results of sinus aspirations in patients on antibiotics. Anesthesiology 2000; 93: 1255–1260.

103. Yousem DM. Imaging of sinonasal inflammatory disease. Radiology 1993; 188:303–314.

104. Fassoulaki A, Pamaouktsoglou P. Prolonged nasotracheal intubation and its association with inflammation of paranasal sinuses. Anesth Analg 1989; 69:50–52.

105. Hansen M, Poulsen MR, Bendixen DK, Hartmann-Andersen F. Incidence of sinusitis in patients with nasotracheal intubation. Br J Anaesth 1988; 61:231–232.

106. Pedersen J, Schurizek BA, Melsen NC, Juhl B. The effect of nasotracheal intubation on the paranasal sinuses. A prospective study of 434 intensive care patients. Acta Anaesth Scand 1991; 35:11–13.

107. Desmond P, Raman R, Idikula J. Effect of nasogastric tubes on the nose and maxillary sinus. Crit Care Med 1991; 19:509–511.

108. Strange C, Wooten S, Schabel S, Heffner J, Sahn S. Radiographic sinusitis following endotracheal intubation. Am Review Resp Dis 1988; 137:63.

109. Jones NS, Cooney TR. Facial pain and sinonasal surgery. Rhinology 2003; 41:193–200.

110. Dal T, Onerci M, Caglar M. Mucociliary function of the maxillary sinuses after restoring ventilation: a radioisotopic study of the maxillary sinus. Eur Arch Otorhinolaryngol 1997; 254:205–207.

111. Lund VJ, Mackay IS. Staging for rhinosinusitis. Rhinology 1993; 31:183–184.

112. Lavigne F, Nguyen CT, Cameron L, Hamid Q, Renzi PM. Prognosis and prediction of response to surgery in allergic patients with chronic sinusitis. J Allergy Clin Immunol 2000; 105:746–751.

113. Brook I, Frazier EH. Correlation between microbiology and previous surgery in patients with chronic maxillary sinusitis. Ann Otol Rhinol Laryngol 2001; 110:148–151.

114. Bhattacharyya N, Kepnes LJ. The microbiology of recurrent rhinosinusitis after endoscopic sinus surgery. Arch Otolaryngol Head Neck Surg 1999; 125:1117–1120.

115. Bhattacharyya N, Gopal HV, Lee KH. Bacterial infection after endoscopic sinus surgery: a controlled prospective study. Laryngoscope 2004; 114:765–767.

116. Cunha BA, Shea KW. Fever in the intense care unit. Inf Dis Clin North Am 1996; 10:185–209.

117. Marik PE. Fever in the ICU. Chest 2000; 117:855–869.

118. Borman KR, Brown PM, Mezera KK, Jhaveri H. Occult fever in surgical intensive care is seldom caused by sinusitis. Am J Surg 1992: 164:412–416.

119. Rice DH. The microbiology of paranasal sinus infections: diagnosis and management. Crit Rev Cl Lab Sci 1978; 9:105–121.

120. Sobin J, Engquist S, Nord CE. Bacteriology of the maxillary sinus in healthy volunteers. Scand J Infect Dis 1992; 24:633–635.

121. Brook I. Aerobic and anaerobic bacterial flora of normal maxillary sinuses. Laryngoscope 1981; 91:372–376.
122. Axelsson A, Brorson JE. The correlation between bacteriology findings in the nose and maxillary sinus in acute maxillary sinusitis. Laryngoscope 1973; 83:2003–2011.
123. Kountakis SE, Skoulas IG. Middle meatal vs. antral lavage cultures in intensive care unit patients. Otolaryngol Head Neck Surg 2002; 126:377–381.
124. Brook I. Discrepancies in the recovery of bacteria from multiple sinuses in acute and chronic sinusitis. Med Microbiol 2004; 53:879–885.
125. Westergren V, Forsum U, Lundgren J. Possible errors in diagnosis of bacterial sinusitis in tracheal intubated patients. Acta Anaesthesiol Scand 1994; 38: 699–703.
126. Westergren V, Lundblad L, Timpka T. Inter-observer variations in assessment from sinoscopy video recordings. Am J Rhinol 1998; 12:159–165.
127. Westergren V, Nilsson M, Forsum, U. Penetration of antibiotics in diseased antral mucosa. Arch Otolaryngol Head Neck Surg 1996; 122:1390–1394.
128. Ceri H, Olson ME, Stremick C, Read RR, Morck D, Buret A. The Calgary Biofilm Device: new technology for rapid determination of antibiotic susceptibilities of bacterial biofilms. J Clin Microbiol 1999; 37:1771–1776.
129. Olson ME, Ceri H, Morck DW, Buret AG, Read RR. Biofilm bacteria: formation and comparative susceptibility to antibiotics. Can J Vet Res 2002; 66:86–92.
130. Chastre J, Fagon J-Y. Ventilator-associated pneumonia: state of the art. Am J Respir Crit Care Med 2002; 165:867–903.
131. Weymuller E, Bishop M. Problems associated with prolonged intubation in the geriatric patient. Otolaryng Clin N Am 1990; 23:1057–1074.
132. Weitzberg E, Lundberg JO. Humming greatly increases nasal nitric oxide. Am J Respir Crit Care Med 2002; 166:131–132.
133. Kerrebijn JDF, Drost HE, Spoelstra HAA, Knegt PP. If functional sinus surgery fails: a radical approach to sinus surgery. Otolaryngol Head Neck Surg 1996; 114:745–747.
134. Meduri GU, Mauldin GL, Wunderink RG, Leeper KV, Jones CB, Tolley E, Mayhall G. Causes of fever and pulmonary densities in patients with clinical manifestations of ventilator-associated pneumonia. Chest 1994; 106:221–235.
135. Holzapfel L. Nasal vs. oral intubation. Minerva Anestesiol 2003; 69:348–352.
136. Adair CG, Gorman SP, Byers LM, Jones DS, Feron B, Crowe M, Webb HC, McCarthy GJ, Milligan KR. Eradication of endotracheal tube biofilm by nebulised gentamicin. Intens Care Med 2002; 28:426–431.
137. Sodhi RNS, Sahi VP, Mittelman MW. Application of electron spectroscopy and surface modification techniques in the development of anti-microbial coatings for medical devices. J Electron Spectrosc 2001; 121:249–264.
138. Nablo BJ, Schoenfisch MH. Antibacterial properties of nitric-oxide releasing sol-gels. J Biomed Mater Res 2003; 67A:1276–1283.
139. Balazs DJ, Triandafillu K, Chevolot Y, Aronsson B-O, Harms H, Descouts P, Mathieu HJ. Surface modification of PVC endotracheal tubes by oxygen glow discharge to reduce bacterial adhesion. Surf Interface Anal 2003; 35:301–309.

140. Balazs DJ, Triandafillu K, Wood P, Chevelot Y, van Delden C, Harms H, Hollenstein C, Matheiu HJ. Inhibition of bacterial adhesion on PVC endotracheal tubes by RF-oxygen glow discharge, sodium hydroxide and silver nitrate treatments. Biomaterials 2004; 25:2139–2151.

141. de Jonge E, Schultz MJ, Spanjaard L, Bossuyt PMM, Vroom MB, Dankert J, Kesecioglu J. Effects of selective decontamination of digestive tract on mortality and acquisition of resistant bacteria in intensive care: a randomized controlled trial. Lancet 2003; 362:1011–1016.

142. Bonten MJM, Brun-Buisson C, Weinstein RA. Selective decontamination of the digestive tract: to stimulate or stifle? Intensive Care Med 2003; 29:672–676.

17

Cystic Fibrosis and Sinusitis

Noreen Roth Henig

*Adult Cystic Fibrosis Center, Advanced Lung Disease Center,
California Pacific Medical Center, San Francisco, California, U.S.A.*

INTRODUCTION

Cystic fibrosis (CF) is the most common fatal genetic disease, but with better understanding of the disease and aggressive treatment, CF patients who once died as infants are living well into adulthood. CF is an autosomal recessive disease that results in multisystem dysfunction, including chronic sino-pulmonary disease, pancreatic exocrine and endocrine insufficiency, hepatobiliary disease, gastrointestinal dysfunction, and male infertility. The classic CF phenotype is a patient diagnosed in infancy as a result of failure-to-thrive or recurrent pneumonias who goes on to have chronic bronchiectasis with difficult-to-treat pathogens and eventually dies of respiratory failure as an adolescent or young adult. Better genotype diagnosis of the disease has shown that there is actually a wide range of CF phenotypes that do not necessarily correlate with the genotype. And, more significantly, better treatment for the manifestations of CF has led to increased survival. In the United States, there are about 30,000 CF patients with almost 40% of them older than 18 years of age. The mean life expectancy is 32 years, and there are increasing numbers of patients in their fifth or sixth decade of life (1,2).

PATHOPHYSIOLOGY OF CF

CF was initially described in 1938 as cystic fibrosis of the pancreas, and within the first fifteen years the pulmonary manifestations of the disease were described (3) and the sweat chloride test was developed for making the diagnosis (4). The myriad of organ involvement in CF, including sinus disease, relates directly to the underlying genetic defect of CF. CF is caused by mutations in a large gene on chromosome 7, which encodes for the 1480 amino acid protein now known as the cystic fibrosis-transmembrane regulator (CFTR) (5). The CFTR is a bidirectional chloride channel that is a member of the ATP-binding cassette transporter family of membrane proteins (6). There are now over 1300 mutations of the CFTR described that fall into five classes of functional defects: (i) premature stop codons, (ii) misfolded proteins that cannot escape the endoplasmic reticulum, (iii) improper activation of the channel once it reaches the cell membrane, (iv) decreased chloride conductance of the channel, and (v) fewer than normal active channels expressed on the cell surface (2).

Exactly how disruption of the CFTR results in the sino-pulmonary manifestations of CF is still under debate. In general, it is accepted that alterations in ion transport across the cell membrane results in altered ionic composition and volume of airway surface fluid. It is also generally accepted that the clinical syndrome is characterized by tenacious respiratory tract secretions, uncontrolled and damaging inflammation, and chronic infection with an unusual set of bacterial pathogens. Two competing hypotheses are proposed for how changes in ionic composition and volume of airway surface fluid actually result in impaired mucociliary clearance of bacteria and heightened inflammation in the respiratory tract. The "low volume" hypothesis contends that water-permeable airway epithelia regulate the volume of the airway surface layer by isotonic transport to maintain optimal function of the mucociliary escalator. The "compositional" hypothesis proposes that airway epithelia regulate airway surface layer salt concentration, which is critical for full function of innate antimicrobial proteins that reside in the airway surface fluid (2,7).

The vast majority of CF patients develop sinus disease, although the true incidence of the disease is not known (8). There is also increasing evidence that suggests that single allelic CFTR mutations are associated with chronic sinusitis in patients without CF (9). This may reflect the activity of CFTR in the nasal and sinus passages.

PATHOPHYSIOLOGY OF CF-RELATED SINUSITIS

Pseudostratified ciliated epithelium lines the nasal cavity, paranasal sinuses, and the tracheobronchial tree. The mucociliary escalator created by this epithelial cell layer performs vital clearance of inorganic and organic inhaled particles. The airway surface liquid that lies atop the epithelial cells and is vital to the mucociliary escalator has two compartments. The sol layer is a fluid layer of lower viscosity that is high in proteins, many with innate antibacterial properties, while the other is a gelatinous layer of higher viscosity that traps inhaled foreign particles. In CF, the mucociliary escalator is impaired despite epithelial cells with normal structure, normal ciliary ultrastructure, and normal ciliary beat frequency. Instead, the underlying defect of CF is attributed to alterations of the airway surface liquid (7).

Alterations of the airway surface liquid contribute to the thick, obstructing mucus and chronic infection that characterizes CF. Impaired chloride conductance from mutated CFTR leads to impaired function of both the sol and gelatinous layers. This results in altered rheology of the mucus itself. It also leads to impairment of endogenous antimicrobial function, possibly by alteration of the osmotic conditions under which the defense proteins work (10). It is postulated by some that this altered airway surface liquid may also be proinflammatory (7).

The result of the derangement of the airway surface liquid leads to the principal components of the pathophysiology of CF: obstruction, inflammation, and infection. Once a patient with CF has become infected, a pathological cycle ensues where obstructing mucus traps bacterial organisms, a brisk neutrophilic response is mounted, and the death of both organisms and inflammatory cells leads to further increase in viscosity of the obstructing mucus, which further traps organisms and attracts neutrophils.

At the gross anatomical level, these microscopic events lead to the obstruction of nasal passages and sinus ostia. Frontal sinuses are often absent or small, attributed to hypopneumatization during formation of the sinuses. Sinonasal polyposis develops in most, although not all, CF patients. Obstructing mucus, polyps, and chronic inflammation can deform the lateral nasal wall, nasal septum, and sinus ostia (11).

Sinonasal polyposis in CF differs from that seen with atopy. In contrast to atopic polyps, CF polyps have thin basement membranes, lack submucosal hyalinization, and are neutrophil- rather than eosinophil-laden. There is also an abundance of acid rather than neutral mucin within CF mucosal glands. These pathological differences are often the first clue that a patient may have CF (12).

MICROBIOLOGY

There is a relatively defined group of pathogens which chronically infect the airways of CF patients (13). These infections are *Haemophilus influenzae, Staphylococcus aureus, Pseudomonas aeruginosa, Stenotrophomonas maltophilia, Achromobacter xylosoxidans*, and *Burkholderia cepacia* complex. There appears to be an age-related prevalence of CF pathogens in both the lower and upper respiratory tracts (Fig. 1). In addition, it is now accepted that the bacterial pathogens in the sinuses are the same as those in the lungs and vice versa. Culturing any of these typical CF organisms from a patient with chronic sinusitis may increase the level of suspicion for CF as an underlying diagnosis. The chronic infection with these organisms, especially

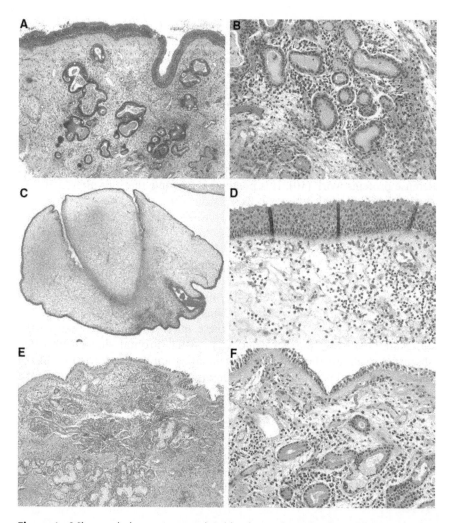

Figure 1 Microsopic images comparing histology of nasal polyps. Panels **A** and **B** represent low power and high power magnification of CF; Panels **C** and **D** represent low and high power of allergic sinusitis and Panels **E** and **F** represent low and high power images of chronic sinusitis. *Source*: Courtesy of Gerald Berrey, M.D.

P. aeruginsosa, is in part achieved by biofilm production by the organisms themselves. Production of biofilms confers relative resistance against anti-biotics and allows the organisms to become permanent infections (14).

Nonbacterial pathogens are also frequently found in the respiratory tract of CF patients. Aspergillus can be found in the transantral aspirates of up to 40% of adult CF patients. Colonization by *Aspergillus* spp. and other fungi is increasingly common with increased use of inhaled antibiotics (15). Because patients with CF are immunocompetent, the fungi remain intraluminal and rarely, if ever, become invasive. Patients with CF-related bronchiectasis are at risk for infection with non-tuberculous mycobacterium (16,17), although the rates of sinus infection are unknown. Pediatric CF patients are not more susceptible to common viral upper respiratory infections than their unaffected siblings (18). However, viral upper respiratory infections may lead to an acute exacerbation of chronic bacterial sinusitis.

Historically, it was thought that there was little correlation between sinus and pulmonary disease (19). The opposite is now believed to be true. Current microbiology techniques and fingerprinting of bacterial genomes reveal that the microbiology of the lower and upper respiratory tract is the same (2). Pathogens that initially infect the upper respiratory tract are aerosolized and inhaled into the lower tract with each breath. Additional communication of infectious agents occurs with postnasal drip. Pathogens that initially infect the lower respiratory tract can infect the upper tract through the same mechanism of aerosolization and inhalation.

CLINICAL OVERVIEW OF CF SINUSITIS

At baseline, patients with CF have chronic sinusitis and bronchiectasis clinically and radiographically. Many CF patients with radiographic evidence of sinusitis are symptom-free. However, when patients present with symptoms of sinusitis, these symptoms are indistinguishable from other etiologies of sinusitis: pain and pressure in the forehead or over the maxillary sinuses, orbital pain, chronic headaches, tooth pain, ear discomfort, postnasal drip, cough aggravated by lying down, persistent need to clear one's throat, hoarseness, and malodorous breath. Many patients suffer from altered sensations of taste and smell, and some have true anosmia. CF patients are chronically infected, often with multiple pathogens. They experience periodic exacerbations of their infections in both their upper and lower respiratory tracts. Often, the term acute or chronic sinusitis is used to distinguish the baseline from symptomatic sinusitis. Exacerbations of infection may present as increased fatigue and malaise rather than as an increased number of sinus or pulmonary symptoms such as increased cough or nasal discharge (20). Fever can occur, but it is often absent in the setting of an acute respiratory tract exacerbation.

The true incidence of sinusitis in CF is not known, but current data suggest that the vast majority of patients develop sinus disease at some time in their lives (8). Symptoms usually present between the ages of 5 and 14 years, although many older patients have undiagnosed or untreated sinus disease. Patients often adapt to their symptoms or carry alternative diagnoses such as migraine headaches. Nasal polyps are the most common manifestation of sinus disease in younger patients, while chronic headaches are more common symptoms in the older CF population.

Imaging studies to diagnose CF-related sinusitis are useful. Plain radiographs can readily identify frontal sinus agenesis or hypoplasia (21). Computed tomography (CT) scans of the sinuses also show abnormal sinus findings in almost all of the CF patients, even those who are asymptomatic. Frontal sinus agenesis and greater than 75% opacification of the maxilloethmoid sinus is considered pathognomonic of CF. Similarly, medial bulging of the lateral nasal wall near the middle meatus and resorption of the uncinate process is highly suggestive of CF (22,23). Recently, a sinus CT scoring system has been proposed, which discriminates between CF and non-CF sinus disease. Nine criteria highlight the most characteristic sinus abnormalities in CF patients, which are grouped as paranasal sinus variants, pneumatization variants, and inflammatory patterns (24) (Table 1). Magnetic resonance imaging (MRI) is useful for both diagnosis and tracking the progression of sinus disease in CF patients. MRI is thought to be more sensitive than CT for visualizing and differentiating soft tissues masses in the paranasal sinuses.

Allergic rhinitis may confound the presentation of CF-related sinusitis. The incidence of allergic rhinitis in CF patients is reportedly the same as in the general population, 20–40% (25). The subset of CF patients who develop nasal polyps have an increased incidence of asthma-like reversible bronchoconstriction, airway hyperreactivity, and positive allergen skin tests (26). However, this is not present in 100% of the CF patients who develop polyposis and the connection, if one exists, is poorly understood. Allergic rhinitis

Table 1 Paranasal Sinus Variants Found Commonly in Patients with CF and Used in a CT Scoring System for Discriminating CF from Non-CF Patients[a]

Paranasal sinus variants
Frontal sinus aplasia
Frontal sinus hypoplasia
Maxillary sinus hypoplasia
Sphenoid sinus hypoplasia
Pneumatization variants
Absence of all of the following:
Agger nasi cells
Haller cells
Pneumatization of the lamellar or bulbous portion of the middle turbinate, nasal bone, crista palli, and anterior clinoid or pterygoid process of the sphenoid bone
Inflammatory patterns
Advanced ethmoidomaxillary disease
Bulging of the laternal nasal wall
Sphenoethmoid recess inflammatory pattern

[a]Revised from Eggesbo HB et al. Proposal of a CT scoring system of the paranasal sinuses in diagnosing cystic fibrosis.
Source: From Ref. 24.

should be diagnosed in addition to CF-related nasal and sinus symptoms in those who have both as the allergic component should be treated as such.

DIAGNOSIS OF CYSTIC FIBROSIS

If CF is suspected in a patient with chronic sinusitis and/or nasal polyposis, the patient should be referred for diagnostic studies (27). The gold standard for making the diagnosis of CF is quantitative pilocarpine iontophoresis, or the "sweat test." A result of a chloride concentration of >60 mmol/L is diagnostic, while a result of 40–59 mmol/L is considered indeterminate but likely to represent CF. The sweat test should be obtained at an accredited testing facility where the test is performed frequently.

The other commonly used diagnostic test for CF is genotyping. Mutation testing is highly specific for CF, but it is not as sensitive as the sweat test. There are now over 1300 identified mutations of the CFTR gene. Approximately 80–85% of CF alleles are detected using standard CF gene mutation testing (28). Testing laboratories may identify the most common 25–29 mutations present in their local population for the standard screen. There are a number of national laboratories that perform expanded CF mutation analysis or actually sequence the gene of the patient suspected of having CF. Increasing the number of genes screened increases the sensitivity for making the CF diagnosis. For an expanded screen of 88 mutations, gene detection sensitivity is as follows: 94% for Caucasians, 97% for Ashkenazi Jews, 72% for Latinos, and 61% for African Americans (29). Mutation screening is less sensitive for Asian and other non-Caucasian populations where there is a higher prevalence of rarer mutations.

Nasal potential differences (NPD) are the third accepted diagnostic test for CF. This test is currently used in research settings primarily, and is only available at a limited number of accredited sites. NPD can be measured directly from the middle nasal turbinate. The basal NPD and the effect of a variety of conductance altering infusates can quite accurately distinguish between patients with and without CF. There are three main characteristics of the NPD associated with CF. First, the basal voltage is raised, reflecting enhanced sodium transport across the relatively chloride-impermeable barrier. Second, with infusion of amiloride, a sodium channel blocker, a larger inhibition of NPD occurs, reflecting an inhibition of the accelerated sodium transport. Third, unlike normal individuals, there is no change in voltage in response to perfusion of a chloride-free solution with isoproterenol, reflecting the absence of CFTR-mediated chloride conductance (Fig. 2).

TREATMENT OF CF-RELATED SINUSITIS

The treatment of CF-related sinusitis is not dissimilar from the treatment of acute and chronic sinusitis in general. As with the pulmonary manifestations of CF, treatment should target the obstruction, infection, and inflammation that characterizes the pathophysiology of the disease. Chronic sinusitis is

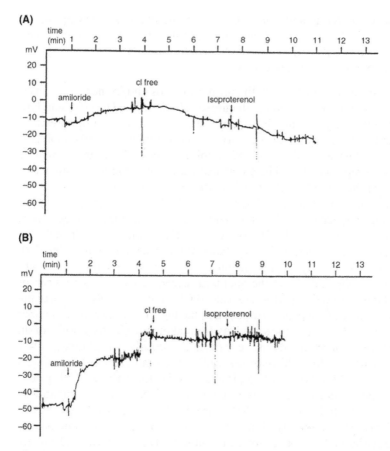

Figure 2   Nasal potential differences in a healthy and a CF patient.

most often treated daily with upper airway clearance and anti-inflammatory agents. Acute exacerbations of chronic sinusitis are treated with systemic antibiotics and often more aggressive upper airway clearance, including surgical debridement, if needed.

Upper Airway Clearance

Clearance of the airways is important for both the upper and lower respiratory tracts. More attention has been focused on airway clearance of the lungs than that of the sinuses; however, the ultimate goal, to remove obstructing mucus, is the same. Upper airway clearance can be achieved by saline flushes, decongestants and mucolytics, and surgical interventions.

  Saline flushing of the nasal passages and sinuses in patients with antrostomies can be taught to patients and done frequently, as much as many times each day. In CF and non-CF sinusitis, symptomatic relief results from mechanical clearance of obstructing mucus (30). It is also suggested that saline flushes may decrease nasal blood flow, resulting in a decongestant effect. There is no controlled study of how best to perform saline flushes. Pre-filled squeeze bottle atomizers are available commercially. Buffered saline solutions can be prepared at home and used with catheter tipped syringes, bulb syringes, Water Piks℠, or a variety of other devices designed to create a high flow irrigant. Flushing of maxillary sinuses through catheters placed following antrostomies is an accepted approach to clearing obstruction in CF. In the original uncontrolled study of 11 CF patients following lung transplantation, the maxillary sinuses were irrigated with tobramycin, which effectively reduced contamination of the transplanted lungs (31). The practice of routine (usually monthly) sinus irrigation with tobramycin is now also performed in CF patients who are not transplant recipients. This practice has been shown to reduce the number of pulmonary exacerbations (32) and the total number of sinus surgeries that patients undergo (33). This was also shown to improve aeration of the sinuses as assessed by MRI (34). Although the practice is routine, it is unclear which component of the monthly flush is most critical—the monthly physician attention to the sinuses, the act of irrigation, or the irrigant. Other antimicrobial irrigants have also been used in patients without any supporting data.

The use of decongestants in CF has not been studied, but both oral and topical decongestants are used in the CF population. Use of decongestants is minimized for fear of rhinitis medicamentosa. Mucolytics such as guaifenesin are often used for symptomatic relief and are thought not to be detrimental. Clinically, guaifenesin is more effective for thinning nasal secretions than pulmonary secretions. Daily use by nebulization of the mucolyic dornase alpha (recombinant DNase) is recommended for all CF patients (35). It is unknown what effect, if any, this has on nasal secretions.

Antihistamines, the cornerstone of allergy-induced rhinitis and sinusitis treatment, were once believed to be contraindicated in patients with CF as they were believed to further dessicate the already thick secretions (36). Clinically, this has not been observed and CF patients who also suffer from allergic rhinitis respond readily to antihistamines. Intranasal cromolyn is used by some practitioners, although there is no data to support its use for CF-related sinusitis.

Antimicrobial Therapy

Antibiotics are the cornerstone of treating infective sinusitis, especially CF-related sinusitis. Nasal swabs, transantral aspirations, and sputum cultures can identify infecting pathogens. Because pathogens are never eradicated in CF, cultures taken months and even years previously are valuable in guiding the selection of antibiotics. Similarly, in vitro sensitivity-testing with a panel of antibiotics should be performed. Systemic antibiotics should be at high doses to increase the concentration of antibiotic in the nares, sinuses, and airways where the pathogens live. The ideal duration of therapy for acute on chronic sinusitis is unknown, but the usual treatment is three to six weeks (8,36).

Antibiotics are given systemically or locally via inhalation or maxillary irrigation. Systemic antibiotics are preferred since exacerbations of upper and lower airway disease occur simultaneously. Nebulized aminoglycosides given thrice weekly are shown to decrease bacterial colonization and decrease inflammation in non-CF sinusitis patients (37). The recommended treatment for CF patients chronically infected with *P. aeruginosa* is twice daily inhalation of tobramycin solution (TOBI®) (38). It is believed that when used with a jet nebulizer as prescribed, TOBI penetrates the maxillary sinuses. Thus, through the course of routine CF care, a reduction of pathogens in the maxillary sinuses does occur.

Anti-Inflammatory Agents

Targeting inflammation in CF has been shown to improve lung function and lower the rate of decline of the forced expiratory volume in one second in the lungs. To date, systemic agents such as prednisone (39,40) and high dose ibuprofen (41) have proven to be beneficial, but these specific agents are limited by toxicity. Nasal steroids are shown to effectively reduce inflammation in non-CF chronic sinusitis (42), and have had variable results in the CF population (8,28,43,44). Regular use of nasal steroids is shown to diminish the size of nasal polyps. Post-polypectomy use of nasal steroids is shown to prevent recurrent formation of nasal polyps. Although no conclusive data exist to support the recommendation, use of inhaled nasal steroids is considered to be a first-line treatment for CF-related sinusitis (36).

Targeting leukotrienes has been another approach to decreasing inflammation in CF. Patients with CF are recognized as having high circulating leukotriene levels (high LTB4), as well as high cysteinyl leukotrienes (45). Leukotriene receptor antagonists are a group of anti-inflammatory agents shown to reduce the symptoms of allergic rhinitis in patients without CF. These agents are used commonly in patients with CF, especially those with asthma-like symptoms or allergic rhinitis.

Macrolide antibiotics are shown to have anti-inflammatory properties distinct from their antimicrobial properties. Regular use of azithromycin in CF is shown to improve pulmonary function and decrease the number of pulmonary exacerbations in CF (46). In a non-CF population, macrolide antibiotic therapy was shown to shrink nasal polyps and reduce the concentration of interleukin-8 in nasal lavage (47).

EXPERIMENTAL THERAPIES

A number of experimental therapies are being explored for the treatment of CF, which will likely benefit the chronic rhinosinusitis as well as the systemic disease. Gene therapy to correct the underlying CFTR defect is the ultimate solution for CF, although many obstacles to this type of therapy remain. The nares and sinus cavities are the usual targets of gene therapy transfer studies (48). A variety of vectors, including adenovirus, liposomes, and adeno-associated virus, have been explored. In one study of an adeno-associated viral vector with a CFTR cassette applied to the nasal mucosa, NPD were corrected and the occurrence of sinusitis was halved during the first month (49). The barriers to gene therapy include rapid turnover of respiratory epithelium, immunogenic response to the vector, and appropriate transcription, translation, and expression of the functional gene.

SPECIAL CONSIDERATIONS

Lung Transplantation and CF-Related Sinus Disease

Lung transplantation is the treatment of choice for CF patients with end-stage lung disease. In general, it is considered a life-extending treatment for carefully selected patients. Lung transplant recipients are immunosuppressed for life. Although the historic concern is that immunosuppression could worsen the chronic sinusitis of CF, experientially most patients with CF do not experience an increase from baseline in sinusitis symptoms, possibly due to the anti-inflammatory effects of the drugs. Instead, the concern is that chronic bacterial infection of the sinuses can result in bacterial infection of the new lungs, and that repeated injury to the lungs results in chronic allograft rejection, otherwise known as obliterative bronchiolitis. In the early 1990s, functional endoscopic sinus surgery with antrostomies was put forth as a method to prevent early bacterial infection, and at certain transplant centers, CF patients were required to undergo sinus evaluation preoperatively (31). This practice is not universally accepted at all lung transplant centers, although more recent data from a center that requires aggressive sinus care post-transplantation suggest that attention to the sinuses does result in fewer episodes of tracheobronchitis and a trend toward less obliterative bronchiolitis (50).

Anesthesia

CF patients referred for otolaryngologic surgery should undergo the same preoperative evaluation for general anesthesia as other patients (51). In general, it is preferable to avoid general anesthesia with endotracheal intubation, if feasible. If patients are intubated, every effort should be made to extubate them as quickly as possible. CF patients can clear their own secretions far more effectively with cough and expectoration than with endotracheal suctioning. Even patients with advanced lung disease generally tolerate general anesthesia if proper precautions are taken.

CONCLUSION

In the last 60 years, CF has evolved from an uncharacterized disease of the pancreas that killed infants to a well-described disease with survival well into adulthood. This incredible accomplishment resulted from multidisciplinary science, as well as from multidisciplinary clinical care. There is increasing recognition of the need to attend to the upper respiratory tract to the same degree as the lower respiratory tract. Otolaryngologists will likely care for increasing numbers of CF patients in the coming years as the population increases and the treatment of sinus disease moves to the forefront.

REFERENCES

1. Cystic Fibrosis Foundation 2003 Registry, www.cff.org.
2. Gibson RL, Burns JL, Ramsey EW. Pathophysiology and management of pulmonary infections in cystic fibrosis. Amer Jo Resp Crit Care Med 2003; 168:918–951.
3. diSant'Agnese PA. The pulmonary manifestations of flbrocystic disease of the pancreas. Diseases of the Chest 1955; 27:654–670.
4. diSant'Agnese PA, Darling MD, Perera G, Shea E. Abnormal electxolye composition of sweat in cystic fibrosis of the pancreas. Clinical significance and relationship to disease. Pediatrics 1953; 12:549–563.
5. Zielenski J, Rozmahel R, Bozon D, Kerem B, Grzelezik Z, Riordan JR, Rommens J, Tsui LC. Genomic DNA sequence of the cystic fibrosis transmembrane regulator (CFTR) gene. Genomics 1991; 10:214–228.
6. Hyde SC, Emley P, Hartshorn, et al. Structural model of ATP-binding proteins associated with cystic fibrosis, multidrug resistance, and bacterial transport. Nature 1990; 346:362–365.
7. Donaldson SH, Boucher RC. Update on pathogenesis of cystic fibrosis lung disease. Curr Op Pulm Med 2003; 9:486–491.
8. Ramsey B, Richardson MA. Impact of sinusitis in cystic fibrosis. J Allergy Clin Immunol 1992; 90:547–553.
9. Wang X, Moylan B, Leopold DA, Kim J, Rubenstein RC, Togias A, Proud D, Zeitlin PL, Cutting GI. Mutation in the gene responsible for cystic fibrosis and predisposition to chronic rhinosinusitis in the general population. JAMA 2000; 284:1814–1819.
10. Smith JJ, Travis SM, Greenberg EP, Welsh MJ. Cystic fibrosis airway epithelia fail to kill bacteria because of abnormal airway surface fluid. Cell 1996; 85:229–236.
11. Tandon R, Derkay C. Contemporary management of rhinosinusitis and cystic fibrosis. Curr Op Otolaryng & Head and Neck Surg 2003; 11:41–44.
12. Gysin C, Alothman GA, Papsin BC. Sinonasal disease in cystic fibrosis: Clinical characteristics, diagnosis, and management. Ped Pulm 2000; 30:481–489.
13. Burns JL, Emerson J, Stapp JR, Yim DL, Kirzewinski J, Louden L, Ramsey BW, Clauser CR. Microbiology of sputum from patients at cystic fibrosis centers in the United States. Clin Infect Dis 1998; 27:158–163.
14. Parsek MR, Singh PK. Bacterial biofilms: an emerging link to disease pathogenesis. Annual Rev. Microbiology 2003; 57:677–701.
15. Bargon J, Dauletbaev N, Kohler B, Wolf M, Poselt HG, Wagner TO. Prophylactic antibiotic therapy is associated with an increased prevalence of *Aspergillus* colonization in adult cystic fibrosis patients. Respir Med 1999; 93:835–838.
16. Olivier KN, Weber DJ, Wallace RJ, Faiz AR, Lee JH, Zhang Y, Brown-Elliot BA, Handler A, Wilson RW, Schecter MS, Edwards LJ, Chakraborti S,

Knowles MR, Nontuberculous Mycobacterium in Cystic Fibrosis Study Group. Nontuberculous mycobacteria I: multicenter prevalence study in cystic fibrosis lung disease. Am J Respir Crit Care Med 2003; 167:810–812.

17. Olivier KN, Weber DJ, Lee JH, Handler A, Tudor G, Molino PL, Tomashefski F, Knowles MR, Nontuberculous Mycobacteria in Cystic Fibrosis Study Group. Nontuberculous mycobacteria I: nested cohort study of impact on cystic fibrosis lung disease. Am J Respir Crit Care Med 2003; 167:835–840.

18. Ramsey BW, Gore EJ, Smith AL, Cooney MK, Redding GJ, Foy H. The effect of respiratory viral infections on patients with cystic fibrosis. Am J Dis Child 1989; 143:662–668.

19. Shapiro ED, Milmoe GJ, Wald ER, Rodnan JB, Bowen AD. Bacteriology of the maxillary sinuses in patients with cystic fibrosis. J Infect Dis 1982; 146: 589–593.

20. Rosenfeld M, Emerson J, Williams-Warren J, Pepe M, Smith A, Montgmorey AB, Ramsey B. Defining a pulmonary exacerbation in cystic fibrosis. J Pediatr 2001; 139:359–365.

21. Ledesma-Medina J, Osman MZ, Girdany BR. Abnormal paranasal sinuses in patients with cystic fibrosis of the pancreas. Pediatr Radiol 1980; 9:61–66.

22. Brihaye P, Clement PA, Dab I, Desprechin B. Pathological changes of the lateral nasal wall in patients with cystic fibrosis. Int J Pediatr Otorhinolaryngol 1994; 141–143.

23. April MM, Zinreich J, Baroody FM, Naclerio RM. Coronal CT scan abnormalities in children with chronic sinusitis. Laryngoscope 1993; 103:985–990.

24. Eggsbo HB, Sovik S, Dolvik S, Eiklid K, Kolmannskog F. Proposal of a CT scoring system of the paranasal sinuses in diagnosing cystic fibrosis. Eur Radiology 2003; 13:1451–1460.

25. Davidson TM, Murphy C, Mitchell M, Smith C, Light M. Management of chronic sinusitis in cystic fibrosis. Laryngoscope 1995; 105:354–358.

26. Crockett DM, McGill TJ, Healy GB, Friedman EM, Skalked LJ. Nasal and paranasal sinus surgery in children with cystic fibrosis. Ann Otol Rhinol Laryngol 1987; 96:367–372.

27. The Diagnosis of Cystic Fibrosis: consensus statement. In: *Clinical Practice Guidelines for Cystic Fibrosis*. Cystic Fibrosis Foundation, Vol. VII, Section I, 1996.

28. Stern RC. The diagnosis of cystic fibrosis. New Engl Jour Med 1997; 7:487–491.

29. Carrier rates and detection rates by ethnic background, www.genzvmegenetics.com. 2005.

30. Brown CL, Graham SM. Nasal irrigations: good or bad? Current Opinion in Otolaryngology & Head & Neck Surgery 2004; 12:9–13.

31. Lewiston N, King V, Umetsu D, Starnes V, Marshall S, Kramer M, Thodore J. Cystic fibrosis patients who have undergone heart–lung transplantation benefit from maxillary sinus antrostomy and repeated sinus lavage. Transplantation Proceedings 1991; 23:120–08.

32. Davidson TM, Murphy C, Mitchell M, Smith C, Light M. Management of chronic sinusitis in cystic fibrosis. Laryngoscope 1995; 105:354–358.

33. Moss RB, King VV. Management of sinusitis in cystic fibrosis by endoscopic surgery and serial antimicrobial lavage reduction in recurrence requiring surgery. Arch Otolaryngol Head Neck Surg 1995; 121:566–572.

34. Graham SM, Launspach JL, Welsh MJ, Zabner J. Sequential magnetic resonance imaging analysis of the maxillary sinuses: implications for a model of gene therapy in cystic fibrosis. J Laryngol Otol 1999; 113:329–335.
35. Shak S, Capon D, Hellmis R, Marster SA, Baker CL. Recombinant human DNase reduces viscosity of cystic fibrosis sputum. Proc Natl Acad Sci USA 1990; 87:9188–9192.
36. Hui Y, Gaffhey R, Crysdale WS. Sinusitis in patients with cystic fibrosis. Eur Arch Otorhinolaryngol 1995; 252:191–196.
37. Kobayashi T, Baba S. Topical use of antibiotics for paranasal sinusitis. Rhinology 1992; 14:77–81.
38. Ramsey BW, Pepe MS, Quan JM, Otto KL, Montgomery AB, William-Warren J, Vasiljev KM, Borowitz D, Bowman CC, Marshall BC, Marshall S, Smith AL. Intermittent administration of inhaled tobramycin in patients with cystic fibrosis. Cystic Fibrosis Study Group. N Engl J Med 1999; 340:23–30.
39. Aurbach HS, Williams M, Kirkpatrick JA, Colton HR. Alternate day prednisone reduces morbidity and improves pulmonary function in cystic fibrosis. Lancet 1985; 2:686–688.
40. Konstan MW. Therapies aimed at airway inflammation in cystic fibrosis. Clin Chest Med 1998; 19:505–513.
41. Konstan M, Byard P, Huppel C, Davis PB. Effect of high dose ibuprofen in patients with cystic fibrosis. N Engl J Med 1995; 332:848–854.
42. Bateman ND, Fahy C, Woolford TJ. Nasal polyps: still more questions than answers. J Laryngol Otol 2003; 117:1–9.
43. Cepero R, Smith RJ, Catlin FI. Cystic fibrosis—An otolaryngologic perspective. Otolaryngol Head Neck Surg 1987; 97:356–360.
44. Hadfield PJ, Rowe-Jones JM, Mackay IS. A prospective treatment trial of nasal polyps in adults with cystic fibrosis. Rhinology 2000; 38:63–65.
45. Cromwell O, Morris HR, Walport MJ, Taylor GW. Identification of leukotriene D and B in sputum from cystic fibrosis patients. Lancet 1981; 2:164–165.
46. Saiman L, Marshall BC, Mayer-Hamblett N, Burns JL, et al. Azithromycin in patients with cystic fibrosis chronically infected with *Pseudomonas aeruginosa*. JAMA 2003; 290:1749–1756.
47. Yamada T, Fujieda S, Mori S, Yamamoto T, Saito H. Macrolide treatment decreased the size of nasal polyps and IL-8 levels in nasal lavage. Am J Rhinol 2000; 14:143–148.
48. Graham SM, Launspach JL. Utility of the nasal model in gene transfer studies in cystic fibrosis. Rhinology 1997; 35:149–153.
49. Wagner JA, Nepomuceno IB, Shah N, Messner AH, Moran ML, Norbash AM, Moss RB, Wine JJ, Gardner P. Maxillary sinusitis as a surrogate model for CF gene therapy clinical trials in patients with antrostomies. J Gene Med 1999; 1:13–21.
50. Holzmann D, Speich R, Kaufmann T, Laube I, Russi EW, Simmen D, Weder W, Boehler A. Effects of sinus surgery in patients with cystic fibrosis after lung transplantation: A 10-year experience. Transplantation 2004; 77: 134–136.
51. Karlet MC. An update on cystic fibrosis and implications for anesthesia. AANA J 2000; 68:141–148.

18

Chronic Rhinosinusitis With and Without Nasal Polyposis

Joel M. Bernstein

Departments of Otolaryngology and Pediatrics, School of Medicine and Biomedical Sciences, Department of Communicative Disorders and Sciences, State University of New York at Buffalo, Buffalo, New York, U.S.A.

INTRODUCTION

Chronic rhinosinusitis (CRS) has been the subject of much debate, as the Rhinosinusitis Task Force convened to confront the difficult issues related to rhinosinusitis, including definition, staging, and basic research (1). In general, the definition of CRS has been based entirely on clinical criteria in which there is evidence of a chronic inflammatory state in the nose and paranasal sinuses for at least 12 weeks (1). Although in most cases this may be the result of untreated acute bacterial rhinosinusitis, the diagnostic criteria were still clinical and offered little explanation of the underlying pathophysiology.

CRS appears to be a clinical syndrome in which a number of factors play a role. These factors include bacteria, allergy, superantigen, congenital anatomical factors in the lateral wall of the nose and septum, biofilm, and fungi (1). The factors associated with CRS can be divided into three categories, which are outlined in Table 1. These three categories include systemic host factors, local host factors, and environmental factors (1). These factors contribute to the pathogenesis of CRS or are simply associated with CRS.

Chronic inflammation is *axiomatic* to the definition of CRS. Therefore, like other chronic inflammatory diseases of, for example, the lung, bowel, and joints, the development and persistence of chronic inflammation require

Table 1 Factors Associated with CRS

Systemic host factors	Local host factors	Environmental factors
Allergy	Anatomic	Microorganisms
Immunodeficiency	Neoplasm	Noxious chemicals
Genetic/congenital	Acquired mucociliary dysfunction	Medications
Mucociliary dysfunction		Trauma
Endocrine		Surgery
Neuromechanism		

knowledge of the involvement of inflammatory mediators, cytokines, and adhesion molecules on the surface of lymphocytes, macrophages, eosinophils, and neutrophils. The counter receptors on the surface of venules, which result in attachment of these inflammatory cells to the vascular endothelium, also need to be identified. Finally, an understanding of chemokines is required to explain the migration of these inflammatory cells into the milieu of the mucosa of the paranasal sinuses and nasal polyps.

The 2003 CRS Task Force redefined the clinical definition of the symptoms associated with CRS (1), which had already been described by Lanza and Kennedy (2) in 1997 and divided into major and minor factors that are summarized in Table 2. The presence of discolored nasal discharge, nasal polyps or polypoid mucosal swelling associated with other endoscopic findings of edema or erythema of the middle meatus, and edema or erythema of the ethmoid bulla were the physical findings that may be associated with CRS.

The 2003 CRS Task Force also defined the radiographic findings of CRS and established that isolated or diffuse mucosal thickening, bone changes, and air fluid levels had to be present for such a diagnosis (1). Magnetic resonance imaging (MRI) was not recommended, but plain films, particularly the Waters' view, demonstrating mucosal thickening of greater than 5 mm or complete opacification of the maxillary sinuses were determined to be indicative of CRS.

Table 2 Factors Associated with the Diagnosis of Chronic Rhinosinusitis

Major factors	Minor factors
Facial pain/pressure	Headache
Facial congestion	Fever
Nasal blockage	Halitosis
Nasal discharge	Fatigue
Hyposmia/anosmia	Dental pain
Postnasal discharge	Cough
	Ear pain/fullness

Many questions regarding CRS have still been unanswered; these include the necessity of antibiotics, the need for antifungal medication, and the role of topical applications (i.e., antifungals, antibacterials, and topical diuretics). The understanding of the inflammatory pathways that may lead to chronic inflammation of the paranasal sinuses is required so that a logical form of medical or surgical therapy can be undertaken. The exact mechanism producing the chronic inflammatory state in CRS is just beginning to become unraveled. This chapter will summarize the epidemiology, etiology, pathogenesis, clinical symptomatology, complications, microbiology, and molecular biology of CRS with and without nasal polyposis. New ideas for therapeutic intervention based on principles of pathogenesis and molecular biology associated with CRS with massive nasal polyposis are considered. Finally, the chapter will conclude with a differential diagnosis of nasal masses.

POTENTIAL ETIOLOGIES FOR THE EARLY STAGES OF CRS

The most important initial phase of CRS is mucosal irritation. The schematic representation of the potential alterations in the nasal mucosa that may occur after insult by bacteria, virus, allergen, air pollution, superantigen, or fungi is shown in Figure 1. These entities may cause upregulation of intercellular adhesion molecule 1 (ICAM-1) or other cytokines. HLA-DR molecules may be upregulated on the epithelial surface, which can then play a role in a specific immune response with the subsequent recruitment of either TH_1 or TH_2 cells and the eventual release of specific cytokines.

Granulocyte-macrophage–colony stimulating factor (GM-CSF), interleukin (IL-8), and tumor necrosis factor (TNF-α) may all be released by this upregulated epithelium and have an effect on macrophage, mast cells, eosinophils, and neutrophils. In addition, INF-γ released by TH_1 cells may also enhance the production of ICAM-1 on the surface of the respiratory epithelium.

The concept of superantigens as a possible cause of the initial triggering event in the etiology of CRS with massive nasal polyposis has been studied in our laboratory (3). We have demonstrated that *Staphylococcus aureus* accounts for about 60% of cultures of the lateral wall of the nose, even in the absence of this organism in the nasal vestibule. These organisms always produce exotoxins, which may act as superantigens. Superantigens may upregulate lymphocytes by attaching to the variable β region of the T cell receptor (TCR) of lymphocytes. Lymphocytes are present in the mucosa of the lateral wall of the nose. Such upregulation may also result in an increase of both TH_1 and TH_2 cytokines, which will be subsequently described in detail.

Initially, then, the first phase of chronic inflammation of the paranasal sinuses is an active upregulation of the immune response in the epithelium of the lateral wall of the nose.

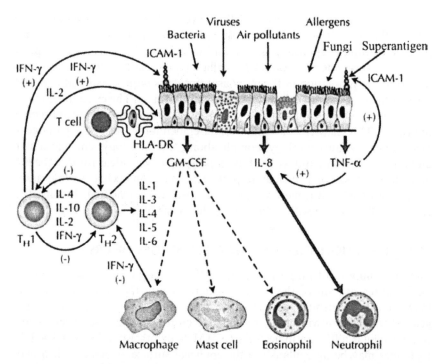

Figure 1 Schematic representation of the potential alterations in respiratory epithelium
that may occur after insult by bacteria, virus, allergen air pollution, and fungus. Thereafter, upregulation of ICAM-1 or other cytokines may occur. Most importantly, HLA-
DR molecules may be upregulated on the epithelial surface, which can play a role in a
specific immune response with the subsequent recruitment of either TH1 or TH2 cells
and their eventual release of specific cytokines. *Abbreviations*: GM-CSF, granulocyte-
macrophage–colony stimulating factor; ICAM-1, intercellular adhesion molecule-1;
IFN-γ, interferon-gamma; TNF-α, TNF-α.

MICROBIOLOGY

The Rhinosinusitis Task Force has reviewed the literature on the microbiology
of CRS, with and without prior surgery (1). Numerous studies of the bacterial
flora in CRS reported the recovery of mixed polymicrobial flora of gram-positive
and gram-negative aerobic and anaerobic bacteria (Chapter 18). However, the
results have varied depending on patient's age and selection criteria, chronicity
of the disease, site of cultures, and specimen transport and culture techniques
(Table 3).

Aerobes represent 50% to 100% and anaerobes 0% to 100% of the microbial isolates (4–8). The predominant aerobes include coagulase-negative
*Staphylococcus, S. aureus, Streptococcus pneumoniae, Streptococcus viridans,
Haemophilus influenzae, Corynebacterium,* and *Moraxella catarrhalis. Fusobacterium, Provotella, Peptostreptococcus,* and *Propionibacterium* spp. are

Table 3 Bacteriology of Chronic Rhinosinusitis

No prior surgery	No prior surgery
Aerobes – 75–100%	Anaerobes – 0–25%
Coagulase-negative *Staphylococcus*	*Fusobacterium sp.*
Staphylococcus aureus	*Provotella sp.*
Streptococcus pneumoniae	*Peptostreptococcus sp.*
Streptococcus viridans	*Proprionibacterium sp.*
Haemophilus influenzae	Prior surgery
Corynebacterium sp.	*Pseudomonas sp.*
Moraxella catarrhalis	*Klebsiella sp.*
	Enterobacter sp.
	Coagulase-negative *Staphylococcus*
	Staphylococcus aureus

Source: Adapted from Ref. 1.

the most common anaerobes. *Pseudomonas, Klebsiella, Enterobacter* spp., coagulase-negative Staphylococcus, *S. aureus*, and the above anaerobic bacteria were all recovered from individuals who had prior surgery (5).

There is abundant evidence that anaerobic bacteria play an important role in both acute and CRS. However, their isolation depended on culture techniques, and unfortunately most studies have not used optimal techniques for their recovery (4–6).

The role of anaerobic bacteria in CRS has been demonstrated in several studies reviewed by Nord (8). The potential ability of beta-lactamase–producing aerobic and anaerobic bacteria to protect penicillin-susceptible organisms by the production of beta-lactamase was illustrated by Brook et al. (9), and Finegold et al. recovered anaerobes from 48% of adults with chronic maxillary sinusitis (10). Brook et al. illustrated that there are differences in the distribution of organisms in single patients who suffer from infections in multiple sinuses, and emphasized the importance of obtaining cultures from all infected sinuses (11).

Adenovirus and respiratory syncytial virus (RSV) have been demonstrated in CRS using the polymerase chain reaction (12). Sinus mucosal biopsies from 20 patients undergoing endoscopic sinus surgery were sterilely collected.

One specimen tested positive for RSV and another for adenovirus by viral culture and immunofluorescence.

EPIDEMIOLOGY OF CRS WITH MASSIVE NASAL POLYPOSIS

The epidemiology of nasal polyposis has been reviewed by a number of investigators. Settipane concluded that nasal polyps are found in about 36% of patients with aspirin-intolerance, 20% of those with cystic fibrosis, 7% of those with asthma, and 0.1% of normal children (13). Other conditions associated with nasal polyps are tabulated in Table 4 and include Churg-Strauss

Table 4 Diseases that may be Associated with Massive Nasal Polyposis

With eosinophilia	Without eosinophilia
Bronchial asthma	Cystic fibrosis
Allergic rhinitis	Primary ciliary dyskinesia
Allergic fungal sinusitis	Chronic nonallergic rhinitis
Aspirin intolerance	Young's syndrome
Churg–Strauss syndrome	

syndrome (CSS), allergic fungal sinusitis, ciliary dyskinetic syndrome, and Young's syndrome.

Settipane demonstrated that nasal polyps were statistically more common in nonallergic patients than in allergic patients (13). Furthermore, nasal polyposis was more common in nonallergic asthma versus allergic asthma patients (13% vs. 5%, $p < 0.01$). About 40% of patients with surgical polypectomies had recurrences. Further investigations by this group demonstrated a family history of nasal polyposis, suggesting a hereditary factor (14).

Similar results were obtained in a recent study that investigated the prevalence of nasal polyposis in 3817 Greek patients with chronic rhinitis and asthma and found nasal polyps in 4.2% of the patients (15). The prevalence of nasal polyps increased with age in both sexes. Its prevalence was 13% in patients with nonallergic asthma, 2.4% in patients with allergic asthma, 8.9% in patients with nonallergic rhinitis, and 1.7% in patients with allergic rhinitis. These results appear to confirm the fact that the absence of IgE-mediated hypersensitivity is more common in patients with nasal polyps.

Nasal polyps appeared to be present more frequently in nonallergic patients than allergic patients and in patients with perennial allergy than patients with seasonal allergy.

Johansson et al. provided the most recent review of the prevalence of nasal polyps in adults (16). This study comprised 1900 inhabitants over the age of 20 years stratified for age and gender.

The prevalence of nasal polyps was 2.7%, and the polyps were more frequent in men, the elderly, and asthmatics.

It appears that most epidemiological studies suggest that nasal polyps occur in less than 5% of the total population, are frequently associated with bronchial asthma and tend to increase with age, and are twice as common in patients who do not have allergy than patients with allergy. There appears to be some evidence that over the age of 40, bronchial asthma associated with nasal polyposis is more common in females.

Fritz et al., who sought to understand the basis of nasal polyposis association with allergic rhinitis, hypothesized that the expression of unique genes was associated with nasal polyposis phenotype (17). After examining 12,000 human genes transcribed in the nasal mucosa in patients with allergic rhinitis with and without nasal polyposis, they identified 34 genes which were differentially expressed between the patient groups. The greatest differential expression identified by the array analysis was for a group of genes associated with neoplasia, including mammaglobin, a gene transcribed 12-fold higher in patients with polyps compared with control patients with rhinitis alone. These data suggested that nasal polyposis involves deregulated cell growth by gene activation in some ways similar to a neoplasm. In addition, mammaglobin, a gene of unknown function associated with breast neoplasia, might be related to polyp growth.

THE CLINICAL DIAGNOSIS OF NASAL POLYPOSIS

The most common symptoms of nasal polyposis include nasal obstruction, hyposmia, nasal discharge, and very often watery rhinorrhea (Table 5). Although adequate diagnosis cannot be obtained by taking a history alone, clinical examination of the nose may often reveal nasal polyposis with the unaided eye. However, endoscopic examination of the nose is imperative and often reveals nasal polyps in the lateral wall of the nose lateral to the middle turbinate, as seen in Figure 2.

Polyps appear as pale, gray, watery solid masses, which are significantly lighter in color than the normal, vascular pink mucosa of the inferior and middle turbinates. Nasal polyposis usually is bilateral, although unilateral nasal polyposis is often seen in allergic fungal sinusitis.

Currently, the best imaging procedure of the paranasal sinuses for the identification of both nasal polyposis and chronic membrane thickening is computerized tomograph (CT) scanning in both the coronal and axial planes (Figs. 3 and 4). The basic and supplementary diagnostic tools for the diagnosis of CRS with or without nasal polyposis are summarized in Table 6. Although MRI is usually not indicated for the diagnosis of CRS, but in some cases where a unilateral mass is found in the nose, MRI can be useful to investigate the presence of mycosis or neoplasm. The presence of abundant eosinophils in nasal cytology may establish whether or not topical corticosteroids would be useful. Nasal biopsy is sometimes indicated, particularly in

Table 5 Symptoms of Nasal Polyposis

Nasal obstruction
Watery rhinorrhea
Postnasal discharge
Anosmia
Nasal pressure
Fatigue
Snoring

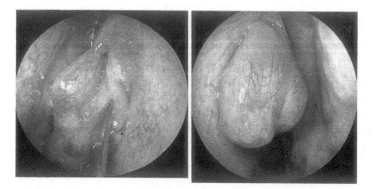

Figure 2 Endoscopic view of the left and right nasal cavity showing polyposis extending from the left middle meatus (*left*) and the right middle meatus (*right*). On the left side of the picture, the forceps is pointing at a large polypoid mass in the lateral wall of the nose completely obstructing the opening of the maxillary sinus.

patients with a unilateral mass in which a neoplasm is suspected. The presence of a unilateral mass will be reviewed later in this chapter.

The most common location of nasal polyps is the lateral wall of the nose. Larsen and Tos have emphasized that nasal polyps are truly derived from the ethmoid portion of the nose, that is, the mucosa lateral to the middle turbinate (18). Polyps most often arise from the areas of mucosa near the natural ostia of the maxillary and ethmoid sinuses. As these polypoid inflammatory growths enlarge, they block the openings of the sinuses and produce total

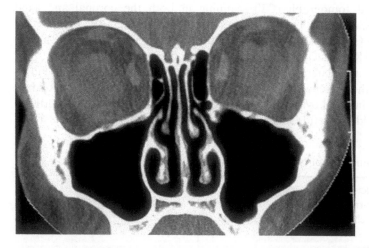

Figure 3 Normal computerized axial tomogram of the paranasal sinuses showing a very patent infundibulum on the left and right side with normal ethmoids and normal maxillary sinuses. There is absolutely no thickened membrane in any of the sinuses.

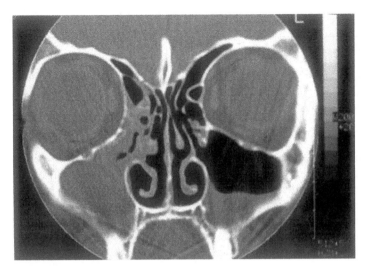

Figure 4 A classical case of bilateral ethmoid and maxillary sinusitis with an air fluid level in the floor of the left maxillary sinus. The ethmoids on the left and the frontal ethmoidal recess on the left are normal. There is complete obstruction of the osteomeatal complex on the right side.

obstruction and subsequent development of acute and eventually CRS. Medical or surgical therapy directed at their removal must then be considered.

Although polypoid swellings of the maxillary, ethmoid, frontal, and sphenoid sinuses may occur, these are less common than the nasal polyps mentioned earlier, which arise lateral to the middle turbinate.

The potential complications of nasal polyposis include nasal obstruction, obstructive sleep apnea, epistaxis, anosmia, and the rare case of bone erosion (Table 7). Hyperteleorism can also result from the benign growth of nasal polyps into the ethmoids, compressing and destroying the lamina papyracea. Malignant transformation of benign nasal polyposis is extremely rare.

Postnasal discharge, which is a common symptom of obstructive nasal polyposis, can aggravate bronchial asthma. The mechanism responsible for

Table 6 Basic and Supplementary Diagnostic Tools for Nasal Polyposis

Basic diagnostic tools	Supplementary diagnostic tools
Case history and clinical examination	Allergy diagnosis
Endoscopy of the nasal cavity	MRI can for certain diagnoses (mycosis, tumor)
CT scan in coronal and axial planes	Nasal cytology
	Nasal biopsy

Table 7 Complications of Nasal Polyposis

Purulent sinusitis
Epistaxis
Rare bone erosion
Hyperteleorism
Very rare malignant transformation

---

the development of asthma from CRS has been debated. Triggered nerves in an affected sinus may result in both parasympathetic stimulation of the bronchial tree and smooth muscle contraction (19). Removal of nasal polyposis and the resulting improvement in the condition of the paranasal sinuses often lead to marked improvement in the symptomatology and the treatment of chronic bronchial asthma (19).

MEDICAL AND SURGICAL THERAPY OF NASAL POLYPOSIS

Because nasal obstruction is a major complaint of patients with nasal polyposis, therapy is directed towards relieving nasal obstruction. Furthermore, knowledge of the specific etiology of nasal polyps, if known, such as an allergic fungal sinusitis, will determine specific treatment. As nasal polyposis is the end result of a variety of pathological processes, the goals of treatment are to relieve nasal blockage, restore olfaction, and improve sinus drainage.

Topical corticosteroids are the mainstay of medical treatment. There is little evidence that a particular topical steroid has better efficacy than any other. Oral corticosteroid therapy is also extremely effective, but caution is advised because of the significant side effects if these oral corticosteroids are used either too often or for long periods of time. If massive nasal polyposis is present, it is most likely that medical therapy will fail. However, oral steroids occasionally may even be effective in such cases, particularly in restoring an improved quality of life to the patient. When topical and oral steroid therapy fail in CRS with massive nasal polyposis, endoscopic surgery can be very successful, especially when accompanied with aggressive postoperative treatment with a number of new topical agents (Table 8). The use of topical steroids, topical diuretics, and topical antibacterial agents can result in symptom-free patients for many years.

The technique of endoscopic sinus surgery is beyond the scope of this chapter, but in general, recurrence rates after endoscopic sinus surgery for severe polyposis may be significant, particularly in patients with asthma. However, there have been only few studies that correlated the combined use of topical steroids, topical diuretics, topical antibacterials, and topical antifungals. Therefore, revision surgery rates and recurrence rates, although higher in patients with massive polyposis and with bronchial asthma, need

Table 8 Topical Therapy Following Endoscopic Surgery for Massive Nasal Polyposis

Topical reagent	Mechanism of action
Topical corticosteroids	Anti-inflammatory activity
Topical diuretics (amiloride or furosemide)	Blocks apical or lateral sodium channels and decreases water uptake by mucosal cells
Topical antibacterials or antifungals	Kills bacterial or fungal flora in nasal mucus
Anti-leukotriene drugs (monteleukast)	Inhibits LTC3 and LTC4 in nasal mucosa
Saline irrigation	Removes blood or mucous crusts

to be revisited with more aggressive use of postoperative topical agents as shown in Table 8. In the case of massive nasal polyposis, modern surgical techniques often have to be performed.

To better understand the chronic inflammatory disease associated with CRS with nasal polyposis and the efficacy of both medical and surgical therapy, a thorough knowledge of the molecular biology of the inflammatory response in CRS with nasal polyposis is required.

The molecular biological events that may lead to the development of the chronic inflammatory disorder leading to massive nasal polyposis can be divided into three phases.

PATHOGENESIS OF CRS

Molecular Biology of Nasal Polyposis

Phase 1: Mucosal Irritation

The events that cause initial mucosal irritation in the lateral wall of the nose involve bacteria, viruses, air pollutants, allergens, fungi, and superantigen release from various microorganisms.

Structural abnormalities such as markedly deviated septum, Haller cells, or marked pneumatization of the middle turbinates can also result in mucosal irritation at the level of the osteomeatal complex. There is increasing evidence that the airway epithelium, which has traditionally been regarded as a physical barrier preventing the entry of inhaled noxious particles into the submucosa, plays an active role as a "metabolically active" physical–chemical barrier (Fig. 1). It may be capable of expressing and generating increased amounts of (1) inflammatory eicosanoids, which are potent cell activators and chemoattractants; (2) pro-inflammatory cytokines, which have profound effect on growth, differentiation, migration, and activation of inflammatory cells; (3) specific cell adhesion molecules, which play a vital role in "inter-tissue trafficking" of the inflammatory cells; and (4) major histocompatability complex (MHC, Class II antigens), which plays an important role in antigen presentation to and subsequent activation of the T cells (20). More recent studies of the response of airway epithelial cells to nonallergic stimuli suggested that these may induce synthesis of inflammatory cytokines. For example, cultured human bronchial epithelial cells exposed to nitric oxide and *H. influenzae* demonstrated that these agents significantly increase synthesis of GM-CSF, IL-8, and TNF-α by epithelial cells in vitro (21,22).

Stimulation of epithelial cells by various agents may lead to the generation of different cytokine profiles and subsequent activation of specific inflammatory cells. Thus, the very early development of CRS in the lateral wall of the nose, with or without nasal polyps, may be the result of stimulation of the epithelium by aerodynamic changes, allowing irritants to metabolically or physically alter or injure the surface epithelium. Once the surface epithelium is injured, a cascade of inflammatory changes may occur. The expression of TNF-α is particularly important in airway inflammation because it is a cytokine with significant influence on epithelial cell permeability (23). Expression of IL-8, a major neutrophil and eosinophil chemotactic factor, and ICAM-1, a member of the immunoglobulin supergene family, may also result from the presence of TNF-α (24,25).

ICAM-1 has been shown to act as both the ligand and the counter-receptor for leukocyte function antigen-1 (LFA-1) expressed on leukocytes (26), and consequently plays a vital role in the recruitment and migration of inflammatory cells to the sites of inflammation in the airways. Furthermore, studies of nasal and bronchial tissues in patients with nasal polyps, perennial–seasonal allergic rhinitis, and asthma have suggested that the expression of ICAM-1 may be upregulated in the airway epithelium (27).

Studies investigating the expression of the MHC Class II antigens have demonstrated that, in accordance with the findings in other cell types, human airway epithelial cells have the ability to express the HLA-DR antigens and the genes encoding these antigens (28). The ability of airway epithelial cells to express HLA-DR antigens, however, suggests that these cells may play a potentially important role in antigen processing, presentation, or both, and possibly involve in immunoregulation through recognition, activation, and proliferation of specific T-lymphocyte types (TH_1 or TH_2), which produce specific cytokine profiles. These cytokines, such as IL-2, interferon-γ, IL-4, and IL-5, have been demonstrated in nasal polyps (29,30). It is therefore possible to speculate that the earliest change in the lateral wall of the nose that may give rise to chronic inflammation or nasal polyposis is the activation or dysfunction of the epithelial cells themselves, resulting in attraction, maintenance, and activation of various inflammatory cells into the epithelium. It is conceivable that if the TH_2 cell-associated pathway is activated, then the transcriptional expression in synthesis of GM-CSF, IL-4, and IL-5 will affect predominantly eosinophil, mast cell, and macrophage function. Moreover, nonallergic stimuli such as air pollutants, bacteria (endotoxin), and viruses can directly affect epithelial cells to increase synthesis of GM-CSF, IL1-β and TNF-α and also to promote TH$_1$ cell-associated pathways, resulting in decreased synthesis of IL-3, IL-4, and IL-5 (31). The overall effect would be to enhance migration and activation of neutrophils in particular, and to attenuate migration and activation of other inflammatory cell types.

A superantigen hypothesis for CRS and nasal polyposis is appealing because one of the most common bacterial species found in the nasal mucus in CRS is *S. aureus* (32). In all of the cases studied so far, these bacteria produced enterotoxins, and the corresponding variable-β region of the T-cell receptor was upregulated (32). These data suggest that the initial injury to the lateral wall of the nose may be the result of toxin-producing staphylococci. Other microorganisms including fungi may also act as superantigens. The superantigen may play a role as an initial trigger in the development of mucosal inflammation in the lateral wall of the nose.

Phase 2: TNF-α and Interleukin-1β

The second phase in the development of chronic inflammation in the lateral wall of the nose and nasal polyposis relates to the activity of TNF-α and IL-1β. The message and the product of these two cytokines are found in the epithelium and endothelium of both nasal polyps and mucosa of CRS (Figs. 5 and 6) (33). The most important function of these two cytokines is upregulation of the expression of endothelial adhesion molecules involved in inflammatory reactions. The cytokines and secretagogues that induce self-surface expression of endothelial adhesion molecules include very late antigen-4 (VLA-4) on the surface of eosinophils, MAC-1 on the surface of macrophage, and LFA-1 on the surface of neutrophils (34–36). The corresponding endothelial markers, which are upregulated and act as counter receptors for these specific adhesion molecules, are vascular cell adhesion molecule-1 (VCAM-1) and ICAM-1. Figure 7 shows a schematic diagram of the attachment of an inflammatory cell to the endothelial cell of a venule in a nasal polyp.

VLA-4 specifically attaches to VCAM-1, and LFA-1 specifically attaches to ICAM-1. The movement of the cell along the endothelium from the trailing edge to the leading edge is shown in Figure 7 and is responsible for migration of the cell along the endothelial cell border. The aforementioned in vitro studies and animal experiments have demonstrated that a distinct set of adhesion molecules is important for adherence of eosinophils to the endothelium and their subsequent extravasation.

In the multistep model of leukocyte recruitment, it is proposed that chemoattractants play a dual role by triggering integrin activation and directing leukocyte migration. Several cysteine–cysteine chemokines, such as eotaxin and RANTES (regulated upon activation, normal T-cell expressed and secreted), have been shown to attract and activate eosinophils in vitro and

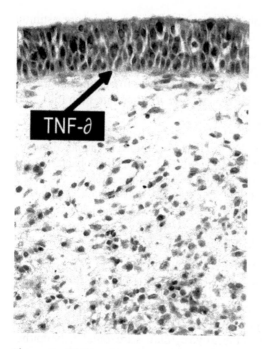

Figure 5 High power photomicrograph (peroxidase–antiperoxidase 400×) of the surface epithelium of a nasal polyp. The arrow points to basal cells, which have the product of TNF-α. The entire epithelium has the product of TNF-α. TNF-α is also found in eosinophils in the lamina propria. *Abbreviation*: TNF-α, tumor necrosis factor.

to recruit eosinophils into inflammatory lesions with little effect on neutrophils (37,38) (Fig. 8).

RANTES also induces selective trans-endothelial migration of eosinophils in vitro (37,38). Moreover, LFA-1 appears to have a higher affinity for ICAM-1 (39). That these chemoattractants can discriminate between leukocyte subsets contributes significantly to the understanding of preferential recruitment of particular cell types in various inflammatory reactions. Finally, increasing evidence supports the notion that cytokines released from activated CD4$^+$ T cells are largely responsible for the local accumulation and activation of eosinophils in allergy-related disorders (40). These T cells produce a particular set of cytokines (TH$_2$ profiles); of these, IL-4 and IL-13 are believed to play a role in the preferential extravasation of eosinophils through selected induction of VCAM-1, whereas IL-5, GM-CSF, and IL-3 are responsible for eosinophil activation and prolonged survival (41). The interaction of VLA-4 on eosinophils and VCAM-1 on venule and endothelial cells is responsible for the specific localization of the eosinophil on the vascular endothelial cell in the nasal polyp. The presence of VLA-4 on the eosinophil and VCAM-1 on the venule endothelial cell

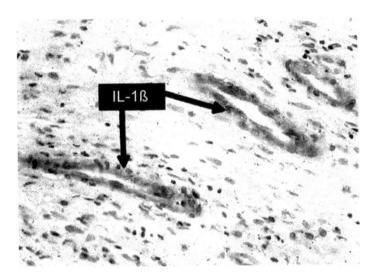

Figure 6 High-power photomicrograph (peroxidase–antiperoxidase 600×) of the lamina propria of a nasal polyp showing the presence of interleukin-1β in the endothelial cells (*Arrows*) of small venules.

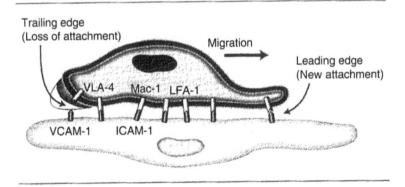

Figure 7 A schematic diagram of the attachment of an inflammatory cell to the endothelial cell of a venule in a nasal polyp. Very late antigen-4 specifically attaches to VCAM-1, and leukocyte function antigen-1 specifically attaches to ICAM-1. The movement of the cell along the endothelium from the trailing edge to the leading edge is shown and is responsible for the migration of the cell along the endothelial cell border. *Abbreviations*: ICAM-1, intercellular adhesion molecule-1; VCAM-1, vascular cell adhesion molecule-1.

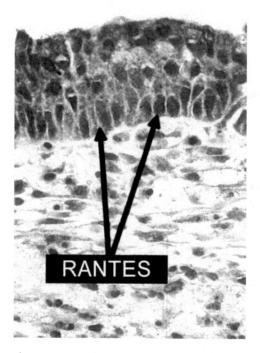

Figure 8 Photomicrograph of RANTES in the epithelium of a nasal polyp as well as in eosinophils in the submucosa (peroxidase–antiperoxidase 800×).

are shown in Figures 9 and 10. Once this slowing of eosinophil migration occurs in the blood flow of the nasal polyp or the nasal mucosa, the chemokines, RANTES, and eotaxin are most likely responsible for the trans-epithelial migration of these eosinophil cells into the lamina propria of the chronic inflammatory tissue in CRS.

These studies suggest that the eosinophil is the predominant cell in the nasal polyp where up to 80% of the inflammatory cells are eosinophils (42). In many tissue sections, there are massive sheets of eosinophils totally filling the lamina propria as the single or solitary inflammatory cell. (Fig. 11)

One of the most important phenomena that occurs within the lamina propria of the nasal polyp is the autocrine upregulation of cytokines that are responsible for the protracted survival of these cells. At least three cytokines are responsible for the decreased apoptosis of eosinophils (41). This mechanism has an effect on the long-term survival of eosinophils and their activation. These three cytokines are IL-3, GM-CSF, and most importantly IL-5. IL-5 appears to have the most active effect in promoting the survival of eosinophils in the nasal polyp. In addition to the production of these eosinophil-promoting cytokines in the epithelium and endothelium of the nasal polyp, the eosinophil itself can respond by producing similar

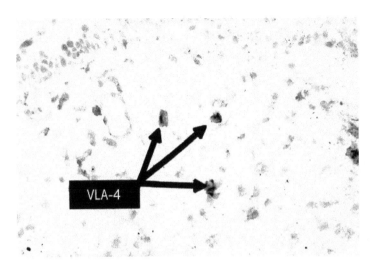

Figure 9 High-power photomicrograph of very late antigen-4 (VLA-4) on the surface of eosinophils in the lamina propria of a nasal polyp (peroxidase–antiperoxidase 600×).

cytokines in an autocrine-upregulated fashion. This vicious cycle of autocrine upregulation enhances the recruitment of even more eosinophils into the nasal tissue so that the chronic inflammatory state of eosinophilia is maintained.

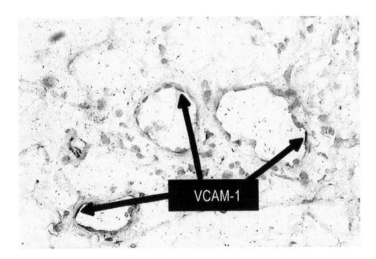

Figure 10 High-power photomicrograph of vascular cell adhesion molecule-1 (VCAM-1) on the tips of the endothelial cells of small venules in the lamina propria of a nasal polyp (peroxidase–antiperoxidase 800×).

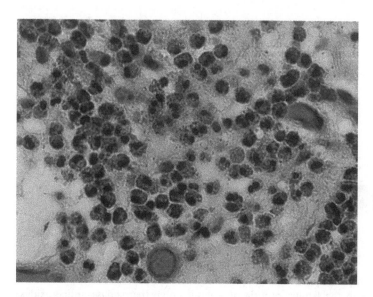

Figure 11 Lamina propria of a nasal polyp in which *Staphylococcus aureus* enterotoxin was present. High-power photomicrograph showing massive accumulation of both eosinophils and degranulating eosinophils (magnification, 600×; hematoxylin and eosin).

Phase 3: Eosinophils and Major Basic Protein

Most research has concentrated on the potential damage to the epithelium caused by inflammatory mediators of eosinophils, particularly that of major basic protein (MBP) (33). Research also focused on the potential role of MBP on sodium and chloride flux in the epithelium of the polyp epithelial cell. Eosinophil cationic protein has been shown to stimulate airway mucus secretion, whereas eosinophilic MBP inhibits the secretion (43). The first study on the role of MBP and its effect on chloride secretion demonstrated that MBP increases net chloride secretion (44).

The role of MBP on net sodium and chloride flux in an animal model of a salt-depleted rat colon demonstrated that MBP significantly increases the net sodium flux into the interior of the epithelial cell (Bernstein and Choshniak, personal communication). Although there was a large movement of chloride both in and out of the cell, there was no significant net flux of chloride. The short-circuit current appeared to be significantly increased with MBP compared with the control. In addition, amiloride, a respiratory epithelial apical sodium channel inhibitor, was able to decrease not only the short-circuit current, but also the amount of sodium flux into the cell. The results of these animal studies are summarized in Figure 12. The use of topical amiloride as an agent in the prevention of edema in recurrent nasal polyposis might be considered as a possible adjunct to steroids.

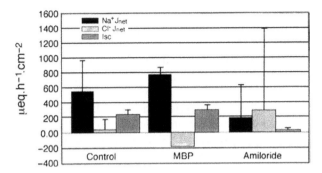

Figure 12   The effect of MBP and amiloride on net flux of sodium$^+$ and chloride$^-$ in a salt-depleted rat colon model. MBP has a significant effect on net sodium flux and amiloride has a marked decreased effect on both the sodium flux as well as the short-circuit current. *Abbreviation*: MBP, major basic protein.

In addition to the substantial accumulation of eosinophils in chronic inflammation in the lateral wall of the nose and nasal polyps, the number of lymphocytes is also significantly increased in CRS inflammation (Fig. 13). Most of the cells that are found in nasal polyps are T cells (29,30). The TCR

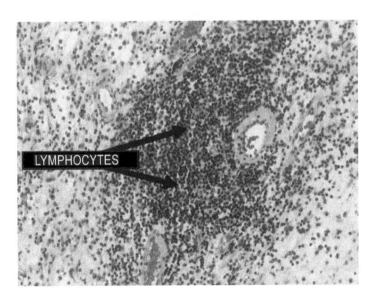

Figure 13   High-power photomicrograph of the lamina propria of the nasal polyp in which *Staphylococcus* enterotoxin was identified in the adjacent mucus. There is a massive lymphocytic infiltrate around a small venule. Most of these lymphocytes are T cells (magnification, 200×; hematoxylin and eosin).

functions in both antigen-recognition and signal transduction, which are crucial initial steps in antigen-specific immune responses. TCR integrity is vital to the induction of optimal and efficient immune responses, including the routine elimination of invading pathogens and the elimination of modified cells and molecules. It has recently been shown that there is an impairment of TCR function in T cells isolated from hosts with various chronic pathologies including cancer, autoimmune, and infectious diseases (45). Preliminary data (Bernstein et al., personal communication) showed that T cells extracted from nasal polyps also possess a defective TCR in comparison with the patient's peripheral blood and that of peripheral blood of normal adult controls.

A common immuno-pathological hallmark of many inflammatory diseases is a T cell invasion and accumulation in the inflamed tissue. Although the exact molecular and micro-environmental mechanisms governing such cellular invasion and tissue retention are not known, some key immunological principles might be at work. Transforming growth factor-β is known to modulate some of these processes including homing, cellular adhesion, chemotaxis, and finally T cell activation, differentiation, and apoptosis (46). The chronicity of T-cell-driven-inflammation may lead to a T cell adaptive immune response. It is suggested therefore that the T lymphocytes that are present in the nasal polyp, as in the chronic inflammation associated with CRS, actually may not be active but may be anergic, which may maintain the inflammatory response in these tissue sites.

Medical Treatment of CRS with Massive Nasal Polyposis Based on the Molecular Biology of Inflammation

Eosinophil and lymphocytic infiltration into the lateral wall of the nose are the characteristic histological findings in patients with CRS and massive nasal polyposis. The previous description of the phases of inflammation has emphasized the interaction of cytokine molecules responsible for the development of the increased numbers and survival of eosinophils and lymphocytes. Therefore, a logical approach to the medical treatment of this inflammatory disorder can only be objectively considered when a complete understanding of this cytokine network has been established.

Hypothetically, antibodies directed against cytokines responsible for the accumulation of lymphocytes and eosinophils in chronic inflammation could be considered in the treatment of CRS with massive nasal polyposis and other chronic inflammatory disorders in which these cells are present. These diseases would include allergic rhinitis, bronchial asthma, allergic fungal sinusitis, Churg–Strauss syndrome (CSS), and, particularly, aspirin-intolerance, which is associated with CRS with nasal polyposis. The list of antibodies directed against cytokines that have been used in both human

Table 9 Anti-Cytokine Antibodies that Have Hypothetical Use in the Treatment of CRS with Massive Nasal Polyposis

Anti-cytokine	Potential mechanism
Anti-TNF-α	Downregulates inflammatory cytokines
Anti-IL1-β	Downregulates inflammatory cytokines
Anti-VLA-4	Decreases attachment of eosinophils to vascular endothelium
Anti-VCAM-1	Decreases attachment of eosinophils to vascular endothelium
Anti-RANTES	Decreases attraction of eosinophils into lamina propria
Anti-eotaxin	Decreases attraction of eosinophils into lamina propria
Anti-IL-5[51]	Decreases survival of eosinophils
Anti-IL-3	Inhibits eosinopoesis
Anti-GM-CSF	Inhibits eosinophil survival
Anti-IL-12[52,53]	Inhibits TH1 cytokines

and animal experiments are tabulated in Table 9. In these tables, the anticytokine and its potential mechanisms are reviewed.

Although these hypothetical strategies may be interesting for the researcher and clinician alike, a more practical approach to the medical treatment of CRS with and without nasal polyposis is depicted in Table 10. A review of this table is essential for the clinician. Antibiotic therapy using pharmacokinetic and pharmacodynamic principles is problematic in the disease that is now called CRS. The presence of bacteria, even though documented in many cases, does not necessarily prove that they are causing the inflammation, although it is certainly possible.

As most experts in rhinology agree today that chronic inflammation is the major problem in CRS with or without nasal polyposis, the use of specific anti-inflammatory drugs is critical. Corticosteroids are the most commonly used anti-inflammatory agents in the treatment of CRS, particularly with nasal polyposis. The mechanism of action of corticosteroids is related to their ability

Table 10 Medical Management of CRS with Massive Nasal Polyposis

Antibiotic therapy using pharmacokinetic–pharmacodynamic principles
Topical and/or systemic corticosteroids
Anti-leukotriene therapy (local or systemic)
Macrolide therapy as anti-inflammatory
Therapy directed against biofilm
Topical diuretic therapy
Anti-allergy therapy (anti-IgE therapy)

to enter cells because of their lipophilicity. Following entrance into the cell, the steroid binds to a steroid receptor where it alters the proteins secreted by that cell. Therefore, corticosteroids can downregulate the synthesis of proteins that are synthesized in eosinophils, basophils, mast cells, T cells, B cells, and even antigen-presenting cells.

Antileukotriene therapy has been considered useful in the treatment of both allergic rhinitis and nasal polyposis. This drug may be particularly useful in the aspirin-sensitive patient who has CRS with nasal polyposis. Although there is an abundant evidence of increasing resistance to macrolides by *S. pneumoniae*, erythromycin and clarithromycin have no bactericidal activity against *H. influenzae*, and there has been growing evidence supporting their effect against neutrophils and some inflammatory cytokines. During the past five decades, there has been an increasing interest in the potential anti-inflammatory effects of macrolide antibiotics. Low-dose macrolide therapy has dramatically increased survival in patients with diffuse panbronchiolitis (47). This has led to further investigation into the potential use of macrolides in chronic lung diseases with an inflammatory component. The effect of macrolides in the downregulation of inflammatory mediators and cytokines in CRS with or without nasal polyposis remains to be established.

Microorganisms are able to adhere to various surfaces and to form a three-dimensional structure known as biofilm. In biofilms, microbial cells show characteristics and behaviors different than those of plankton cells. Once a biofilm has been established on the surface, the bacteria harbored inside are less exposed to the host's immune response and less susceptible to antibiotics. There have as yet been very few studies on biofilm in CRS. However, there have been several studies on the behavior of bacteria on the mucous membrane of the middle ear in experimental animals suggesting particularly that nontypable *H. influenzae* may be involved in biofilm formation (48). The concept of biofilms in CRS needs more study, but if present, may be one of the reasons why bacteria continue to colonize the sinuses in chronic inflammatory disease.

Topical diuretic therapy with furosemide is a beneficial therapy in the postoperative management of CRS with nasal polyposis (49).

Anti-IgE therapy is a new therapeutic tool used by allergists for the neutralization of IgE and the inhibition of IgE synthesis (50). Monoclonal anti-IgE therapy may be a rational approach when allergy is a major trigger in the patient with IgE-mediated hypersensitivity.

Diseases Associated with Nasal Polyposis

Although nasal polyposis most frequently occurs in adults with bronchial asthma who have either allergic rhinitis or nonallergic rhinitis, there are other diseases which can be associated with nasal polyposis. A brief summary of these diseases is discussed below (Table 4).

Cystic Fibrosis

Nasal polyposis associated with cystic fibrosis occurs in young children and young adults. It is the only disease in which nasal polyposis occurs in children under the age of five. The histopathology of nasal polyposis in cystic fibrosis, however, is quite different than that in noncystic fibrosis. Lympho-plasmacytic cells are predominant, and eosinophils, though present, are not common. Furthermore, the disease arises from the sinuses and encroaches upon the lateral wall of the nose, which is opposite that of the noncystic fibrosis patient where the disease arises in the lateral wall of the nose and compresses the sinus ostia. The prevalence of nasal polyps in cystic fibrosis varies between 20% and 40%. An inverse relationship exists between nasal polyposis in cystic fibrosis and pulmonary function; a better pulmonary function is generally present in patients with cystic fibrosis who have nasal polyposis (54).

Allergic Fungal Sinusitis

Allergic fungal sinusitis is probably the only well-documented sinusitis that is related to fungal elements, specifically those that produce an IgE-mediated response. McClay et al. reported one of the largest studies of the clinical presentation of allergic fungal sinusitis in children (55). One of the characteristic findings in allergic fungal sinusitis is the presence of obvious bony facial abnormalities, proptosis, unilateral asymmetric sinus disease, bony extension on CT scan, and fungi on culture. Bipolaris and curvilaria are equally recovered from both adults and children, whereas adults have a greater incidence of aspergillus. Children have more obvious facial skeletal abnormalities, unilateral sinus disease, and asymmetrical disease than adults. The treatment of allergic fungal sinusitis, in addition to a combination of surgery and systemic or topical corticosteroids, also includes immunotherapy to pertinent fungal and nonfungal antigens.

NARES Syndrome

Perennial rhinitis without allergy has recently been named nonallergic rhinitis with eosinophilia syndrome (NARES). The symptoms include nasal hyper-reactivity involving sneezing, rhinorrhea, and nasal obstruction. Nasal endoscopy and sinus CT reveal an evolution towards nasal polyposis in some patients. In general, this disease is not associated with intolerance to aspirin, and some investigators suggest that NARES may be a precursor to the triad of nasal polyposis, chronic sinusitis, and bronchial asthma (56).

Church-Strauss Syndrome (CSS)

CSS is a rare multiple organ disease that belongs to the group of systemic granulomatous vasculitis. The initial symptoms are often bronchial asthma and allergic rhinitis; later in the course of the disease, the patients exhibit lung, heart, and kidney manifestations. There have been approximately

200 cases published worldwide. The patients in general are on steroid therapy and often have nasal polyposis and bronchial asthma. Occasionally, cytotoxic drugs are necessary (57).

Aspirin-Intolerance

Aspirin-intolerance is associated with non-IgE-mediated nasal polyposis, chronic sinusitis, and bronchial asthma. Occasionally, other drugs can also be associated with aspirin-intolerance; they include alcohol, metabisulfites, benzoates, tartrazine, and codeine. All of these chemicals may be linked to nonallergic eosinophilic rhinitis with the possible development of nasal polyposis (58).

Primary Ciliary Dyskinesia

The syndrome of cilia dyskinesia is known as a heterogeneous ciliary dysfunction caused by morphological defect of the dynein arms, the nexin links, the radial spokes, and the transposition of micro tubules (59). This disease is usually associated with chronic broncho-pulmonary infections and nasal polyposis resistant to therapy and is usually diagnosed by electron microscopic evaluation of the ultra-structure of the mucosal cilia. Usually it is associated with disorders of the ciliated epithelium of other parts of the body and is often misdiagnosed as cystic fibrosis. However, in ciliary dyskinesia, unlike cystic fibrosis, there is no evidence of a defect in sodium and chloride transport along the apical surface of the cell.

Young's Syndrome

Young's syndrome is part of primary ciliary dyskinesia and is characterized by repeated airway infections and congenital epididymis obstruction (60). Sperm analyses reveal absence of spermatozoa, although spermatogenesis in testes biopsies may be normal. Mucociliary clearance is impaired and patients often have recurrent sino-bronchial disease with rare reports of nasal polyposis (61).

Differential Diagnosis of Unilateral and Bilateral Masses in the Nasal Cavity

Although nasal polyps are the most common inflammatory growth in the nose of adults and some children, the presence of a unilateral nasal mass should alert the clinician to the many benign sinonasal lesions that can occur in this area. The nose and sinuses represent one of the regions of greatest histological diversity in the body with any tissue capable of producing benign and malignant tumors that can mimic nasal polyposis. In addition, certain congenital and anatomical conditions may simulate a polyp, emphasizing the need for preoperative imaging even when only a biopsy is being considered.

Conversely, benign nasal polyposis may be associated with both significant bone skull base erosion and, in exceptional cases, intracranial invasion.

Benign Lesions in Adults

Anatomic

Pneumatization of the middle turbinate (concha bullosa) can produce a large mass in the nose which might simulate a fleshy polyp or tumor. This pneumatization may be present on one or both sides, but its true nature can be determined by palpation and, if any confirmation is required, by CT scanning (Table 11).

Tumors

Inverted Papilloma

These are the most common true nasal tumors, arising within the middle meatus from where extension may occur into the nasal cavity and any of the sinuses (62). The tumor has been a source of concern owing to its reportedly high recurrence rate and occasional association with malignant transformation. The recurrence rate may be related to inadequate removal, whereas the malignant transformation rate ranges from 0% to 55% in the literature, almost owing to a failure to recognize the presence of squamous cell carcinoma at the time of removal. The true potential for malignant transformation in large well-done series is less than 5%. However, inverted

Table 11 Benign Tumors Simulating Nasal Polyps

Anatomic
  Concha bullosa

Tumors
  Epithelial
    Papilloma (inverted, everted, cylindric)
    Minor salivary (pleomorphic adenoma)

  Mesenchymal
    Neurogenic (meningioma, schwannoma, neurofibroma)

  Vascular (hemangioma, angiofibroma)
  Fibro-osseous (ossifying fibroma)
  Muscular (leiomyoma, angioleiomyoma)

Granulomatous/inflammatory
  Wegener's granulomatosis
  Sarcoidosis
  Crohn's disease

papilloma may also occur in association with nasal polyposis, be bilateral, and infiltrate adjacent bone. This has led to diagnostic and management problems in the past and reinforces the need for submission of all tissue removed at surgery for histopathological examination.

Angiofibroma

Juvenile angiofibroma occurs almost exclusively in male children or adolescents who present with nasal obstruction and epistaxis (63). This may be combined with dacrocystitis, otitis media with effusion, swelling of the cheek, and, occasionally, visual loss. The tumor arises within the spehnopalatine foramen present in the nasal cavity and nasopharynx from where it may extend into the sphenoid. The lesion will spread laterally through the pterygopalatine region compressing the back wall of the maxillary sinus to dumb-bell into the infratemporal fossa, and from there may affect the orbit via the infra-orbital fissure. Biopsy of the lesion may result in life-threatening hemorrhage, but fortunately a combination of CT and MRI allows both the diagnosis and extent of the lesion to be determined accurately.

A number of other benign tumors may occur in the nose, all of which are extremely rare and in which a combination of biopsy and imaging will determine the histology, extent, and the most appropriate surgical approach for excision. These benign tumors involve other papillomas and minor salivary gland tumors, for example, pleomorphic adenomas. They may also involve benign mesenchymal tumors such as fibro-osseous-ossifying fibroma, vascular hemangioma, schwannomas, neurofibromas, and meningioma.

Inflammatory Granulomatous Conditions

Diseases such as Wegner's granulomatosis (64), sarcoidosis, and very rarely Crohn's disease (65) may present with granulomatous changes within the nose and the sinuses. It is exceptional, however, for these to simulate nasal polyps, and they are usually manifested by a friable granular mucosa associated with crusting and bleeding, pansinusitis, and ultimately loss of nasal structure and support.

Any malignant tumor may mimic nasal polyposis as could mucinous adenocarcinoma, which may effect both ethmoid labyrinths and produce bilateral lesions. Squamous cell carcinoma is the most common malignant neoplasm of the sinonasal region. However, the whole spectrum of histological types of tumors may occur of which the most common simulating localized nasal polyps are adenocarcinoma, olfactory neuroblastoma, and malignant melanoma (Table 12).

Differential Diagnosis of a Nasal Mass in Children

The differential diagnosis of a unilateral mass in the nose of a child includes congential lesions such as encephalocoele, glioma, dermoid cyst, and naso-

Table 12 Malignant Lesions Simulating Nasal Polyps

Epithelial
Squamous cell carcinoma
Adenocarcinoma
Adenoid cystic carcinoma
Acinic cell carcinoma
Mucoepidermoid carcinoma
Olfactory neuroblastoma
Malignant melanoma
Metastatic tumors (e.g., kidney, breast, pancreas)
Mesenchymal tumors
Lymphoma
Rhabdomyosarcoma
Chondrosarcoma
Ewing's sarcoma

lacrimal duct cyst and lesions such as craniopharyngioma, hemangioma, neurofibroma, and rhabdomyosarcoma. Imaging prior to any intervention is mandatory; optimally a combination of CT and MRI is aimed at defining the skull base defect and at determining the most appropriate surgical approach. When true nasal polyposis occurs cystic fibrosis must be suspected until proven otherwise (Table 13).

CONCLUSIONS

Nasal polyps are common, effecting almost 5% of the population. Their cause, however, remains unknown and is not the same in all patients. They have a clear association with asthma, aspirin-intolerance, cystic fibrosis, and chronic, nonallergic rhinosinusitis. Histologically, they contain large quantities of

Table 13 Differential Diagnosis of a Nasal Mass in a Child

Congenital
Encephalocoele
Glioma
Dermoid cyst
Nasolacrimal duct cyst
Neoplasia
Benign
Craniopharyngioma
Hemangioma
Neurofibroma
Malignant
Rhabdomyosarcoma

extracellular fluid, mast cell degranulation, and massive eosinophilic infiltration as well as lymphocytic infiltration. While this appearance suggests an allergic etiology, there is little conclusive evidence to support this. However, preliminary evidence suggests that in the absence of systemic allergy, a local allergic process could be the cause (66).

The definition of CRS with and without nasal polyposis continues to be evolving and requires understanding of a broader range of etiologies and pathogenesis in addition to bacterial or viral infections. We need to know whether the inflammation is of infectious or noninfectious origin. Although allergic fungal sinusitis is a well-defined clinical entity, the ubiquitous nature of fungal spores in the nasal mucus makes the role of fungal infection in patients without allergic fungal sinusitis difficult to determine, and currently the role of this condition in nasal polyposis remains unclear.

Endoscopic or microscopic sinus surgery of nasal polyps is considered only after failure of appropriate medical treatment. Excellent results can be achieved by functional endoscopic sinus surgery that utilizes endoscopic guidance or three-dimensional microscopic control with microdebriders. Furthermore, with the use of the currently available therapies, the results of surgery can be long-lasting.

Therapeutic options include pharmaco-therapies and surgery. The pharmaco-therapeutic approach includes antibiotics, systemic and topical steroids, and possibly antifungals and novel anti-inflammatory therapies such as the use of antibodies directed against a number of inflammatory cytokines, antileukotrienes, and low-dose macrolide therapy. In the case of massive nasal polyposis, modern surgical techniques will still have to be performed before the above-mentioned therapeutic options will be possible.

REFERENCES

1. Benninger ME, Ferguson BJ, Hadley JA, Hamilos DL, Jacobs M, Kennedy DW, Lanza DC, Marple BF, Osguthorpe JD, Stankiewicz JA, Anon J, Denneny J, Emanuel I, Levine H. Adult chronic rhinosinusitis: definitions, diagnosis, epidemiology, and pathophysiology. Otolaryngol Head Neck Surg 2003; 129L:S1–S32.
2. Lanza DC, Kennedy DW. Adult rhinosinusitis defined. Otolaryngol Head Neck Surg 1997; 117:S1–S7.
3. Bernstein JM, Ballow M, Schlievert PM, Rich G, Allen C, Dryja D. A superantigen hypothesis for the pathogenesis of chronic hyperplastic sinusitis with massive nasal polyposis. Am J Rhinol 2003; 17:321–326.
4. Brook I. Microbiology and antimicrobial management of sinusitis. Otolaryngol Clin North Am 2004; 37:253–266.
5. Brook I, Frazier EH. Correlation between microbiology and previous sinus surgery in patients with chronic maxillary sinusitis. Ann Otol Rhinol Laryngol 2001; 110:148–151.
6. Wald ER. Microbiology of acute and chronic sinusitis in children and adults. Am J Med Sci 1998; 316:13–20.

7. Bhattacharyya N. The role of infection in chronic rhinosinusitis. Curr Allergy Asthma Rep. 2002; 2:500–506.

8. Nord CE. The role of anaerobic bacteria in recurrent episodes of sinusitis and tonsillitis. Clin Infect Dis 1995; 20:1512–1524.

9. Brook I, Yocum P, Frazier EH. Bacteriology and beta-lactamase activity in acute and chronic maxillary sinusitis. Arch Otolaryngol Head Neck Surg 1996; 122:418–422.

10. Finegold SM, Flynn J, Rose FV, Jousimes-Somer H, Jakielaszek C, McTeague M, Wexler HM, Berkowitz E, Wynne B. Bacteriologic findings associated with chronic bacterial maxillary sinusitis in adults. Clin Infect Dis 2002; 35:428–433.

11. Brook I. Discrepancies in the recovery of bacteria from multiple sinuses and acute and chronic sinusitis. J Med Microbiol 2004; 53:879–885.

12. Ramadan HH, Farr RW, Wetmore SJ. Adenovirus and respiratory syncytial virus in chronic sinusitis using polymerase chain reaction. Laryngoscope 1997; 107:923–925.

13. Settipane GA. Epidemiology of nasal polyps. Allergy Asthma Proc 1996; 17: 231–236.

14. Greisner WA, Settipane GA. Hereditary factor for nasal polyps. Allergy Asthma Proc 1996; 17:283–286.

15. Grigoreas C, Vourdas D, Petalas K, Simeonidi S, Demeroutis I, Tsioulos T. Nasal polyps in patients with rhinitis and asthma. Allergy Asthma Proc 2002; 23:169–174.

16. Johansson L, Akerlund A, Holmberg K, Melen I, Bende M. Prevalence of nasal polyps in adults: Skovde population-based Study. Ann Otol Rhinol Laryngol 2003; 112:625–629.

17. Fritz SB, Terrell JE, Conner ER, Kukowska-Latallo JF, Baker JR. Nasal mucosal gene expression in patients with allergic rhinitis with and without nasal polyps. J Allergy Clin Immunol 2003; 112:1057–1063.

18. Larsen PL, Tos M. Origin of nasal polyps: an endoscopic autopsy study. Laryngoscope 2004; 114:710–719.

19. Slavin RG. Sinusitis in adults and its relation to allergic rhinitis, asthma, and nasal polyps. J Allergy Clin Immunol 1988; 82:950–956.

20. Holling TM, Schoote N, vanDenElsen PJ. Function and regulation of MHC class II molecules in T-lymphocytes: of mice and men. Hum Immunol 2004; 65: 282–290.

21. Opdahl H, Haugen T, Hagberg IA, Aspelin T, Lyberg T. Effects of short-term nitrogen monoxide inhalation on leukocyte adhesion molecules, generation of reactive oxygen species, and cytokine release in human blood. Nitric Oxide J 2000; 4:112–122.

22. Khair OA, Devalia JL, Abdelaziz MN, et al. Effect of erythromycin on *Haemophilus influenzae* endotoxin-induced release of IL-6, IL-8 and sICAM-1 by cultured human bronchial epithelial cells. Eur Respir J 1995; 9:1451–1457.

23. Mitseyama H, Kambe F, Murakami R, Cao X, Ishiguro N, Seo H. Calcium signaling pathway involving calcineurin regulates interleukin-8 gene expression through activation of NF-kappa B in human osteoblast-like cells. J Bone Miner Res 2004; 19:671–679.

24. Lu L, Chen SS, Zhang JQ, Ramires FJ, Sun Y. Activation of nuclear factor-kappa B and its proinflammatory mediator cascade in the infected rat heart. Biochem Biophys Res Commun 2004; 321:879–885.
25. DeCesaris P, Starace D, Sarace G, Fillippini A, Stefanini M, Ziparo E. Activation of Jun N-terminal kinase/activated protein kinase pathway by tumor necrosis factor-α leads to intercellular adhesion molecule-1 expression. J Biochem 1999; 274:278–282.
26. Maeda K, Kai K, Hayashi T, Hasegawa K, Matsumura T. Intercellular adhesion molecule-1 (ICAM-1) and lymphocyte function associated antigen-1 (LFA-1) contributes to the elimination of equine herpes virus type I (EHV-1) from the lungs of intranasally infected BALB/c mice. J Comp Pathol 2004; 130:162–170.
27. Rogala B, Namyslowski G, Marowka-Kata K, Gawlik R, Gabriel A. Concentration of s-ICAM-1 in nasal polyp tissue. Med Sci Monitor 2000; 6:1109–1112.
28. Papon JF, Coste A, Gendron MC, Cordonnier C, Wingerstmamm L, et al. HLA-DR and ICAM-1 expression and modulation in epithelial cells from nasal polyps. Laryngoscope 2002; 112:2067–2075.
29. Sanchez-Segura A, Brieva JA, Rodriguez C. T lymphocytes that infiltrate nasal polyps have a specialized phenotype and produce a mixed TH1/TH2 pattern of cytokines. J Allergy Clin Immunol 1998; 102:953–960.
30. Bernstein JM, Ballow M, Rich G, Allen C, Swanson M, Dmochowski J. Lymphocyte subpopulations and cytokines in nasal polyps: is there a local immune system in the nasal polyp? Otolaryngol Head Neck Surg 2004; 130(535):526–535.
31. Khatami S, Brummer E, Stevens DA. Effects of granulocyte-macrophage colony stimulating factor (GM-CSF) in vivo on cytokine production and proliferation by spleen cells. Clinical Exp Immunol 2001; 125:198–201.
32. Bernstein JM, Ballow WM, Schlievert PM, Rich G, Allen C, Dryja D. A superantigen hypothesis for the pathogenesis of chronic hyperplastic sinvsitis with massive polyposis. Am J Rhinol 2003; 17:321–326.
33. Bernstein JM. The molecular biology of nasal polyposis. Curr Allergy Asthma Rep 2001; 1:262–267.
34. Bocchino V, Bertorelli G, D'Ippolito R, Castagnaro A, Zhuo X, Grima P, DiComite V, Damia R, Olivieri D. The increased number of very late activation antigen-4-positive cells correlates with eosinophils and severity of disease in the induced sputum of asthmatic patients. J Allergy Clin Immunol 2000; 105:65–70.
35. Benimetskaya L, Loikej D, Khaled Z, Loike G, Silverstein SC, Cao L, el Koury J, Cai TQ, Stein CA. Mac-1 (CD11b/CD18) is an oligodeoxynucleotide-binding protein. Nat Med 1997; 3:412–420.
36. Lum AF, Green C, Lee GR, Staunton DE, Simon SI. Dynamic regulation of LFA-1 activation and neutrophil arrest on intercellular adhesion molecule-1 (ICAM-1) in shear flow. J Biol Chem 2002; 277:20660–20670.
37. Kakazu T, Chihara J, Saito A, Nakajima S. Effect of cytokine RANTES on induction of activated eosinophils. Jpn J Thoracic Dis 1995; 33:1226–1232.
38. Gorski P, Wittczak T, Walusiak J, Palczynski C, Ruta U, Kuna P, Alam R. Eotaxin but not MCP-3 induces eosinophil influx into nasal fluid in allergic patients. Allergy 2002; 57:519–528.

39. Lum AF, Green CE, Lee GR, Staunton DE, Simon SI. Dynamic regulation of LFA-1 activation and neutrophil arrest on intercellular adhesion molecule (ICAM-1) in shear flow. J Bio Chem 2002; 277:2660–2670.
40. Douglas IS, Leff AR, Sperling AI. CD4+ T-cell and eosinophil adhesion is mediated by specific ICAM-3 ligation and results in eosinophil activation. J Immunol 2000; 164:3385–3391.
41. Carlson M, Peterson C, Venge P. The influence of IL-3, IL-5, and GM-CSF on normal human eosinophil and neutrophil C3b-induced degranulation. Allergy 1993; 48:437–442.
42. Bernstein JM, Gorfien J, Noble B, Yankaskas JR. Nasal polyposis: immunohistiochemistry and bioelectrical findings (a hypothesis for the development of nasal polyps). J Allergy Clin Immunol 1997; 99:165–175.
43. Lundgren JD, Davey RT Jr, Lundgren B, Mullol J, Marom Z, Logun C, Baraniuk J, Kaliner MA, Shelhamer JH. Eosinophil cationic protein stimulates and major basic protein inhibits airway mucus secretion. J Allergy Clin Immunol 1991; 87:689–698.
44. Jacoby DE, Ueki JF, Witticombe JH, Loegering DA, Gleich GJ, Nadel JA. Effect of human eosinophil major basic protein on ion transport in the dog tracheal epithelium. Am Rev Respir Dis 1988; 137:13–16.
45. Baniyash M. TCR zeta-chain downregulation: curtailing an excessive inflammatory immune response. Nat Rev Immunol 2004; 467:675–687.
46. Luethviksson BR, Gunnlaugsdottir B. Transforming growth factor-β as a regulator of site-specific T-cell inflammatory response. Scan J Immunol 2003; 58:129–138.
47. Jaff A, Bush A. Anti-inflammatory effects of macrolides in lung disease. Ped Pulmonol 2001; 31:464–473.
48. Ehrlich GD, Veeh R, Wang X, Costerton JW, Hayes JD, Hu FZ, Daigle BJ, Ehrlich MD, Post JC. Mucosal biofilm formation on middle-ear mucosa in the chinchilla model of otitis media. JAMA 2002; 287:1710–1715.
49. Passali D, Bernstein JM, Passali FM, Damiani V, Passali GC, Bellusi L. Treatment of recurrent chronic hyperplastic sinusitis with nasal polyposis. Arch Otolaryngol Head Neck Surg 2003; 129:656–659.
50. Bez C, Schubert R, Kopp M, Ersfeld Y, Rosewich M, Kuehr J, Kamin W, Berg AV, Wahu U, Zielen S. Effect of anti-immunoglobulin E on nasal inflammation in patients with seasonal allergic rhino conjunctivitis. Clin Exp Allergy 2004; 34:1079–1085.
51. Leckie MJ. Anti-interleukin-5 monoclonal antibodies: pre-clinical evidence in asthma models. Am J Respir Med 2003; 2:245–259.
52. Stobie L, Gurunathan S, Prussin C, Sacks DL, Glaichenhaus M, Wu CY, Seder RA. The role of antigen and IL-12 in sustaining TH1 memory cells in vitro: IL12 is required to maintain memory/effector TH1 cells sufficient to mediate protection to an infectious parasite challenge. Proc Natl Acad Sci USA 2000; 97:8427–8432.
53. Bryan SA, O'Connor BJ, Matti S, Leckie MJ, Kanabar V, Khan J, Warrington SJ, Renzetti L, Rames A, Bock JA, Boyce MJ, Hansel TT, Holgate ST, Barnes PJ. Effects of recombinant human interleukin-12 on eosinophils, airway hyperresponsiveness and the late asthmatic response. Lancet 2000; 356:2149–2153.

54. Cimmino M, Cavalieri M, Nardone M, Plantulli A, Orefice A, Esposito V, Raia V. Clinical characteristics and genotype analysis of patients with cystic fibrosis and nasal polyposis. Clin Otolaryngol Allied Sci 2003; 48:125–132.

55. McClay JE, Marple B, Kapadia L, Biavatim J, Nussenbaum B, Newcomer M, Manning S, Booth T, Schwade N. Clinical presentation of allergic fungal sinusitis in children. Laryngoscope 2002; 112:565–569.

56. Moneret-Vautrin DA, Hsieh V, Wayoff M, Guyot JL, et al. Non-allergic rhinitis with eosinophilia syndrome; a precursor of the triad: nasal polyposis, intrinsic asthma and intolerance to aspirin. Ann Allergy 1990; 64:513–518.

57. Trittel C, Moller J, Euler HH, Werner JA. A differential diagnosis in chronic polypoid sinusitis (Churg–Strauss Syndrome). Laryngol Rhinol Otol 1995; 74: 577–580.

58. Moneret-Vautrin DA, Wayoff N, Bonn C. Mechanisms of aspirin intolerance. Annales I Oto-Laryngologie et de Chirurgie Cervico-Faciale 1985; 102:357–363.

59. Becker B, Morganroth K, Reinhardt D, Irlilch G. The dyskinetic cilia syndrome in childhood. Modifications of ultra-structural patterns. Respiration 1984; 46: 180–186.

60. DeIongh R, Ing A, Rutlend J. Mucociliary function, ciliary ultra-structure, and ciliary orientation in Young's Syndrome. Thorax 1992; 47:184–187.

61. Balbani AP, Marone SA, Butugan O, Saldiva PH. Young's syndrome: recurrent respiratory tract infections and azoospermia. Revista DaAssociacao Medica Brasileria 2000; 46:88–89.

62. Tsunoda R, Takooda S, Nishijima W, Ogawa M, Terada S. Inverted papillomas in the nose and paranasal sinuses. Nippon Jibiinkoka Gakkai Kaiho (J Otorhinolaryngol Soc Jpn) 1994; 97:912–918.

63. Jamal MN. Imaging and management of angiofibroma. Eur Arch Otorhinolaryngol 1994; 251:241–245.

64. Verschuur HP, Struyvenberg PA, van Benthem PP, van Rossum M, Hiemstra I, Hordijk GJ. Nasal discharge and obstruction as presenting symptoms of Wegner's granulomatosis in childhood. Ped Otorhinolaryngol 1993; 27:91–95.

65. Ernst A, Preyer S, Plauth M, Jenss H. Polypose pansinusitis als eine ungewohnliche-extraintestinale manifestation des morbus Crohn. HNO 1993; 41:33–36.

66. Bachert C, Gevaert P, Holtappls G, Johansson SG, vanCauwenberge P. Total and specific IgE in nasal polyps is related to local eosinophilic inflammation. J Allergy Clin Immunol 2001; 107:607–614.

19

Sinusitis of Odontogenic Origin

Itzhak Brook

Departments of Pediatrics and Medicine, Georgetown University School of Medicine, Washington, D.C., U.S.A.

John Mumford

Department of Periodontics, Naval Postgraduate Dental School, Bethesda, Maryland, U.S.A.

INTRODUCTION

Sinusitis of odontogenic source accounts for about one-tenth of all cases of maxillary sinusitis (1). The maxillary sinus is situated between the nasal and the oral cavities and is, therefore, the most susceptible of all sinuses to invasion by pathogenic bacteria through the nasal ostium or the oral cavity. Sinusitis originating from odontogenic source differs in its pathophysiology, microbiology, and management from sinusitis from other causes. It usually occurs when the Schneidarian membrane is disrupted by conditions such as those infections originating from maxillary teeth, maxillary dental trauma, odontogenic pathology of maxillary bone, or iatrogenic causes such as dental extractions, maxillary osteotomies in orthognathic surgery, and placement of dental implants (2). The treatment of sinusitis of odontogenic source often requires management of the sinus infection as well as the odontogenic source.

PATHOPHYSIOLOGY

The maxillary sinus emerges in the third fetal month and starts growing into the adjacent maxilla in the fifth fetal month. The final growth of the maxillary sinus occurs between 12 and 14 years of age and concurs with the formation of the permanent teeth and growth of the upper jaw alveolar process (3). Before the sinus reaches adult size, there is considerable distance between the sinus floor and the maxillary teeth apices. However, when the growth of the maxillary sinus is completed, its volume reaches 15 to 20 mL and it is surrounded by the orbital floor, the lateral nasal walls, and the dento-alveolar portion of the maxilla. It can even extend into the palatine and zygomatic bones.

Continued expansion and pneumatization of the maxillary sinus can persist throughout the life of dentate individuals, which may induce inferior displacement of the floor of the sinus in the direction of the maxillary posterior teeth roots (4). The maxillary teeth roots may protrude into the sinus cavity, resulting in surrounding of the apical aspects of the dental roots by the sinus mucoperiosteum (5,6).

A significant difference in the height of the sinus floor exists between dentulous and edentulous individuals. In individuals with maxillary tooth loss, pneumatization can progress inferiorly and create a recess in the part of the alveolar bone between the remaining teeth that was occupied before by the lost tooth. In the completely edentulous person, the sinus can expand and extend into the alveolar bone, occasionally leaving only thin alveolar bone between the sinus and the oral cavity (4). The placement of the dental implants in such patients requires preprosthetic surgical procedures such as alveolar ridge augmentation with bone grafting and sinus membrane elevation.

The roots of the maxillary premolar and molar teeth are situated below the sinus floor. The second molars' roots are the closest to the sinus floor, followed by the roots of the first molar, third molar, second premolar, first premolar, and canine (1). In contrast, the roots of the central and lateral incisors are not close to the maxillary sinus. The apex of the maxillary second molar root is the closest to the sinus floor (mean distance of 1.97 mm) and the apex of the buccal root of the maxillary first premolar is the furthest from the sinus floor (mean distance of 7.5 mm) (7). These short distances explain the easy extension of an infectious process from these teeth and the maxillary sinus.

The thickness of the lateral wall of the maxilla, which forms the anterior wall of the sinus, is 2 to 5 mm. The labial levator and the orbicularis oculi muscle attach to this wall above the infraorbital foramen and direct the spread of infection from the maxillary teeth to the maxillary sinus.

The incidence of sinusitis associated with odontogenic infections is very low despite the high frequency of dental infections. The floors of the sinus and nose are composed of very dense cortical bone and are most probably an effective barrier that rarely allows for direct penetration of odontogenic infections into the maxillary sinus or nasal floor. The weakness of the lateral wall of the maxilla can be penetrated more readily than the floor of the sinus, explaining why most odontogenic infections are manifested more often as soft tissue vestibular or facial space infections and not as sinusitis. However, odontogenic infections can drain into the sinus, especially in individuals whose dental roots are proximal to the floor of the maxillary sinus.

The closeness of the maxillary teeth to the antrum, which is especially evident in a pneumatized sinus, can sometimes leave only the mucoperiosteum (Schneidarian membrane) separating the sinus cavity from the roots of the tooth. The majority of maxillary sinus infections associated with odontogenic source occur as sequelae of dental caries that lead to pulpitis and dental abscess formation. Another rare, but possible, origin of pulpitis may occur as a result of severe periodontal disease. As bone loss progresses, it may involve a lateral canal or the apex of the tooth. Periodontal pathogens may then secondarily infect the pulpal tissues leading to a retrograde pulpitis (8). The bacterial virulence factors such as the enzymes collagenase, lysosomes, and toxins can enhance invasion and tissue breakdown. The odontogenic infections can perforate into the alveolar bone through the root-tip foramina at the apex of the tooth. The odontogenic infections can spread through the thin maxillary buccal alveolar bone into the buccal soft tissue. Infections originating from either the palatal root of the maxillary molars or the lateral incisor roots can sometimes spread subperiosteally and dissect into the hard palate. Odontogenic infections can also reach the orbit through the sinus or by alternative routes (9).

Iatrogenic dental causes can also account for maxillary sinusitis. Routine root canal therapy can initiate periapical inflammation at the floor of the sinus and instrumentation can even introduce bacteria into the sinus cavity, both of which can propagate rhinosinusitis (10). Other iatrogenic causes are displacement of a maxillary tooth root tip into the sinus that occurs during extraction, extrusion of materials used in root canal therapy into the sinus, and perforation of the sinus membrane during exodontias, periodontal surgery, or implant placement. During tooth extraction, significant forces are placed on the alveolar bone. Widely divergent roots, carious teeth, or heavily restored teeth may make the extraction more difficult because the roots tend to fracture under luxation. The remaining roots can sometimes be removed only by careful removal of alveolar bone surrounding them; at times, this process may remove thin bone separating sinus membrane from the oral cavity with a resultant exposure of the sinus.

The apical force employed on the roots during extraction can displace the root into the maxillary sinus. The presence of a periapical cyst, granuloma, or periapical infection that had eroded the surrounding bone can enable easier displacement of the tooth. An entire tooth can be displaced into the sinus, especially during removal of a maxillary third molar (wisdom tooth). Removal of teeth around a lone-standing molar can lead to alveolar bone resorption resulting in thinning of the alveolar bone between the oral cavity and the sinus. When that lone-standing molar is eventually extracted, alveolar bone or maxillary tuberosity fracture with concomitant oro-antral communication can occur. The risk of this occurring may increase if the tooth is ankylosed to the alveolar bone, where the periodontal ligament has become mineralized and fused to the bony socket.

Severe intrabony defects between teeth or within the furcation of maxillary teeth resulting from severe periodontal disease can also encroach on the sinus floor. The elimination of the periodontal pocket and arresting the disease process require the removal of periodontal pathogens from the diseased root surfaces and may require osseous resection of the intrabony defect. The sinus can be inadvertently exposed during resection of the intrabony defects or instrumentation of the diseased root surfaces within the involved furcation. Dental implant placement involving sinus lift procedures are becoming more commonplace for the replacement of missing maxillary posterior teeth. Although the reported incidence of infection is low, sinusitis can occur as a result of contamination of the sinus cavity by oral pathogens (11). Figures 1 and 2 demonstrate inadvertent sinus membrane perforation while performing a closed sinus lift in conjunction with dental implant placement. Other oral and maxillofacial surgery or dental procedures, such as maxillary orthognathic surgery, preprosthetic surgery,

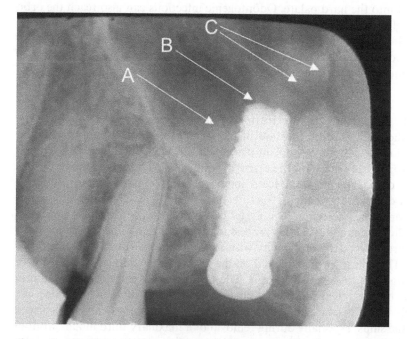

Figure 1 Maxillary sinusitis secondary to perforation of sinus membrane. Arrow A demonstrates the extent of the graft material within the maxillary sinus. Arrow B demonstrates the implant perforation of the sinus membrane. Arrow C demonstrates the graft material expressed beyond the sinus membrane.

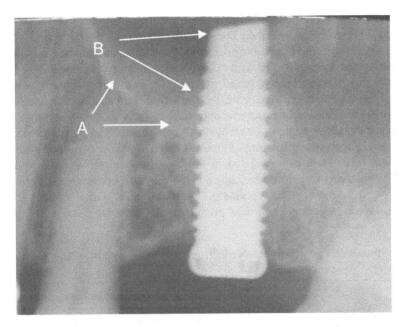

Figure 2 Perforation of the maxillary sinus during implant placement. Arrow A demonstrates the floor of the maxillary sinus. Arrow B demonstrates the implant perforating and extending into the maxillary sinus.

and the placement of implants without sinus lift procedures, have been implicated as causing sinusitis (12–14).

Oro-antral fistula can also be responsible for the development of maxillary sinusitis, especially of a chronic nature. These fistula are defined as an osteo-mucosal communication between the oral cavity and either the sinus or the nasal cavity. They are generally iatrogenic and occur following dental procedures such as extractions, removal of an intramaxillary cyst, or external maxillary sinus surgery. They can also be due to persistent apico-dental infection that forms a fistula into the antrum, necrosis of a maxillary tumor, and follow a surgical correction of cleft palates and lips.

MICROBIOLOGY

Streptococcus pneumoniae, Haemophilus influenzae, and *Moraxella catarrhalis* are the most common pathogens implicated in acute sinusitis (15), whereas anaerobic bacteria can be isolated from up to 67% of patients who have chronic infection (16,17). However, anaerobes were isolated from approximately 5% to 10% of patients with acute sinusitis, mostly from those who developed maxillary sinusitis secondary to odontogenic infection (15). It has been reported that sinusitis resulting from pathogenic bacteria originating from the oral cavity most commonly include Streptococci, anaerobic gram-positive cocci

(Peptostreptococci), and anaerobic gram-negative rods (fusobacteria, bacteroides) (11). We recently described our experience over a 30-year period of studying the aerobic and anaerobic microbiology of acute and chronic maxillary sinusitis that was associated with odontogenic infection (18). Aspirates of 20 acutely and 28 chronically infected maxillary sinuses that was associated with odontogenic infection were processed for aerobic and anaerobic bacteria (Table 1). A total of 37 isolates were recovered from the 20 cases of acute maxillary sinusitis (1.85/specimen), 16 aerobic and facultatives, and 21 anaerobic. Aerobic and facultative organisms alone were recovered in two specimens (10%), anaerobes only were isolated in 10 (50%), and mixed aerobic and anaerobic bacteria were recovered in eight (40%). The predominant aerobes were α-hemolytic streptococci (5), Microaerophilic streptococci (4), and *Staphylococcus aureus* (2). The predominant anaerobic bacteria were

Table 1 Predominant Bacteria Recovered from 48 Patients with Maxillary Sinusitis with an Odontogenic Origin[a]

	Number of isolates	
Bacteria	Acute sinusitis ($N=20$)	Chronic sinusitis ($N=28$)
Aerobic bacteria		
α-Hemolytic streptococci	5	7
Microaerophilic streptococci	4	5
Streptococcus pneumoniae	1	
Streptococcus pyogenes	1	2
Staphylococcus aureus	2 (2)	5 (5)
Staphylococcus epidermidis	1 (1)	1 (1)
Haemophilus influenzae	1	–
Subtotal aerobes	16 (3)	21 (6)
Anaerobic bacteria		
Peptostreptococcus species	12	16
Veilonella parvulla	3	2
Eubacterium species	1	2
Propionibacterium acne	2	3
Fusobacterium species	2 (1)	2
Fusobacterium nucleatum	7 (2)	10 (4)
Bacteroides species	4 (1)	5
Bacteroides fragilis group	–	2 (2)
Prevotella melaninogenica species	12 (5)	27 (9)
Porphyromonas asaccharolytica	6 (1)	7 (4)
Subtotal anaerobes	50 (10)	77 (19)
Total	66 (13)	98 (25)

[a]Number within parentheses indicates β-lactamase–producing bacteria.
Source: From Ref. 18.

anaerobic gram-negative bacilli (22), *Peptostreptococcus* spp., and *Fusobacterium* spp. (9). A total of 127 isolates were recovered from the 28 cases of chronic maxillary sinusitis (4.5 per patient): 50 aerobic and facultatives and 77 anaerobic. Aerobes and facultatives were recovered in three instances (11%), anaerobes only in 11 (39%), and mixed aerobic and anaerobic bacteria were recovered in 14 (50%). The predominant aerobes were α-hemolytic streptococci (7), microaerophilic streptococci (4), and *S. aureus* (5). The predominant anaerobes were anaerobic gram-negative bacilli (36), *Peptostreptococcus* spp. (16), and *Fusobacterium* spp. (12). No correlation was found between the predisposing odontogenic conditions and the microbiological findings.

These findings illustrate the unique microbiology of acute and chronic maxillary sinusitis associated with odontogenic infection, where anaerobic bacteria predominate in both types of infections. *S. pneumoniae, H. influenzae,* and *M. catarrhalis,* the predominate bacteria recovered from acute maxillary sinusitis not of odontogenic origin (15,19), were mostly absent in acute maxillary sinusitis that was associated with an odontogenic origin. In contrast, anaerobic bacteria predominated in both acute as well as chronic sinusitis. However, the number of both aerobic and anaerobic isolates in infected sinuses associated with odontogenic origin was similar in chronic sinusitis and acute sinusitis. A higher number of aerobic and anaerobic organisms per specimen were also found in chronic ethmoid, frontal, maxillary, and sphenoid sinusitis that were not associated with an odontogenic origin as compared to acute infections in these sinuses (19).

The most common anaerobic isolates recovered in this study in acute and chronic infection were *Peptostreptococcus* spp., *Fusobacterium* spp., pigmented *Prevotella,* and *Porphyromonas* spp., all members of the oropharyngeal flora (20). These organisms also predominate in periodontal and endodontal infection (21–23). The high recovery rate of these anaerobic bacteria in maxillary sinusitis of odontogenic origin is similar to the findings in chronic maxillary, ethmoid, frontal, and sphenoid sinusitis where these organisms also predominate (15–17,19).

Dental infections are generally mixed polymicrobial aerobic and anaerobic bacterial infections caused by the same families of oral microorganisms made of obligate anaerobes and gram-positive aerobes (21). Because anaerobic bacteria are part of the normal oral flora and outnumber aerobic organisms by a ratio of 1:10 to 1:100 at this site (20), it is not surprising that they predominant in odontogenic infections. There are at least 350 morphological and biochemically distinct bacterial species that colonize the oral and dental ecologic sites. The microorganisms recovered from odontogenic infections generally reflect the host's indigenous oral flora.

The polymicrobial nature of dental infections was evident in many studies (21–23). A study that evaluated the microbiology of 32 periapical abscesses highlighted the polymicrobial nature and importance of anaerobic bacteria in this infection (Table 2) (22). Seventy-eight bacterial isolates,

Table 2 Predominate Bacteria Isolates Recovered from 32 Perapical Abscesses

Bacteria	Number of isolates
Aerobic bacteria	
α-Hemolytic streptococcus	11
Streptococcus faecalis	3
Streptococcus milleri	3
Staphylococcus aureus	1
Haemophilus parainfluenzae	2
Subtotal aerobes	23
Anaerobic bacteria	
Peptostreptococcus species	18
Veilonella parvulla	2
Eubacterium species	2
Fusobacterium species	9
Bacteroides fragilis group	2
Prevotella melaninogenica	3
Prevotella oralis	4
Prevotella oris-buccae	2
Prevotella intermedia	2
Porphyromonas gingivalis	7
Subtotal anaerobes	55
Total	78

Source: From Ref. 22.

55 anaerobic, and 23 aerobic and facultative, were recovered. Anaerobic bacteria only were present in 16 (50%) patients, aerobic and facultatives in 2 (6%), and mixed aerobic and anaerobic flora in 14 (44%). The predominant isolates were *Peptostreptococcus, Bacteroides, Prevotella*, and *Porphyromonas* spp., mainly *Porphyromonas gingivalis*. The major aerobic pathogen was streptococci and there were few gram-negative organisms.

The association between periapical abscesses and sinusitis was established in a study of aspirate of pus from five periapical abscesses of the upper jaw and their corresponding maxillary sinusitis (23). Polymicrobial flora was found in all instances where the number of isolates varied from two to five. Anaerobes were recovered from all specimens. The predominant isolates were *Prevotella, Porphyromonas, Peptostreptococcus* spp., and *Fusobacterium nucleatum*. Concordance in the microbiological findings between the periapical abscess and the maxillary sinus flora was found in all instances. These findings confirm the importance of anaerobic bacteria in periapical abscesses and demonstrate their predominance in maxillary sinusitis that is associated with them. The concordance in recovery of organisms in paired infections illustrates the dental origin of the infection with subsequent extension into the maxillary sinus. The proximity of the maxillary molar teeth to the floor of the maxillary sinus allows such a spread.

Certain organisms were only present at one site and not the other (23). The discrepancies in isolation of certain organisms generally not recovered from infected sinuses, such as *P. gingivalis, Streptococcus sanguis,* and *Streptococcus milleri,* suggests that these organisms do not thrive well in the sinus cavity. These organisms were also not recovered in the infected sinuses in this report. However, other organisms such as *Peptostreptococcus* spp., *Prevotella intermedia,* and *Fusobacterium* spp. were isolated in both sites. These organisms were also recovered in the infected sinuses in this report.

The higher frequent recovery of anaerobes in chronic sinusitis associated with an odontogenic origin may be related to the poor drainage and increased intranasal pressure that develops during inflammation (24). This can reduce the oxygen tension in the inflamed sinus (25) by decreasing the mucosal blood flow and depressing the ciliary action (26). The lowering of the oxygen content and the pH of the sinus cavity supports the growth of anaerobic organisms by providing them with an optimal oxidation-reduction potential (27).

SYMPTOMS

Dental pain, headache, and anterior maxillary tenderness can be present in conjunction with sinusitis-like symptoms such as nasal congestion and discharge with or without a postnasal drip. However, there may be minimal sinusitis symptoms and dental pain because there is no osteomeatal obstruction and the sinus stay open. This allows for the pressure in the tooth to be relieved as the infection drains superiorly into an open sinus space. The clinical symptoms gradually increase as the sinusitis worsens.

Dental symptoms may vary from an acute pain that is associated with an exposed dental nerve to a dull pain originating from a dental infection extending into the bone around the apex of a root. The pain can also originate from periodontal disease, gum disease involving the supporting hard and soft tissues around teeth. Dental aches and increased sensitivity of several adjacent maxillary teeth frequently occur on patients with acute sinusitis who do not suffer from an odontogenic problem. What makes the diagnosis more difficult is that referred pain from symptomatic teeth to adjacent structures is also common.

Obtaining history of past sinus disease, oro-antral communication, allergic rhinitis, or foreign body displacement into the sinus cavity can assist in making the correct diagnosis. It is often difficult to determine whether the patient's symptoms originate from the sinus or an odontogenic source, and this dilemma may lead to the performance of unnecessary root canal therapy or tooth extraction. Performance of a thorough dental and sinus evaluation that utilizes adequate radiological studies can assist in establishing the correct diagnosis.

DIAGNOSIS

The diagnosis of sinus disease of odontogenic origin is based on thorough dental and medical examinations that include the evaluation of the patient's symptoms and past medical history, and correlating them with the present physical findings. Physical examination includes inspection of the buccal soft tissue, the vestibule for swelling, and the erythema. In addition, determination of current or past symptoms of a toothache, persistent sensitivity to percussion and/or thermal changes, tooth mobility, recent dental procedures (including root canals, periodontal surgery, or implant placement), and a periapical radiograph should be considered, even though this finding is rarely seen in association with maxillary sinusitis. Soft tissue swelling is rarely caused by maxillary sinusitis because of the absence of anastomosing veins connected to the overlying subcutaneous tissue, even though lengthy chronic sinusitis may eventually erode the wall of the sinus causing a visible intraoral soft tissue swelling (28).

An apical root that is diseased can be the nidus for a bacterial sinusitis. Palpation of the anterior maxilla can produce a dull pain and careful percussion of the maxillary teeth can reveal if the pain can be localized to one or more teeth. Assessment of the vitality of the teeth using electric or thermal pulp testing can aid in the diagnosis. Otolaryngological evaluation using rhinoscopy, nasal and sinus endoscopy, and aspiration of sinus contents for cytological and microbiological assessments can further assist in making the correct diagnosis.

Radiological imaging is an important tool in establishing the correct diagnosis. Whereas a periapical radiograph is the image preferred in determining a dental abscess or periodontal disease, the panoramic radiographic view is very helpful for evaluating the relationship of the maxillary teeth and periapical pathology to the maxillary sinus (Fig. 3A and B). In addition, the panoramic view is helpful in identifying the presence of pneumatization, pseudocysts, and the location of displaced roots, teeth, or foreign bodies inside the maxillary sinus. A Water's view plain-film radiograph is an acceptable alternative to a panoramic radiograph. However, the CT scan is the golden standard for adequate maxillary sinus imaging because of the ability to visualize bone and soft tissue and obtain thin sections and multiple views. Axial and coronal sinus CT views can demonstrate the relationship of a periapical abscess to a sinus floor defect and the diseased tissues and determine the exact location of a foreign body within the maxillary sinus. Delayed retrieval of a foreign body from the maxillary sinus may require additional imaging studies, such as a CT scan, especially when the position cannot be verified by plain radiographs or if significant sinus disease is involved.

MANAGEMENT

The association between an odontogenic condition and maxillary sinusitis warrants a thorough dental examination of patients with sinusitis.

(A)

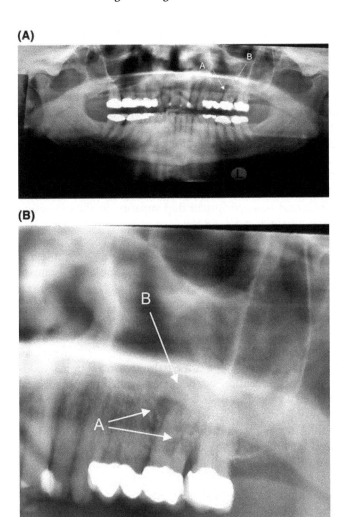

(B)

Figure 3 (**A**) Maxillary sinusitis secondary to dental abscess. Arrow A demonstrates the floor of the maxillary sinus. Arrow B demonstrates the periapical abscess extending into the maxillary sinus. (**B**) Enlarged view.

Concomitant management of the dental origin and the associated sinusitis will insure complete resolution of the infection and may prevent recurrence and complications.

A combination of medical and surgical approaches is generally required for the treatment of odontogenic sinusitis. Elimination of the source of the infection (e.g., removal of an external dental root from the sinus cavity, removal of failed endosseous implants in communication with the sinus cavity, extraction, or root canal therapy of an infected tooth) is necessary to prevent recurrence of the sinusitis.

When displacement of a root or entire tooth into the sinus has occurred, removal of the root tip through the socket is indicated. However, if no perforation of the sinus membrane has occurred and the dental root fragment is not infected and is 3 mm or less, the root can be left in place (29). Sinus precautions and medical treatment including decongestants and antibiotics are employed. The patient should be closely monitored for signs of sinus infection until the anatomical defect heals completely.

Removal of the dental root tip is indicated when it is infected or when its size is greater than 3 mm (29). The surgical removal is performed by reflection of a full-thickness mucoperiosteal flap superior to the extraction socket or in the canine-premolar recess. Bone is removed to form a window in the buccal alveolar process and the root tip is retrieved. This technique is advantageous to extraction through widening the extraction socket, especially in the posterior maxillary areas (second and third molars). Removal through the extraction socket can result in creating a large oro-antral communication. If the primary closure with a buccal flap fails, more significant flap advancement can be used. In instances where retrieval of the root or tooth is unsuccessful, treatment with antibiotics and decongestants is administered, and sinus precaution instructions are employed. Retrieval can be postponed, and is eventually performed through a modified Caldwell-Luc approach. A new application of the lateral wall sinus lift surgical approach to the maxillary sinus can also be used for the retrieval of root fragments and foreign objects (30).

A low rate of infection is associated with sinus lift procedures, where bone grafts are placed into the maxillary sinus cavity; however, in patients who develop sinus infections, removal of the graft material and the implant is required (11).

Endoscopic techniques have been developed in recent years for the treatment of chronic maxillary sinusitis of dental origin. The procedure evolves the creation of an antrostomy window through which the irreversibly diseased tissue, polyps, and foreign materials are removed (31).

The management of oro-antral communication that can complicate dental surgery includes primary closure of the defect and adequate medical treatment. A defect smaller than 5 mm will usually heal spontaneously with normal blood clot formation and routine mucosal healing (32). However, utilization of a resorbable barrier to cover and protect the defect during the initial stages of healing may be indicated. Primary closure is necessary if the defect is greater than 5 mm. Surgery should be performed in a disease-free sinus environment with the infection under control.

Although odontogenic therapy and surgical drainage are of primary importance, administration of antimicrobial therapy is an essential part of the management of patients with serious odontogenic infections and their complications. Similarly, the management of sinusitis includes proper anti-microbial therapy and surgical drainage when improvement is delayed or absent. Oral administration of antibiotics that are effective against oral flora and sinus pathogens for 21 to 28 days is required. Additionally administered are systemic nasal decongestants, local nasal decongestant for two to three days, moisturizing nasal drops, and saline sprays.

A growing number of anaerobic gram-negative bacilli (i.e., pigmented *Prevotella* and *Fusobacterium* spp.,) have acquired resistance to penicillin through the production of the enzyme β-lactamase (33). This has also been observed in our recent report (18), where 10 β-lactamase–producing bacteria (BLPB) were recovered from 7 (35%) specimens of acute sinusitis and 25 BLPB were recovered from 21 patients (75%) with chronic sinusitis. Penicillin was considered the drug of choice for the therapy of such infections because of the susceptibility of most oral pathogens; however, the growing resistance of these strains limits the use of this drug.

The recovery of penicillin-resistant organisms in patients with maxillary sinusitis associated with an odontogenic origin may require the administration of antimicrobial agents also effective against these organisms. These include clindamycin, cefoxitin, a carbapenem (i.e., imipenem, meropenem), or the combination of a penicillin and a β-lactamase inhibitor (21). Metronidazole should be administered with an agent effective against the aerobic or facultative streptococci. Alternative therapy for penicillin-allergic patients have been reported and include cefaclor, trimethoprim–sulfamethoxazole, and clindamycin (11).

SUMMARY

Odontogenic sinusitis is a well-recognized condition and accounts for approximately 8% to 12% of cases of maxillary sinusitis. An odontogenic source should be considered in individuals with symptoms of maxillary sinusitis with a history of odontogenic infection, dento-alveolar surgery, periodontal surgery, or in those resistant to conventional sinusitis therapy. Diagnosis usually requires a thorough dental and clinical evaluation including appropriate radiographs. The most common causes of odontogenic sinusitis include dental abscesses and periodontal disease that had perforated the Schneidarian membrane, irritation and secondary infection caused by intra-antral foreign bodies, and sinus perforations during tooth extraction or endosseous implant placement, with or without sinus lift procedures. An odontogenic infection is a polymicrobial aerobic–anaerobic infection with anaerobes outnumbering the aerobes. The most common isolates include anaerobic streptococci and gram-negative bacilli, and enterobacteriaceae. Surgical and dental treatment of the odontogenic pathological conditions combined with medical therapy is indicated. When present, an odontogenic foreign body should be surgically removed. Surgical management of oro-antral communication is indicated to reduce the likelihood of causing chronic sinus disease. The management of odontogenic sinusitis includes a three- to four-week course of antimicrobials effective against the oral flora pathogens.

REFERENCES

1. Maloney PL, Doku HC. Maxillary sinusitis of odontogenic origin. J Can Dent Assoc 1968; 34:591–603.
2. Kretzschmar DP, Kretzschmar JL. Rhinosinusitis: review from a dental perspective. Oral Surg Oral Med Oral Pathol Oral Radiol Endod 2003; 96:128–135.
3. Abubaker A. Applied anatomy of the maxillary sinus. Oral Maxillofac Clin N Am 1999; 11:1–14.
4. Sicher H. The viscera of head and neck. Oral Anatomy. St Louis (MO): CV Mosby, 1975:418–424.
5. Kelley HC, Kay LW. The maxillary sinus and its dental implications. Dental Practice Handbook. Bristol (UK): John Wright and Sons 1975:1–13.
6. Skillern RH. Maxillary sinus. The Catarrhal and Suppurative Diseases of the Accessory Sinus of the Nose. Philadelphia: JB Lippincott, 1947:104–125.
7. Eberhardt JA, Torabinejad M, Christiansen EL. A computed tomographic study of the distances between the maxillary sinus floor and the apices of the maxillary posterior teeth. Oral Surg Oral Med Oral Pathol Oral Radiol Endod 1992; 73:345.
8. Simon J, Glick D, Frank A. The relationship of endodontic–periodontic lesions. J Periodont 1972; 43:202–208.
9. Mehra P, Caiazzo A, Bestgen S. Odontogenic sinusitis causing orbital cellulitis: a case report. J Am Dent Assoc 1999; 130:1086–1092.
10. Watzek G, Bernhart T, Ulm C. Complications of sinus perforations and their management in endodontics. Dent Clin North Am 1997; 41:563–583.
11. Misch C. The pharmacologic management of maxillary sinus elevation surgery. J Oral Implantol 1992; 18:15–23.
12. Ueda M, Kaneda T. Maxillary sinusitis caused by dental implants: report of two cases. J Oral Maxillofac Surg 1992; 50:285–287.
13. Timmenga N, Raghoebar GM, Boering G, Weissenbruch RV. Maxillary sinus function after sinus lifts for the insertion of dental implants. J Oral Maxillofac Surg 1997; 55:936–939.
14. Regev E, Smith R, Perrott D, Pogrel M. Maxillary sinus complications related to endosseous implants. Int J Maxillofac Implants 1995; 10:451–461.
15. Nash D, Wald E. Sinusitis. Pediatr Rev 2001; 22:111–117.
16. Brook I. Bacteriology of chronic maxillary sinusitis in adults. Ann Otol Rhinol Laryngol 1989; 98:426–428.
17. Nord CE. The role of anaerobic bacteria in recurrent episodes of sinusitis and tonsillitis. Clin Infect Dis 1995; 20:1512–1524.
18. Brook I. Microbiology of acute and chronic maxillary sinusitis associated with an odontogenic origin. Laryngoscope 2005; 115:823–825.
19. Brook I. Microbiology and antimicrobial management of sinusitis. Otolaryngol Clin North Am 2004; 37:253–266.

20. Socransky SS, Manganiello SD. The oral microbiota of man from birth to senility. J Periodontol 1971; 42:485–496.
21. Brook I. Microbiology and management of endodontic infections in children. J Clin Pediatr Dent 2003; 28:13–17.
22. Brook I, Frazier EH, Gher ME. Aerobic and anaerobic microbiology of periapical abscess. Oral Microbiol Immunol 1991; 6:123–125.
23. Brook I, Frazier EH, Gher ME. Microbiology of periapical abscesses and associated maxillary sinusitis. J Periodontol 1996; 67:608–610.
24. Drettner B, Lindholm CE. The borderline between acute rhinitis and sinusitis. Acta Otolaryngol (Stockh) 1967; 64:508–513.
25. Carenfelt C, Lundberg C. Purulent and non-purulent maxillary sinus secretions with respect to pO_2, pCO_2 and pH. Acta Otolaryngol (Stockh) 1977; 84: 138–144.
26. Aust R, Drettner B. Oxygen tension in the human maxillary sinus under normal and pathological conditions. Acta Otolaryngol (Stockh) 1974; 78:264–269.
27. Carenfelt C. Pathogenesis of sinus empyema. Ann Otol Rhinol Laryngol 1979; 88:16–20.
28. Rafetto L. Clinical examination of the maxillary sinus. Oral Maxillofac Surg Clin N Am 1999; 11:35–44.
29. Gonty A. Diagnosis and management of sinus disease. In: Peterson LJ, ed. Philadelphia: J.B Lippincott 1992:225–266.
30. Uckan S, Buchbinder D. Sinus lift approach for the retrieval of root fragments from the maxillary sinus. Int J Oral Maxillofac Surg 2003; 32:87–90.
31. Lopatin A, Sysolyatin SP, Sysolyatin PG, Melnikov MN. Chronic maxillary sinusitis of dental origin: is external surgical approach mandatory? Laryngoscope 2002; 112:1056–1059.
32. Laskin D. Management of oroantral fistula and other sinus-related complications. Oral Maxillofac Clin North Am 1999; 11:155–164.
33. Brook I, Calhoun L, Yocum P. Beta-lactamase-producing isolates of Bacteroides species from children. Antimicrob Agents Chemother 1980; 18:164–166.

20

Fungal Sinusitis

Carol A. Kauffman

*Division of Infectious Diseases, University of Michigan Medical School,
Veterans Affairs Ann Arbor Healthcare System, Ann Arbor, Michigan, U.S.A.*

INTRODUCTION

Fungal sinusitis spans a wide clinical spectrum that includes acute fulminant invasive infection in immunocompromised hosts, chronic infection in individuals who are not immunosuppressed, and allergic disease. Current classification schemes separate fungal sinusitis into four categories. The definitions of the four major forms of fungal sinusitis are as follows:

- Acute invasive fungal sinusitis—rapid invasion of fungi through the mucosa of the nasal cavity or sinuses into soft tissues and blood vessels of the face, orbit, and cavernous sinus accompanied by hemorrhagic infarction and necrosis
- Chronic invasive fungal sinusitis—subacute to chronic infection characterized by invasion through the mucosa of the sinuses leading to destruction of the bony structures of the sinuses and orbit and subsequent spread to the brain
- Mycetoma—masses of fungal hyphae that grow in the sinus cavity but do not invade through the mucosa, also termed a fungus ball
- Allergic fungal sinusitis—allergic response of the host to colonization of the sinuses by certain molds; this is not an infectious process

The fungi causing sinusitis are almost always molds; it is exceedingly uncommon to see fungal sinusitis caused by yeast-like organisms. The molds

419

that cause fungal sinusitis are ubiquitous in the environment; thus, exposure is quite common and disease is primarily determined by the status of the host. Local factors, such as nasal polyps and the presence of atopy in the host, are important in the development of allergic fungal sinusitis. Acute invasive infection occurs almost entirely in markedly immunosuppressed patients. The clinical manifestations of the four forms of fungal sinusitis differ, as might be expected, as does the approach to treatment. Not unexpectedly, overlap can occur with these four syndromes in some patients.

EPIDEMIOLOGY

The Organisms

The fungi most commonly found to cause invasive sinusitis belong to the genus *Aspergillus* (1–5) (Table 1). *Aspergillus fumigatus* and *Aspergillus flavus* cause most infections, while other species of *Aspergillus* have uncommonly been associated with invasive infection (2,6,7). Patients with chronic invasive sinusitis in the United States are usually infected with *A. fumigatus* (3); however, in the Middle East and India, chronic sinusitis is almost always due to *A. flavus* (8,9).

Other hyaline or non-pigmented filamentous fungi, in addition to *Aspergillus* species, are the causative agents of all forms of fungal sinusitis. Typical molds from this group that cause sinusitis include *Fusarium* species, *Pseudallescheria boydii* (*Scedosporium apiospermum*), and *Paecilomyces* species (2,10–14). In markedly immunosuppressed hosts, especially those who are neutropenic, acute invasion is the rule. In the older, non-immunosuppressed host, chronic invasion occurs with these fungi. Mycetoma and,

Table 1 Fungal Sinusitis: Risk Factors and Most Common Etiological Agents

Clinical syndrome	Risk factors	Usual organisms
Acute invasive fungal sinusitis	Hematologic malignancy Transplant recipient Diabetes with ketoacidosis Deferoxamine therapy HIV infection Corticosteroids	*Aspergillus* Zygomycetes
Chronic invasive fungal sinusitis	Diabetes mellitus	*Aspergillus*
Mycetoma (fungus ball)	Corticosteroids Chronic sinusitis	*Aspergillus* Dematiaceous fungi
Allergic fungal sinusitis	Atopy, nasal polyps	Dematiaceous fungi *Aspergillus*

rarely, allergic fungal sinusitis have also been described in association with the non-*Aspergillus* hyaline molds (15–17).

Dematiaceous or pigmented molds are the major cause of allergic fungal sinusitis, but can also cause mycetoma, chronic invasive infection, and uncommonly, acute invasive infection in immunocompromised hosts (17–20). Infection with these fungi is also known as phaeohyphomycosis. Organisms in this group include *Bipolaris, Curvularia, Alternaria, Exserohilum,* and *Cladosporium* (21,22).

The zygomycetes, *Rhizopus, Mucor, Rhizomucor,* and less commonly, *Absidia* and *Cunninghamella,* are prominent pathogens causing acute invasive fungal sinusitis (23–25). The zygomycetes rarely cause any of the other types of fungal sinusitis.

The Host

Almost without exception, acute invasive fungal sinusitis is seen in immunocompromised hosts (Table 1). The groups at highest risk include those with hematological malignancies, those receiving a solid organ or hematopoietic stem cell transplant, insulin-dependent diabetics, those treated with deferoxamine for iron overload states or with corticosteroids for a variety of diseases, and patients with HIV infection (2,4,6,10,12–14,23,26–35).

Patients with hematological malignancies are at risk for invasive fungal sinusitis primarily while they are neutropenic; those with prolonged severe neutropenia are at most risk (2,23,26,29). The addition of corticosteroids and broad-spectrum antibiotic therapy contribute to the risk of developing invasive sinusitis. Among those who have received a hematopoietic stem cell transplant, the greatest risk is in the immediate post-transplant period before engraftment and late after transplant with the development of graft-versus-host disease (GVHD) that almost always requires intensive immunosuppression (4,13,27,30).

Solid organ transplant recipients are at less risk for invasive fungal sinusitis than those who have received a hematopoietic stem cell transplant. However, those who require intensive immunosuppression for graft rejection and those who have concomitant cytomegalovirus (CMV) infection are at increased risk (33–36). Interestingly, lung transplant recipients who have higher rates of pulmonary infection with *Aspergillus* than recipients of other organs rarely manifest invasive fungal sinusitis (35).

Corticosteroids are a cofactor for fungal invasion in many of the patients in the risk groups just described, but, when used alone, they also appear to place patients at risk for acute invasive sinusitis (32).

In addition to the above risk groups, several unique populations have an increased risk of developing acute invasive sinusitis due to zygomycetes. Diabetics are especially at risk for infection when they are insulin-dependent and develop ketoacidosis (25). Ketoacidosis appears to be important because of its detrimental effects on neutrophil chemotaxis, phagocytosis, and killing (37), essential for defense against the zygomycetes. Use of the iron chelator, deferoxamine, for removing excess iron that accumulates with multiple transfusions, places patients at risk for infection with certain zygomycetes, most notably *Rhizopus* species (31). *Rhizopus* is able to link to deferoxamine, using it as a siderophore to obtain iron, a necessary growth factor.

In contrast to acute invasive sinusitis, most patients with chronic invasive fungal sinusitis are not immunosuppressed. The patients are usually older and may have non-insulin dependent diabetes mellitus (3,5,18,38). Corticosteroids are frequently used as initial therapy before the correct diagnosis is made and undoubtedly contribute to the progression of disease, but not to its initial development (38). There is usually no obvious exposure to the infecting fungus.

Primary paranasal granuloma is a form of chronic invasive fungal sinusitis that is seen in healthy young men who have no underlying illness. This disease is described almost entirely from rural semi-arid areas of the Middle East or the Indian subcontinent (8,9,39).

The situation with sinus mycetoma is similar to that of chronic invasive fungal sinusitis in that the patients who develop mycetomas are not immunosuppressed. However, there is almost always a history of recurrent episodes of sinusitis and, in some, a history of nasal polyps (1,16,40).

The typical patient with allergic fungal sinusitis is young or middle-aged and has no underlying immunosuppression or other chronic systemic diseases. These patients do have a history of atopy manifested by rhinitis and/or asthma, recurrent sinusitis, and nasal polyposis that can be severe (17,41).

PATHOGENESIS

Acute invasive sinusitis is characterized by rapid spread into the bony structures of the sinuses and orbit and subsequent progression in a matter of days to involve the major vessels in the cavernous sinus and the brain (1,6,23). The organisms that cause this syndrome have the propensity to invade blood vessels causing thrombosis, hemorrhage, and tissue infarction. Patients with neutropenia have a minimal host response and death ensues quickly (42). Those who are not neutropenic have a more vigorous host response, but because of host factors such as ketoacidosis or deferoxamine therapy, or organism factors, especially when a zygomycete is involved, host defenses are ineffective and thrombosis, tissue necrosis, and rapid death ensue (24,31).

Chronic invasive fungal sinusitis contrasts with the acute form in that it progresses slowly over weeks to months, and the host response is a mixture of necrotizing and granulomatous inflammation (1,3,8,18). The difference in the pathogenesis of this infection from that of acute invasive sinusitis is related to the normal numbers of functioning neutrophils and macrophages that are present. The invading fungi, primarily *Aspergillus*, are the same in both forms of sinusitis. Destruction of the bony structures of the sinuses is usual. The mass of hyphae and the inflammatory response frequently extend into the posterior aspect of the orbit, impinge on the optic nerve, and may extend into the brain.

Primary paranasal granuloma is similar in pathogenesis, but described mostly in reports from Sudan, other Middle Eastern countries, and India (8,9). The host response is granulomatous. The few differences that exist between primary paranasal granuloma and chronic invasive sinusitis probably reflect the rapidity with which the diagnosis is made, host differences, and perhaps the dominant role played by *A. flavus* in primary paranasal granuloma.

Mycetoma formation is similar to that noted in pulmonary mycetomas, which develop in existing cavitary pulmonary lesions (43). The maxillary sinuses are almost always involved (40). The fungi are able to grow luxuriantly, forming a mass of hyphae that expands and can cause necrosis of adjacent bony structures. However, invasion through the mucosa and growth in the bone does not occur. Obstruction of drainage from the sinus creates many of the symptoms and signs.

The pathophysiology of allergic fungal sinusitis has not been clearly elucidated. However, it is clear that this disease happens almost entirely in atopic individuals and that sensitization to fungal antigens is crucial for the development of symptoms and signs. Two different theories exist. One theory relates the pathogenesis to a type I immediate hypersensitivity response involving eosinophils and IgE (44), and the other relates disease to antigen–antibody complexes, triggering cytokine release (17,41). Whichever mechanism initiates the hypersensitivity response, the end result is edema, which obstructs sinus drainage, thus allowing further proliferation of fungi and increased inflammatory reaction. Although the condition may begin in one sinus, frequently many or all sinuses are involved as the disease progresses.

One of the cardinal features of allergic fungal sinusitis is the production of allergic mucin, a substance that has been described as peanut butter–like because of its tenacious character; this substance fills and obstructs the sinuses. Microscopically, allergic mucin is composed of eosinophils, Charcot–Leyden crystals, cellular debris, and hyphae (41). Neutrophils and macrophages are absent.

Clinical Manifestations

Patients with acute invasive fungal sinusitis almost always have sinus or facial pain that is out of proportion to the physical findings. In addition, headache, purulent or bloody rhinorrhea, decreased smell and taste, and visual changes are frequently noted. Fever is common and these patients appear acutely ill. On physical examination, facial asymmetry, periorbital swelling, and dusky-colored or black lesions on the nasal mucosa or the palate can be seen; tenderness over the sinuses, hypesthesia of the palate or nasal mucosa, and absence of bleeding on light abrasion of the nasal mucosa can be elicited. As the infection progresses, symptoms related to ophthalmic and central nervous system invasion occur; these include stroke, mental status changes, cranial nerve palsies, proptosis, ophthalmoplegia, chemosis, and blindness.

Chronic invasive fungal sinusitis is usually manifested by facial pain and swelling, but the acuity of the presentation is much less than that noted with acute invasive sinusitis (3). Fever is usually absent and the patients do not appear acutely ill. When the orbit is involved, ptosis, blurring of vision, and diplopia occur. This can progress to the orbital apex syndrome with proptosis, ophthalmoplegia, and visual loss. Additionally, there may be loss of smell, nasal congestion, and discharge. Physical examination findings include unilateral facial swelling, ptosis, proptosis, periorbital edema, ophthalmoplegia, nasal discharge, and facial tenderness. The major differential is between tumor and infection.

Patients with mycetoma usually complain of purulent, often foul-smelling nasal discharge, nasal congestion, and facial pain. The maxillary sinuses are involved in almost all cases; mycetomas are reported uncommonly in the frontal sinuses (16,40). On examination of the nares, nasal obstruction is sometimes noted and unilateral foul-smelling, purulent nasal secretions are found.

Most patients with allergic fungal sinusitis have had symptoms of chronic and recurrent nasal congestion and discharge of semi-solid nasal crusts for years before the diagnosis is made. They are usually known to have had recurrent nasal polyposis. Facial pain and fever are uncommon. Initial consultation may have been sought with an ophthalmologist because of the development of proptosis or diplopia (45). Children frequently present in this manner because the mass of allergic mucin expands more easily into the orbit in children whose bones are incompletely calcified (46). Examination of the nares reveals obstruction to the airway and polyps with or without accompanying changes in the orbit.

DIAGNOSIS

The diagnosis of acute invasive fungal sinusitis in an immunocompromised patient or diabetic is extremely urgent because death can occur in a matter of days. Facial pain or other sinus symptoms in the appropriate host should be considered to be due to invasive fungal infection until proved otherwise. In the at-risk population, urgent consultation with an otolaryngologist is essential. For the other forms of fungal sinusitis, consultation is also essential, but the disease progresses more slowly and the timeliness of diagnosis is not as urgent. In patients with orbital apex syndrome or other orbital

Table 2 Criteria for the Diagnosis of Sinus Mycetoma

Sinus opacification on CT scan
Mucopurulent, cheesy mass separate from mucosa present at surgery or endoscopy
Mass composed of hyphae on histopathologic examination; no allergic mucin found
Chronic low-grade inflammation seen in adjacent mucosa
No fungal invasion of mucosa or bone

Source: Adapted from Ref. 16.

complaints, ophthalmological consultation and biopsy of the orbital mass is essential. Diagnostic criteria have been established in an attempt to standardize the definitions of sinus mycetoma and allergic fungal sinusitis (Tables 2 and 3). However, in the case of allergic fungal sinusitis, there is still no agreement on exact criteria, especially the requirement for evidence of IgE-type immune reactivity to fungal antigens.

Imaging studies have proved to be very useful in differentiating invasive from noninvasive fungal sinusitis and in defining the extent of disease prior to surgery (24,28,42) (Figs. 1–3). A computed tomography (CT) scan dedicated to imaging the sinuses and orbits is the imaging study of choice; a magnetic resonance imaging (MRI) study with gadolinium is more appropriate to assess the extension of infection into the cavernous sinus, meninges, and brain.

The CT scan generally demonstrates thickening or opacification of one or more sinuses and may show air–fluid levels in acute invasive infection. However, a normal CT scan has been reported in as many as 12% of patients with acute infection, reflecting the fulminant nature of the disease (28). Patients with allergic fungal sinusitis usually have opacification of multiple sinuses. Special attention should be directed to the bony walls of the sinuses, looking for thinning or destruction. With acute invasion, bony changes are rarely noted because of the rapidity of spread of the infection; with

Table 3 Criteria for the Diagnosis of Allergic Fungal Sinusitis[a]

No underlying immunosuppressive condition
Presence of atopy; evidence for IgE-type immune reactivity to fungal antigens
Nasal polyposis
Sinus opacification on CT scan
Allergic mucin found at surgery or endoscopy
Fungal hyphae found with allergic mucin on histopathologic examination
No fungal invasion of mucosa or bone

[a]The need for demonstration of a type I immune response to fungal antigens or even the previous existence of atopy and nasal polyposis has been brought into question by some authors. The firmest evidence is the demonstration of allergic mucin in material removed from the sinuses.

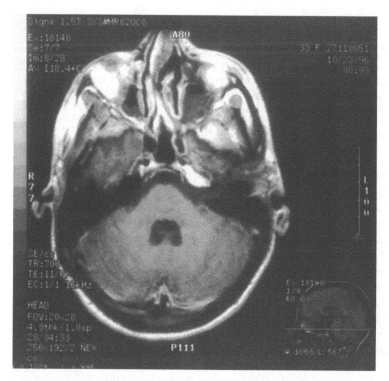

Figure 1 Acute invasive fungal sinusitis due to the zygomycete *Rhizopus* that occurred in a young diabetic woman who had ketoacidosis and who developed the acute onset of facial pain, ptosis, ophthalmoplegia, and loss of vision. Opacification of the left ethmoid sinus with extension into the orbit can be seen on this MRI scan.

chronic invasive disease, bony changes are common (3). Mycetomas and, sometimes, allergic fungal sinusitis can cause pressure necrosis of bone due to the expanding mass of either hyphae or allergic mucin (1).

Endoscopic evaluation is helpful in all patients with fungal sinusitis. In high-risk immunocompromised patients with facial pain, endoscopic evaluation should be performed urgently, even when the CT scan does not show clear-cut changes of acute sinusitis. Examination of the involved sinus in patients with chronic symptoms can help differentiate among invasive infection, mycetoma, and allergic disease. In the case of mycetoma, the mass can be separated from the mucosa; the material is either "cheesy" or firm in consistency. In patients with allergic fungal sinusitis, endoscopic examination documents the presence of darkly colored, thick, sticky allergic mucin filling the involved sinuses and usually the presence of nasal polyposis.

If possible during the endoscopic procedure, biopsy material should be obtained from both mucosa and bone for histopathologic examination and culture. Histological evidence of tissue invasion is necessary to make a diag-

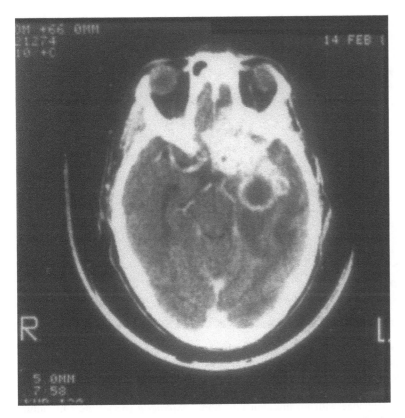

Figure 2 Chronic invasive fungal sinusitis in an elderly woman who had no under-lying illnesses and who developed the gradual onset of worsening facial pain, followed by orbital apex syndrome. The CT scan shows invasion of tissues posterior to the orbit and extension into the frontal lobe with abscess formation. *Aspergilllus fumigatus* was the responsible pathogen.

nosis of invasive sinusitis. However, this is often difficult in neutropenic patients who are also thrombocytopenic; in these cases, lavage can be per-formed for cytological and culture studies. In severely immunocompromised patients, growth of a mold from the sinus is adequate to make a diagnosis of acute invasive fungal sinusitis (47). In mycetoma, well-circumscribed masses of hyphae are present and the integrity of the mucosa is intact. Histopatho-logical examination of material obtained from patients with allergic fungal sinusitis shows hyphae within allergic mucin and no invasion of mucosa or bone (Table 3).

Histopathological examination is very useful in differentiating infection due to the zygomycetes, which show characteristic broad non-septate hyphae from infection due to other filamentous fungi with acutely branching septate

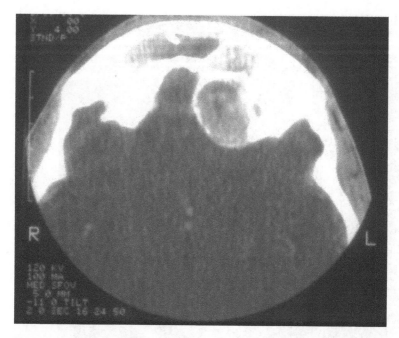

Figure 3 CT scan of a young man who had a long history of recurrent nasal discharge and several previous surgical procedures on his sinuses. The CT scan shows a mass occupying the left frontal sinus with impingement, but no invasion of the left frontal lobe. Histopathological examination showed allergic mucin and pigmented hyphae with no invasion into bone. *Alternaria* species grew in culture of the material removed at surgery.

hyphae (Figs. 4 and 5). In the case of the zygomycetes, culture of material from the sinuses often yields no organisms, but the histopathological picture is distinctive enough to make a diagnosis. However, histopathology alone is inadequate to differentiate among the septate fungi, especially *Aspergillus*, *Pseudallescheria* (*Scedosporium*), and *Fusarium*. Defining the specific organism causing the infection is essential for choosing the appropriate antifungal agent when treating acute or chronic invasive infection.

TREATMENT

The treatment of invasive infection combines aggressive surgical debridement with antifungal agents. Specific risk factors, such as iron chelation therapy or diabetic ketoacidosis, if present, should be eliminated as soon as possible (25). Surgical debridement must remove all necrotic tissue, including the orbit if necessary; the edges of the excision should extend to tissue that bleeds normally. If aggressive surgical debridement cannot be accomplished,

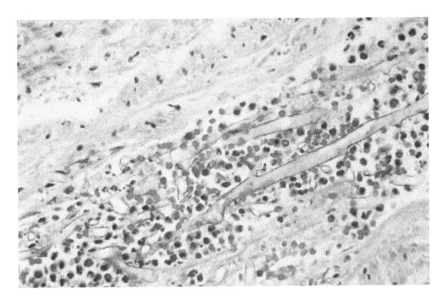

Figure 4 Broad non-septate hyphae typical of that of a zygomycete invading through a blood vessel. This histologic appearance is sufficiently distinctive to make a diagnosis even if the culture yields no growth.

especially in the imunocompromised patient, the outcome is dismal (2,4,6,10, 14,23,28). However, long-term treatment with antifungal agents sometimes succeeds in curing chronic invasive sinusitis even when the entire fungal burden cannot be surgically removed (5,38,39). The difference in outcome is directly related to the relatively intact immune system of the host with chronic invasive infection in contrast to those with acute invasive infection.

Empiric antifungal therapy should be initiated as soon there is a reasonable likelihood that acute invasive fungal sinusitis is present (Table 4). If it is likely that a zygomycete is the cause of the infection, a lipid formulation of amphotericin B should be given (23,48,49). If the likely organism is a species of *Aspergillus*, *Fusarium*, or *Pseudallescheria,* voriconazole is the antifungal agent of choice. Voriconazole is fungicidal for many filamentous fungi and has shown superiority over amphotericin B for invasive aspergillosis (50). Individual case reports document effectiveness for some patients with infections due to *Fusarium* or *Pseudallescheria,* organisms which are generally not susceptible to amphotericin B (51–53). In contrast, the zygomycetes are not susceptible to voriconazole. Frequently, in the high-risk immunocompromised patient, both lipid formulation amphotericin B and voriconazole are given until the culture results are known.

A variety of adjunctive measures have been tried in addition to surgical debridement and antifungal therapy in an attempt to cure acute invasive sinusitis. These include hematopoietic growth factors, such as GM-CSF

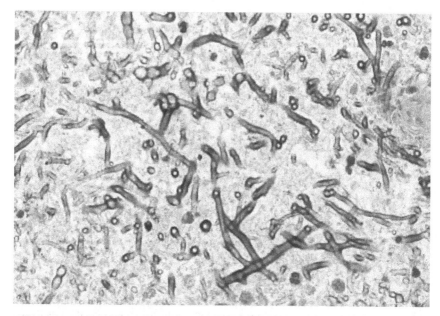

Figure 5 Thinner, septate hyphae characteristic of hyaline molds such as *Aspergillus, Pseudallescheria (Scedosporium)*, and others. The histopathological picture is not specific for any particular organism, and the diagnosis must be established by growth of the organism in culture.

and G-CSF, and hyperbaric oxygen (23,54–56). Most importantly, if host defenses do not return even modestly, as in a profoundly neutropenic patient, none of the measures used will likely be beneficial.

Chronic invasive fungal sinusitis has a high recurrence rate, and very frequently, all infected tissue cannot be removed by surgery without great risk to the patient. For this reason, the management of this disease involves long-term suppressive azole therapy. Itraconazole was previously used for this indication (39), but has been mostly supplanted by voriconazole, which has better anti-*Aspergillus* activity, better absorption of the oral formulation, and superior central nervous system and ocular penetration than itraconazole (57). In cases of chronic fungal sinusitis due to dematiaceous molds, voriconazole is a reasonable choice, but there have been few patients treated and there is more clinical experience with itraconazole at this time (58).

The treatment of mycetoma differs greatly from that of invasive fungal sinusitis. The most important measure to be undertaken is removal of the obstructing inflammatory mass and drainage of the sinus. Performing these procedures through endoscopic surgery has gained in popularity in recent years (40). Radical drainage procedures, previously performed when it was

Table 4 Antifungal Agents Used to Treat Invasive Forms of Fungal Sinusitis

Organism	Agent	Dosage and comments
Zygomycetes (Rhizopus, Mucor)	Lipid formulation AmB (AmBisome or Abelcet)	Begin with 5 mg/kg/day IV. Increase to 10 mg/kg/day on day 2. Give 500 mL saline load prior to infusion. Monitor BUN, creatinine, K^+, Mg^{++} daily
Aspergillus	Voriconazole (preferred)	Load with 6 mg/kg q 12 hr IV on day 1. Then 4 mg/kg q 12 hr IV. When able to take oral medications, 200 mg bid
	Lipid formulation AmB (if voriconazole cannot be used)	5 mg/kg/day IV. Give 500 mL saline load prior to infusion Monitor as noted above
	Itraconazole (2nd line agent)	Load with 200 mg tid oral suspension for 3 days, then 200 mg bid. Use as follow-up agent to AmB or for chronic invasive sinusitis
Hyaline molds (Fusarium, Paecilomyces, Pseudallescheria, etc.)	Voriconazole	See Aspergillus above
Darkly pigmented fungi (Bipolaris, Curvularia, Alternaria, etc.)	Itraconazole	See Aspergillus above. Most experience with this agent for chronic invasive sinusitis
	Voriconazole	400 mg bid orally on day 1. Then 200 mg bid orally. Little experience with this agent to date for chronic invasive sinusitis

Note: The above dosages for agents given intravenously are appropriate for both children and adults. For itraconazole given orally, the dosage is 5 mg/kg/day for children who weigh <40 kg. For voriconazole given orally, the dosage is 100 mg bid for children less than 13 year of age.

thought that there was a high risk of fungal invasion, are now rarely used. Antifungal agents appear to have no role in the treatment of mycetoma (16).

Allergic fungal sinusitis is also treated with surgery rather than antifungal agents. The major goal of surgery is removal of allergic mucin filling the sinus. Generally, a permanent drainage route is also accomplished at the time of surgery (41). Surgery is increasingly performed using endoscopic procedures. Follow-up endoscopic evaluation is very important; it is thought that early removal of recurrent polyps and nasal crusts may help prevent recurrence of the disease.

Follow-up long-term medical management to try to prevent recurrent disease is very important. However, there is much controversy with regard to what constitutes appropriate medical management (59–63). Systemic corticosteroids are of benefit in the postoperative period, but long-term use, not surprisingly, is associated with more risks than benefits. However, all patients should receive long-term intranasal corticosteroids. There are no data showing a benefit in using systemic antifungal agents for this disease. Intranasal instillation of antifungal agents, such as amphotericin B and itraconazole, has been advocated, but there are no studies showing a benefit of this practice. Preparation of solutions of antifungal agents is not standardized; frequently, these solutions are prepared in individual hospital pharmacies. It seems unlikely that antifungal activity is maintained in formulations that are dispensed for the patient to use for sinus irrigation at home. The role of immunotherapy with specific fungal antigens remains controversial, but data have been presented which show that immunotherapy can both decrease reliance on intranasal corticosteroids and decrease the rate of recurrence (63).

CONCLUSIONS

A broad spectrum of pathological changes and clinical manifestations constitute fungal sinusitis. Invasive disease is associated with high morbidity and mortality. The immune status of the host is the most important factor in the development of invasive infection. Highly immunosuppressed individuals and diabetics in ketoacidosis are likely to have acute, rapidly progressive, invasive sinusitis, especially with *Aspergillus* species and the zygomycetes. Immediate aggressive surgical debridement and antifungal therapy are essential for cure. Immunocompetent hosts can develop several chronic forms of fungal sinusitis. Chronic invasive fungal sinusitis requires aggressive surgical debridement and antifungal therapy that may have to be extended to become long-term suppressive therapy. Mycetoma, a localized non-invasive mass of fungal hyphae, can be removed surgically to effect a cure. Finally, allergic fungal sinusitis appears to be a hypersensitivity reaction to fungal antigens rather than actual infection and is treated with surgical debridement and anti-inflammatory agents rather than antifungal agents.

REFERENCES

1. deShazo RD, Chapin K, Swain RE. Fungal sinusitis. N Engl J Med 1997; 337:254–259.
2. Iwen PC, Rupp ME, Hinrichs SH. Invasive mold sinusitis: 17 Cases in immunocompromised patients and review of the literature. Clin Infect Dis 1997; 24: 1178–1184.
3. Washburn RG, Kennedy DW, Begley MG, Henderson DK, Bennett JE. Chronic fungal sinusitis in apparently normal hosts. Medicine (Baltimore) 1988; 67:231–247.
4. Drakos PE, Nagler A, Or R, Naparstek E, Kapelushnik J, Englehard D, Rahav G, Ne'emean D, Slavin S. Invasive fungal sinusitis in patients undergoing bone marrow transplantation. Bone Marrow Transplant 1993; 12:203–208.
5. Stringer SP, Ryan MW. Chronic invasive fungal rhinosinusitis. Otolaryngol Clin N Amer 2000; 33:375–387.
6. Talbot GH, Huang A, Provencher M. Invasive *Aspergillus* rhinosinusitis in patients with acute leukemia. Rev Infect Dis 1991; 13:219–232.
7. Byard RW, Bonin RA, Haq AU. Invasion of paranasal sinuses by *Aspergillus oryzae*. Mycopathologia 1986; 96:41–43.
8. Kameswaran M, Al-Wadei A, Khurana P, Okafor BC. Rhinocerebral aspergillosis. J Laryngol Otol 1992; 106:981–985.
9. Panda NK, Sharma SC, Chakrabarti A, Mann SBS. Paranasal sinus mycoses in north India. Mycoses 1998; 41:281–286.
10. Gucalp R, Carlisle P, Gialanella P, Mitsudo S, McKitrick J, Dutcher J. *Paecilomyces* sinusitis in an immunocompromised adult patient: Case report and review. Clin Infect Dis 1996; 23:391–393.
11. Watters GW, Milford CA. Isolated sphenoid sinusitis due to *Pseudallescheria boydii*. J Laryngol Otol 1993; 107:344–347.
12. Anaissie E, Kantarjian H, Ro J, Hopfer R, Rolston K, Fainstein V, Bodey G. The emerging role of *Fusarium* infections in patients with cancer. Medicine (Baltimore) 1988; 67:77–83.
13. Marr KA, Carter RA, Crippa F, Wald A, Corey L. Epidemiology and outcome of mould infections in hematopoietic stem cell transplant recipients. Clin Infect Dis 2002; 34:909–917.
14. Hunt SC, Miyamoto C, Cornelius RS, Tami TA. Invasive fungal sinusitis in the acquired immunodeficiency syndrome. Otolaryngol Clin N Amer 2000; 33: 335–347.
15. Marple BF, Mabry RL. What we now know about allergic fungal sinusitis. J Respir Dis 2000; 21:23–31.
16. deShazo RD, O'Brien M, Chapin K, Soto-Aguilar M, Swain R, Lyons M, Bryars WC, Alsip S. Criteria for diagnosis of sinus mycetoma. J Allergy Clin Immunol 1997; 99:475–485.
17. Ponikau JU, Sherris DA, Kern EB, Homburger HA, Frigas E, Gaffey TA, Roberts GD. The diagnosis and incidence of allergic fungal sinusitis. Mayo Clin Proc 1999; 74:877–884.
18. Zieske LA, Kopke RD, Hamill R. Dematiaceous fungal sinusitis. Otolaryngol Head Neck Surg 1991; 105:567–577.

19. Dunn JJ, Wolfe MJ, Trachtenberg J, Kriesel JD, Orlandi RR, Carroll KC. Invasive fungal sinusitis caused by *Scytalidium dimidiatum* in a lung transplant recipient. J Clin Microbiol 2003; 41:5817–5819.
20. Ismail Y, Johnson RH, Wells MV, Pusavat J, Douglas K, Arsura EL. Invasive sinusitis with intracranial extension caused by *Curvularia lunata*. Arch Intern Med 1993; 153:1604–1606.
21. Revankar SG, Patterson JE, Sutton DA, PullenR, Rinaldi MG. Disseminated phaeohyphomycosis: Review of an emerging mycosis. Clin Infect Dis 2002; 34: 467–476.
22. Dixon DM, Polak-Wyss A. The medically important dematiaceous fungi and their identification. Mycoses 1991; 34:1–18.
23. Kontoyiannis DP, Wessel VC, Bodey GP, Rolston KVI. Zygomycosis in the 1990s in a tertiary-care cancer center. Clin Infect Dis 2000; 30:851–856.
24. Ferguson BJ. Mucormycosis of the nose and paranasal sinuses. Otolaryngol Clin N Amer 2000; 33:349–365.
25. Sugar AM. Mucormycosis. Clin Infect Dis 1992; 14(suppl 1):S126–S129.
26. Ruess M, Greene JN, Vincent AL, Sandin RL. Invasive *Aspergillus* involving the ethmoidal sinuses in cancer patients: Report of four cases and review of the literature. Infect Dis Clin Pract 1999; 8:323–327.
27. Yuen K-Y, Woo PCY, Ip MSM, Liang RHS, Cjiu EKW, Siau H, Ho P-L, Chen FFE, Chan T-K. Stage-specific manifestation of mold infections in bone marrow transplant recipients: risk factors and clinical significance of positive concentrated smears. Clin Infect Dis 1997; 25:37–42.
28. Gillespie MB, O'Malley BW, Francis HW. An approach to fulminant invasive fungal rhinosinusitis in the immunocompromised host. Arch Otolaryngol Head Neck Surg 1998; 124:520–526.
29. Guiot HF, Fibbe WE, van't Wout JW. Risk factors for fungal infection in patients with malignant hematologic disorders: Implications for empirical therapy and prophylaxis. Clin Infect Dis 1994; 18:525–532.
30. Ribaud P, Chastang C, Latge J-P, Baffroy-Lafitte L, Parquet N, Devergie A, Esperon H, Selimi F, Rocha V, Derouin F, Socie G, Gluckman E. Survival and prognostic factors of invasive aspergillosis after allogeneic bone marrow transplantation. Clin Infect Dis 1999; 28:322–330.
31. Daly AL, Velazquez LA, Bradley SF, Kauffman CA. Mucormycosis: Association with deferoxamine therapy. Am J Med 1989; 87:468–471.
32. Gonzalez-Crespo MR, Gomez-Reino JJ. Invasive aspergillosis in systemic lupus erythematosus. Semin Arthritis Rheum 1995; 24:304–314.
33. Paya CV. Fungal infections in solid-organ transplantation. Clin Infect Dis 1993; 16:677–688.
34. Kanj SS, Welty-Wolf K, Madden J, Tapson V, Baz MA, Davis RD, Perfect JR. Fungal infections in lung and heart-lung transplant recipients: Report of 9 cases and review of the literature. Medicine (Baltimore) 1996; 75:142–156.
35. Flume PA, Egan TM, Paradowski LJ, Detterbeck FC, Thompson JT, Yankaskas JR. Infectious complications of lung transplantation: Impact of cystic fibrosis. Am J Resp Crit Care Med 1994; 149:1601–1607.

36. Mehrad B, Paciocco G, Martinez F, Ojo TC, Iannettoni MD, Lynch JP. Spectrum of *Aspergillus* infections in lung transplant recipients. Chest 2001; 119:169–175.
37. Chinn RY, Diamond RD. Generation of chemotactic factors by *Rhizopus oryzae* in the presence and absence of serum: Relationship to hyphal damage mediated by human neutrophils and effects of hyperglycemia and ketoacidosis. Infect Immun 1982; 38:1123–1129.
38. Bradley SF, McGuire NM, Kauffman CA. Sino-orbital and cerebral aspergillosis: cure with medical therapy. Mykosen 1987; 30:379–385.
39. Gumaa SA, Mahgoub ES, Hay RJ. Post-operative reponses of paranasal *Aspergillus* granuloma to itraconazole. Trans Royal Soc Trop Med Hyg 1992; 86:93–94.
40. Klossek J-M, Serrano E, Peloquin L, Percodani J, Fontanel J-P, Pessey J-J. Functional endoscopic sinus surgery and 109 mycetomas of paranasal sinuses. Laryngoscope 1997; 107:112–117.
41. Marple BF. Allergic fungal rhinosinusitis: Current theories and management strategies. Laryngoscope 2001; 111:1006–1019.
42. deCarpentier JP, Ramamurthy L, Denning DW, Taylor PH. An algorithmic approach to *Aspergillus* sinusitis. J Laryngol Otol 1994; 108:314–318.
43. Judson MA. Noninvasive *Aspergillus* pulmonary disease. Sem Respir Crit Care Med 2004; 25:203–219.
44. Manning SC, Holman M. Further evidence for allergic pathophysiology in allergic fungal sinusitis. Laryngoscope 1998; 108:1485–1496.
45. Carter KD, Graham SM, Carpenter KM. Ophthalmic manifestations of allergic fungal sinusitis. Am J Ophthalmol 1999; 27:189–195.
46. Goldstein MF, Atkins PC, Cogen FC, Kornstein MJ, Levine RS, Zweiman B. Allergic *Aspergillus* sinusitis. J Allergy Clin Immunol 1985; 76:515–524.
47. Ascioglu S, Rex JH, dePauw B, Bennett JE, Bille J, Crokaert F, Denning DW, Donnelly JP, Edwards JE, Erjavec Z, et al. Defining opportunistic invasive fungal infections on immunocompromised patients with cancer and hematopoietic stem cell transplants: An international consensus. Clin Infect Dis 2002; 34:7–14.
48. Strasser MD, Kennedy RJ, Adam RD. Rhinocerebral mucormycosis: Therapy with amphotericin B lipid complex. Arch Intern Med 1996; 156:337–339.
49. Moses AE, Rahav G, Barenholz Y, Elidan J, Azaz B, Gillis S, Brickman M, Polacheck I, Shapiro M. Rhinocerebral mucormycosis treated with amphotericin B colloidal dispersion in three patients. Clin Infect Dis 1998; 26:1430–1433.
50. Herbrecht R, Denning DW, Patterson TF, Bennett JE, Greene RF, Oestman J-W, Kern WV, Marr KA, Ribaud P, Lortholary O, et al. Voriconazole versus amphotericin B for primary therapy of invasive aspergillosis. N Engl J Med 2002; 347:408–415.
51. Nesky MA, McDougal EC, Peacock JE Jr. *Pseudallescheria boydii* brain abscess successfully treated with voriconazole and surgical drainage: Case report and literature review of central nervous system pseudallescheriasis. Clin Infect Dis 2000; 31:673–677.
52. Munoz P, Marin M, Tornero P, Rabadan PM, Rodriquez-Creixems M, Bouza E. Successful outcome of *Scedosporium apiospermum* disseminated infection treated

with voriconazole in a patient receiving corticosteroid therapy. Clin Infect Dis 2000; 31:1499–1501.

53. Consigny S, Dhedin N, Datry A, Choquet S, LeBlond V, Chosidow O. Successful voriconazole treatment of disseminated *Fusarium* infection in an immunocompromised patient. Clin Infect Dis 2003; 37:311–313.

54. Gaviria JM, Grohskopf LA, Barnes R, Root RK. Successful treatment of rhinocerebral zygomycosis: A combined-strategy approach. Clin Infect Dis 1999; 28:160–161.

55. Garcia-Diaz JB, Palau L, Pankey GA. Resolution of rhinocerebral zygomycosis associated with administration of granulocyte-macrophage colony-stimulating factor. Clin Infect Dis 2001; 32:166–170.

56. Ferguson BJ, Mitchell TG, Moon R, Camporesi EM, Farmer J. Adjunctive hyperbaric oxygen for treatment of rhinocerebral mucormycosis. Rev Infect Dis 1988; 10:551–559.

57. Johnson LB, Kauffman CA. Voriconazole: A new triazole antifungal agent. Clin Infect Dis 2003; 36:630–637.

58. Sharkey PK, Graybill JR, Rinaldi MG, Stevens DA, Tucker RM, Peterie JD, Hoeprich PD, Greer DL, Frenkel L, Counts GW, Goodrich J, Zellner S, Bradsher RW, van der Horst CM, Israel K, Pankey GA, Barranco CP. Itraconazole treatment of phaeohyphomycosis. J Am Acad Dermatol 1990; 23: 577–586.

59. Marple BF, Mabry RL. Comprehensive management of allergic fungal sinusitis. Am J Rhinol 1998; 12:263–268.

60. Quraishi HA, Ramadan HH. Endoscopic treatment of allergic fungal sinusitis. Otolaryngol Head Neck Surg 1997; 117:29–34.

61. Kupferberg SB, Bent JP, Kuhn FA. Prognosis for allergic fungal sinusitis. Otolaryngol Head Neck Surg 1997; 117:35–41.

62. Ferguson BJ. What role do systemic corticosteroids, immunotherapy, and antifungal drugs play in the therapy of allergic fungal rhinosinusitis? Arch Otolaryngol Head Neck Surg 1998; 124:1174–1177.

63. Mabry RL, Mabry CS. Allergic fungal sinusitis. The role of immunotherapy. Otolaryngol Clin N Amer 2000; 33:433–440.

Sinusitis in Immunocompromised, Diabetic, and Human Immunodeficiency Virus–Infected Patients*

Todd D. Gleeson and Catherine F. Decker

Division of Infectious Diseases, Department of Internal Medicine, National Naval Medical Center, Bethesda, Maryland, U.S.A.

INTRODUCTION

Over the past several decades, medical advancements in transplantation and in the treatment of immunocompromised patients have led to increased survival in several patient populations including oncology and transplant patients, type 1 diabetics, and human immunodeficiency virus (HIV)-infected patients. Not surprisingly, these patients are at increased risk for infectious complications. As the at-risk population continues to grow, sinusitis has become an increasingly recognized problem in these immunocompromised groups and presents unique challenges to the clinician in both diagnosis and management. Although each group differs in its acquired risk and the various impairments in the immune function, the importance of early recognition, diagnosis, and aggressive combined modality treatment is common to all immunocompromised patients.

The degree of impairment of the immune system is the most important host factor in determining the clinical presentation and course of sinusitis.

_____

*The opinions and assertions contained herein are those of the authors and are not to be construed as official or as reflecting the views of the Department of Defense, the Department of the Navy, or the naval services at large.

The spectrum of sinonasal disease varies from a slow, indolent course in the presence of mild immunocompromise to an acute fulminant course if the immunocompromised state is severe. For example, one investigator reports that recurrent or refractory sinusitis in the outpatient setting may in fact be due to relative immune dysfunction characterized by an unexpectedly high incidence of low immunoglobulin levels and common variable immunodeficiency (1). Conversely, neutropenic patients with invasive fungal rhinosinusitis have a devastating outcome with 100% mortality in the absence of bone marrow recovery (2).

Historically, acute sinusitis has referred to community-acquired bacterial sinusitis. In immunocompromised groups, acute versus chronic sinusitis is not as clearly defined. The chronicity of sinusitis in these immunocompromised groups correlates with immune status and the underlying immunodeficiency. Generally, chronic sinusitis refers to disease extending beyond four weeks in duration. Acute fulminant disease can occur over days in patients with significant immune system impairment. Severely immunocompromised individuals receiving therapy for sinusitis may appear to have a chronic disease characterized by a course that extends to several weeks. However, if treatment is withdrawn prematurely, the sinonasal infection may rapidly worsen, often resulting in a fatal outcome (3,4).

Although sinusitis in the immunocompromised patient may be caused by common pathogens, such as *Haemophilus influenzae* and *Streptococcus pneumoniae*, it more often results from infection with more unusual organisms. This chapter reviews the clinical presentation, diagnosis, and treatment of sinusitis in three groups of immunocompromised hosts: neutropenic patients, diabetic patients, and HIV-infected patients.

SINUSITIS IN NEUTROPENIC PATIENTS

As a result of increasing rates of transplantation and the use of immunosuppressive agents over the past several years, the population at-risk for invasive fungal rhinosinusitis is growing. This disease continues to be a potentially lethal and dreaded infectious complication of chemotherapy or bone marrow transplant-induced neutropenia. It occurs in 2 to 4% of patients undergoing bone marrow transplantation (5,6) and despite therapy, the majority of cases result in death (7). Recovery of the immune system is still the major prognostic factor in patients with this infection.

Predisposing Factors

Several risk factors for sinusitis have been identified in neutropenic patients. Although susceptibility to fungal infections is characteristic of patients with defects in CD4 mediated function, quantitative or qualitative defects in neutrophil function also predispose hosts to the development of fungal infections. Absolute neutrophil counts (ANC) below 500 cells/mL are strongly correlated with the development of invasive fungal disease (8). In bone marrow transplant (BMT) patients, the critical time period for the development of fungal rhinosinusitis is approximately three weeks after transplantation (2). Secondary risk factors include two weeks or more of any of the following: systemic steroid use (seen in up to 50% of patients with a mean dose of 2.22 mg/kg/day prednisone equivalent) (9,10), ANC <500 cells/mm^3 (11), and exposure to multiple broad-spectrum antibiotics (9,10,12,13). In addition, it has been reported that nasal mucosa ciliary dysfunction in BMT patients predisposes to sinusitis (14).

Etiology

Immunocompetent patients are more often infected by gram-positive bacteria, and the most common organisms causing sinusitis in neutropenic patients are gram-negative bacteria, followed by gram-positive bacteria and fungi (15). Bacteria including *Pseudomonas aeruginosa, Enterobacter* species, *Escherichia coli, Serratia marcescens, Haemophilus influenzae, Staphylococcus,* and *Streptococcus* species have all been isolated from sinus cultures in neutropenic patients. *Aspergillus* species are often the causative organisms of invasive fungal rhinosinusitis in the neutropenic host, although *Mucor, Rhizopus*, and *Alternaria* species, and other invasive molds have also been implicated (11,16).

Clinical Presentation

The most common presentation of fungal rhinosinusitis, seen in up to 90% of infected neutropenic patients, is fever unresponsive to 48 hours of appropriate broad-spectrum intravenous antibiotics (2). Most patients have fever and at least one additional finding (17), including sinus tenderness, facial edema, or rhinorrhea. Headache, facial pain, cranial nerve palsies, and visual loss are also seen (11,12,17).

Diagnosis

A thorough rigid nasal endoscopic examination should be performed in any immunocompromised patient with localizing symptoms of sinusitis. Some centers advocate nasal endoscopy for all febrile neutropenic patients who do not respond to 48 hours of appropriate broad-spectrum intravenous antibiotics (12). Endoscopic examination may reveal changes in the nasal mucosa, including discoloration, granulation, or ulceration (10,16,18). White discoloration indicates tissue ischemia secondary to fungal invasion of blood vessels, whereas clinical progression to black discoloration and ulceration is a later finding of tissue necrosis (10). Decreased sensation and decreased mucosal bleeding are also ominous signs (12). These findings on nasal endoscopy may precede rapid facial swelling, nasal symptoms, and systemic dissemination.

The middle turbinate, which acts as the major filter in the nasal airway, is most commonly involved in invasive fungal rhinosinusitis (10,19). Local mucosal disruption, drying secondary to oxygen passing through the nasal cannula, allergy, or changes in the normal flora that can occur with bacterial sinusitis may promote fungi to become invasive (10). In most cases, invasive rhinosinusitis originates in the nasal cavity before extension into the paranasal sinuses. Identifying disease early, when it is still confined to the nasal cavity or middle turbinate, seems to have a positive impact on survival (10). Performing middle turbinate biopsies in all patients at-risk for invasive fungal rhinosinusitis, who have fever unresponsive to 48 hours of broad-spectrum antibiotics or symptoms of rhinosinusitis, or both, may be an effective diagnostic technique to help achieve the goal of early detection (19).

Computed tomography (CT) is the preferred imaging modality in establishing the diagnosis of fungal rhinosinusitis and is more reliable than plain radiography (16,20,21). A fine cut CT scan of the paranasal sinuses not only reveals the presence of sinusitis, but also defines bony architecture as well as intracranial spread or orbital involvement. Although intravenous contrast helps delineate periorbital or dural inflammation, it is not mandatory for most initial evaluations (12). A CT scan showing focal bony erosion should alert the clinician to invasive fungal disease, although a definitive diagnosis rests on histological confirmation. In one series, 12% of patients with invasive fungal rhinosinusitis had a normal CT scan; (12) therefore, imaging cannot replace careful endoscopic nasal evaluation and biopsy.

Magnetic resonance imaging (MRI) may be even more sensitive than CT, and is superior to CT in delineating intracranial extension of disease (8,12). Some postulate that the presence of ferromagnetic elements within fungal concretions may produce a characteristic signal intensity on MRI (20).

Invasive fungal rhinosinusitis is a histopathological diagnosis and is characterized by the mucosal infiltration of mycotic organisms from sinus air spaces to adjacent orbital and intracranial structures. This infiltration results in tissue necrosis, and invasion of blood vessels produces thrombosis and infarction. Fulminant invasive disease occurs primarily in neutropenic patients and BMT recipients, whereas indolent invasive fungal sinusitis is a more slowly destructive disease seen in immunocompetent hosts, diabetics, or patients with AIDS. Biopsy and culture provide proper speciation which can direct therapy, as in the case of infection by *Pseudallescheria boydii*, which is resistant to amphotericin B (12).

Treatment

After endoscopic evaluation and antrostomy, if a bacterial etiology of sinusitis is discovered, gram stain and culture with identification of antibiotic sensitivities of the organism are of major importance for successful treatment of sinusitis in the neutropenic patient (15). Antibiotics that cover both gram-negative and gram-positive organisms should be given empirically, with further modifications directed by culture and sensitivity results of the aspirate (Table 1).

When a diagnosis of invasive fungal rhinosinusitis is made, immediate treatment must be instituted. A successful outcome is contingent on both the recovery of immune function and early medical and surgical intervention (22). Aggressive surgical debridement to clear margins removes devitalized tissues that further support fungal growth, enhances the ability of antifungal drugs to reach infected areas, and provides more time for bone marrow to recover (12,23). Administration of high-dose systemic amphotericin B at a dose of >1.5 mg/kg/d, for a total dose of two grams or more, gives the best chance of survival (10,16,18,20–22). The use of liposomal amphotericin B should be reserved for patients with renal disease. Despite an aggressive-combined modality approach, mortality is still 100% in both intracranial extension of disease and in patients in whom immune function does not recover (12,22) (Fig. 1).

New antifungal drugs may prove superior to amphotericin B in the treatment of invasive aspergillosis, including sinonasal disease. One study reports voriconazole to be superior to amphotericin B in both response rate and survival in the treatment of invasive aspergillosis. Voriconazole also caused fewer drug-related adverse events than amphotericin B (24). Some centers advocate using voriconazole as first-line treatment for invasive *Aspergillus* infections (25).

The administration of growth factors also plays a role in the treatment of neutropenic patients with fungal rhinosinusitis. Patients who respond to granulocyte colony–stimulating factor (GC–SF) are more likely to have a favorable outcome. One study demonstrated that responders to GC–SF were more likely to have contained disease than nonresponders. However, it is unclear if this outcome reflects response to GC–SF or better underlying bone marrow status in survivors (10). Granulocyte transfusions have also been used in invasive fungal rhinosinusitis to enhance immune status and bridge the interval until hematopoietic regeneration occurs (23,26).

Close follow-up with repeated visualization with rigid nasal endoscopy is essential. Patients should have repeat endoscopy in 48 to 72 hours if there is any suspicion for residual disease following the original debridement (12). Neutropenic patients should continue to receive weekly rigid nasal endoscopy until resolution of neutropenia and then monthly for six months thereafter (12). Patients who have had fungal rhinosinusitis are especially susceptible to relapse or reinfection during future episodes of neutropenia (10,27). Patients undergoing chemotherapy or bone marrow transplantation who have had episodes of sinonasal or pulmonary aspergillosis have at least a 50% risk of developing a recurrence during re-induction chemotherapy

Table 1 Recommended Antimicrobial Therapy for Sinusitis in Neutropenic, Diabetic, and HIV-Infected Patients

Host	Etiology	Antimicrobial	Dose	Duration
Neutropenic	Bacterial	Imipenem or Ceftazidime	500 mg IV q6h 2 g IV q8h	Resolution of neutropenia
	Fungal	Amphotericin B[a]	1.5 mg/kg/d IV	2 grams total dose
Diabetic	Bacterial	Cefuroxime	1.5 g IV q8h	14 days minimum
	Fungal	Amphotericin B	1.5 mg/kg/d IV	2 grams total dose
HIV-infected	Bacterial	Ciprofloxacin and Ceftazidime[b]	400 mg IV q12h 2 g IV q8h	14 days minimum
	Fungal	Amphotericin B	1.5 mg/kg/d IV	2 grams total dose
		Common opportunistic pathogens		
	Cryptococcus	Amphotericin B followed by Fluconazole	0.7–1.0 mg/kg/d 400 mg po qd	2 weeks 10 weeks/then suppression
	Nocardia	Trimethoprim–Sulfamethoxazole	15 mg/kg/dIV or PO 75 mg/kg/d IV or PO	6 months minimum
	Cytomegalovirus	Ganciclovir	5 mg/kg IV q12h	21 days induction treatment/maintenance 5 mg/kg IV q d
	Mycobacterium kansasii	Rifampin and Isoniazid and Ethambutol	10 mg/kg/d po 5 mg/kg/d po 15–25 mg/kg/d po	18 months with minimum of 12 months of negative cultures

[a] *Pseudallescheria boydii* requires voriconazole 6 mg/kg IV q12h on day 1, then 200 mg po q12h until neutropenia resolved.
[b] Based on high prevalence of *Pseudomonas* in HIV-infected sinusitis patients, two anti-pseudomonal drugs should be administered empirically.

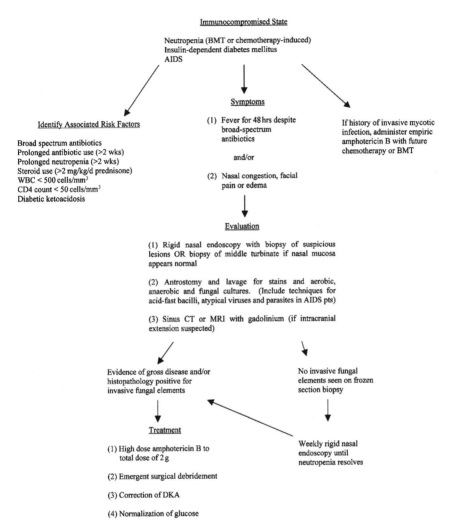

Figure 1 Algorithm for the diagnosis and management of rhinosinusitis in the immunocompromised patient. BMT indicates bone marrow transplant; AIDS, acquired immunodeficiency syndrome; WBC, white blood cell; DKA, diabetic ketoacidosis

or transplantation (28). Hence, antifungal therapy should be empirically initiated with further courses of chemotherapy or bone marrow transplantation in these patients (Fig. 1).

Prevention

Few studies have evaluated primary and secondary prophylaxis of invasive fungal sinusitis with antifungal drugs. One trial of amphotericin nasal spray in a BMT unit reported an incidence of 1.8% of invasive fungal disease, compared to 13.8% in historical controls (29,30). A benefit in using intravenous amphotericin to prevent aspergillosis in BMT patients has not been clearly demonstrated in a sufficient number of controlled trials (30). In patients who have experienced a previous episode of invasive aspergillosis, however, prophylactic intravenous amphotericin during re-induction chemotherapy or bone marrow transplantation decreases the rate of recurrent aspergillosis (30).

SINUSITIS IN DIABETIC PATIENTS

Patients with diabetes mellitus are at an increased risk of developing a variety of infections, including sinusitis. Although the underlying condition of diabetes mellitus cannot be reversed, effective glycemic control improves multiple factors important in the host response to sinusitis.

Predisposing Factors

The proclivity for diabetic patients to develop infections is not unexpected given that hyperglycemia produces qualitative immune dysfunction through impairment of neutrophils. Normalization of glucose and correction of diabetic ketoacidosis are essential in treating and preventing infections in these patients (31,32). Whereas it may be difficult to prove a causal relationship between hyperglycemia and infection, in vitro and clinical evidence support such a relationship. The degree of hyperglycemia has been shown to affect phagocytic function (33), granulocyte adherence (34), chemotaxis (35), and bactericidal function in vitro (36), all of which improve with aggressive glycemic control (37). Hyperglycemia may also impair complement fixation and thereby decrease opsonization. Diabetic microangiopathy may also predispose the diabetic patient to infection (38), however, it has not been specifically reported as a risk factor for sinusitis.

Etiology

Although fungal rhinosinusitis has been well studied in diabetics, diabetic patients are also susceptible to acute bacterial sinusitis that may be recalcitrant if pansinusitis is present. The predominant organisms recovered in bacterial sinusitis in diabetic patients are streptococci and staphylococcal organisms, followed by gram-negative bacteria (38). The increased frequency of sinusitis caused by *Staphylococcus aureus* in this population is not unexpected given the increased *S. aureus* carrier state in diabetic patients requiring insulin (39).

Aspergillus and *Zygomycetes* species are the most common causes of fungal sinusitis in this patient group, whereas *Candida* species are rarely reported (40). The diabetic patient is particularly susceptible to *Rhizopus* infection for many reasons unique to the organism. *Rhizopus* organisms thrive in high glucose, acidic conditions due to an active ketone reductase system, making a patient with diabetic ketoacidosis a prime host. In fact, normal serum inhibits rhizopus growth, whereas serum from patients in diabetic ketoacidosis stimulates growth (41). In addition, due to impaired transferrin binding, diabetic patients also have increased free serum iron that may also promote rhizopus growth (41). The same pathophysiologic mechanism is responsible for the increased susceptibility to *Mucor* found in hemodialysis patients and iron-overloaded patients treated with deferoxamine (42).

Clinical Presentation

The clinical presentation of bacterial sinusitis in the diabetic is not unlike that of the general population, including symptoms of sinus pain, nasal congestion, and purulent discharge. However, invasive fungal rhinosinusitis in the diabetic patient may have as subtle a presentation as in the neutropenic patient, and should be considered in any diabetic who does not respond to antibiotics for bacterial sinusitis. The most common symptoms and signs include fever, followed by nasal ulceration and necrosis, and periorbital or facial swelling. Visual disturbances include decreased vision, cranial nerve palsy, diplopia, and periorbital pain. While patients may only complain of facial numbness or epistaxis, palatal or gingival necrosis may be present (43).

Diagnosis

If fungal rhinosinusitis is suspected, early and rapid diagnosis should be pursued, as in neutropenic hosts, with radiographic and endoscopic examinations. CT is the preferred radiographic modality as it provides more detail than plain films, including landmarks for possible surgical resection. Early radiographs may be normal, whereas bony erosion is seen late in the progression of disease (41). Evidence on CT of infiltration of the periantral fat planes may be the earliest sign of invasive fungal disease (44). Endoscopy should be performed with antral aspiration for aerobic, anaerobic, and fungal cultures.

A definitive diagnosis of invasive fungal rhinosinusitis in the diabetic patient requires histopathological identification of fungal organisms. Mucormycosis may be presumptively diagnosed by identification of ribbon-like hyphae with few or absent hyphal septations and hyphal branching at right angles (41). The etiologic agents of mucormycosis may be seen easily with hematoxylin and eosin tissue stains, and demonstrate invasion of blood vessels (41).

Treatment

For bacterial sinusitis, oral antibiotics directed against the most commonly isolated organisms are appropriate for initial treatment in a diabetic patient without fever, systemic symptoms, or pansinusitis (Table 1). In diabetic patients with pansinusitis, empiric intravenous antibiotics should be used with coverage for both streptococci and *S. aureus*, such as a first- or second-generation Cephalosporin (38). Treatment should be modified according to the gram stain and culture after antral aspiration. Dental apicitis may also be an important nidus of infection of the paranasal sinuses and requires concurrent treatment for effective cure of sinusitis in the diabetic patient (38).

In invasive fungal sinusitis in the diabetic patient, early recognition and diagnosis are paramount. As the extent of disease is dependent on the host response, reversal of diabetic ketoacidosis and glycemic control are essential medical interventions (45). Immediate surgical consultation with surgical debridement to clear margins and systemic administration of amphotericin B optimize chances of recovery.

Prevention

The best preventive strategy for sinusitis in the diabetic population is to achieve excellent glycemic control in the outpatient setting in order to prevent microcirculation damage and immune system impairment. In the inpatient setting, rapid reversal of diabetic ketoacidosis and normalization of glucose help limit extent of disease and improves survival.

SINUSITIS IN HIV-INFECTED PATIENTS

Sinusitis is common throughout all stages of HIV infection (46). Historically, retrospective studies report the incidence of sinusitis in HIV-infected patients in the range of 10% to 20%. However, more recent prospective studies have shown the incidence to be twice as high (60–70%) as in the general population (38.5%) (46–51). Declining immune function marked by decreasing CD4-cell counts is associated with an increased incidence of sinus disease (52).

Predisposing Factors

A number of factors may predispose the HIV-infected patient to sinonasal disease. As in BMT patients, mucociliary clearance abnormalities have been demonstrated in patients infected with HIV (53), particularly with CD4 counts less than 300 cells/mm^3. IgE-mediated allergic disease is more prevalent in HIV-infected patients than in noninfected individuals and can cause mucosal edema and blockage of sinus ostia, resulting in a secondary bacterial infection. Nasopharyngeal lymphoid hypertrophy occurs in 56 to 88% of patients in early HIV infection and decreases in size with immune system impairment (54,55). This local lymphoid hypertrophy may mechanically alter sinus drainage, predisposing to sinusitis. Finally, qualitative and quantitative humoral immunity defects likely predispose HIV-infected patients to sinusitis (56,57).

Etiology

In general, the infecting organisms that cause sinusitis in the HIV-infected patient vary with the degree of immunosuppression. Of the bacterial causes of sinusitis, there is a higher prevalence of *P. aeruginosa* and staphylococcal organisms, which may be due to impaired cellular immunity in HIV infection (58). Specifically, in two large studies, *Pseudomonas* was isolated in 17% of maxillary antral punctures (48,59). Other bacteria recovered include streptococcal organisms, *H. influenzae*, *Klebsiella pneumoniae*, *E. coli*, *Listeria monocytogenes*, *Peptostreptococcus* and other anaerobes, and *Propionibacterium acnes* (46,48,59,60).

While bacterial sinusitis can occur at any stage of HIV infection, sinusitis caused by opportunistic pathogens such as protozoa, fungi, and atypical viruses usually occurs with a CD4 count less than 200 cells/mm^3. A retrospective series of 12 AIDS patients with CD4 counts less than 100 cells/mm^3, who underwent sinus surgery, reported 42% of the patients had unusual or opportunistic infections (60). The risk of fungal sinusitis generally occurs when the CD4 count drops below 150 cells/mm^3 (61). *Aspergillus* is the most common cause of fungal sinusitis in AIDS patients (62,63). Other fungal organisms reported include *Cryptococcus* and *Rhizopus* species. However, given that neutrophil function remains relatively intact in AIDS patients, mucormycosis is not frequently seen (41). Other reported opportunistic pathogens include microsporidia, cryptosporidia, cytomegalovirus (CMV), *Acanthamoeba*, *Nocardia*, and *Mycobacterium kansasii* (46,59,60,64–69). In a prospective series, 20 of 54 HIV-infected patients with evidence of sinusitis on MRI underwent maxillary sinus aspiration. A probable etiologic agent was found in two-thirds of patients. One-third of the infectious organisms were atypical, including CMV and mycobacteriae, and one patient had Non-Hodgkin's lymphoma (46).

Clinical Presentation

While sinusitis in HIV-infected patients is frequently asymptomatic, it can be recurrent and refractory to usual medical management (47,48,70). Symptoms of sinusitis are often nonspecific and may be attributed to other causes. Usually, patients experience fever, headache, nasal congestion, and postnasal drainage. In one retrospective series of HIV-infected patients with sinusitis, the triad of fever, headache, and nasal congestion was present in 68% of patients (48). Other symptoms and signs include facial pain or tenderness, cough, purulent discharge, and cutaneous edema.

Diagnosis

Asymptomatic patients may have incidental radiographic evidence of sinusitis noted on radiographic imaging done for other purposes. Radiographic findings of sinusitis do not correlate with symptoms and may be just as severe and extensive in asymptomatic patients as in those with symptoms (48). One report notes that up to one-third of patients with radiographic evidence of sinusitis had no symptoms (47). Computed tomography (CT) and MRI are the most sensitive imaging modalities for sinusitis in the HIV-infected patient. Radiographically, the majority of cases involve the maxillary and ethmoid sinuses, followed by sphenoid disease, which often is not detected by plain radiographs. The extent of radiographic disease seems to correlate with the degree of immunosuppression. Tarp et al. (46) prospectively reported the findings of MRIs performed on 54 febrile hospitalized HIV-infected patients. Radiographic sinusitis was noted in 54%, with more extensive changes seen in patients with AIDS (22/32 cases compared with 16/38 in HIV-infected without AIDS). HIV-infected patients also tend to have greater opacification of sinuses, as well as multiple sinuses involved. Unilateral, localized disease is unusual (48).

Recognizing that HIV-infected patients have a high rate of infection by unusual organisms, it is imperative to perform aerobic, anaerobic, fungal, viral, and mycobacterial laboratory evaluations and cultures when a sinus aspiration is performed (71). Early culture avoids delay in microbe-specific therapy and should be performed if a patient is not improving with empiric antibiotic therapy for usual bacterial pathogens. Surgical specimens should be evaluated histopathologically for giant cells and viral inclusion bodies of invasive CMV infection, and also should prompt immunohistochemical staining for CMV early antigen (65). In patients with AIDS and refractory cases of sinusitis, electron microscopy should be performed on sinonasal tissue to rule out protozoa such as microsporidia (69). *Acanthamoeba* and *Cryptosporidium* can also be diagnosed histologically (67).

Treatment

Initial antibiotic therapy should be directed against the most common bacterial pathogens and should be modified according to gram stain and culture or identification of opportunistic pathogens (49,59,60,72). Oral amoxicillin/clavulanic acid may be used in the outpatient setting, with escalation of therapy to broad-spectrum intravenous antibiotics if the symptoms do not improve or worsen (72). The status of the immune system of the HIV-infected patient should also be taken into consideration when choosing initial therapy, particularly if the patient has a CD4 count less than 100 cells/mm^3 (72). If the patient shows signs of systemic toxicity, intravenous antibiotics should be the initial treatment, including coverage for *P. aeruginosa* (49,59,72). The combination of two antimicrobial agents with activity against *P. aeruginosa* has been shown to improve mortality in AIDS patients with pseudomonas infection compared to monotherapy (72–74).

A high index of suspicion should be maintained for opportunistic pathogens as etiologies of sinusitis in AIDS patients, including fungi, protozoa, mycobacteria, and viruses, all of which require specific antimicrobial therapy (Table 1).

Decongestants and mucolytic agents are also effective, as is topical steroid, which may be used if there is no evidence of opportunistic infection and if the CD4 count is greater than 50 cells/mm^3 (4). Endoscopic sinus surgery also plays an important role in management, and if necessary can be safely done in all HIV-infected patients regardless of CD4-cell count. HIV-infected patients tolerate the procedure well and recover rapidly (4). Initiation of highly active antiretroviral therapy (HAART) and reconstitution of the immune system and CD4-cell counts is an important adjunct to the surgical and medical management of sinusitis in HIV-infected patients.

Prevention

Although sinusitis is not associated with decreased survival (75), prevention appears to improve morbidity. Prophylaxis against *Mycobacterium avium* and *Pneumocystis carinii* has the added benefit of prevention of bacterial sinusitis. In a large prophylaxis trial, trimethoprim/sulfamethoxazole (TMP/SMX) significantly reduced the risk of bacterial sinusitis (76). TMP-SMX had the added benefit of reducing the risk of any bacterial infection compared to dapsone or aerosolized pentamidine (AP). In a prospective observational study, HIV-infected patients receiving TMP-SMX for *Pneumocystis carinii* prophylaxis (PCP) and clarithromycin for prevention of MAC had a 46% and 44% reduction in the overall risk of infection, respectively. Patients who received both antibiotics decreased the overall risk of infection even further, though this was not statistically significant (58).

CONCLUSION

While sinusitis is a commonly encountered problem, it can be a very severe infection in the immunodeficient patient. One of the most immunocompromising conditions is that of chemotherapy or bone marrow transplantation–induced neutropenia, which can predispose patients to life-threatening invasive fungal rhinosinusitis. Diabetic patients are also an at-risk population for this infection. Modification of risk factors, such as normalization of glucose and reversal of neutropenia, are critical for recovery. Aggressive surveillance, early diagnosis, surgical debridement, and antifungal agents are the mainstay of treatment. HIV-infected patients are also predisposed to sinusitis. The spectrum of their disease may range from asymptomatic to recalcitrant to treatment. With a greater degree of immunosuppression, sinusitis is more severe and opportunistic pathogens are frequently recovered.

REFERENCES

1. Chee L, Graham SM, Carothers DG, Ballas ZK. Immune dysfunction in refractory sinusitis in a tertiary care setting. Laryngoscope 2001; 111:233–235.
2. Kennedy CA, Adams GL, Neglia JP, Giebink GS. Impact of surgical treatment on paranasal fungal infections in bone marrow transplant patients. Otolaryngol Head Neck Surg 1997; 116:610–616.
3. Ferguson BJ. Definitions of fungal rhinosinusitis. Otolaryngol Clin North Am 2000; 33:227–235.
4. Gurney TA, Lee KC, Murr AH. Contemporary issues in rhinosinusitis and HIV infection. Curr Opin Otolaryngol Head Neck Surg 2003; 11:45–48.
5. Choi SS, Milmoe GJ, Dinndorf PA, Quinones RR. Invasive aspergillus sinusitis in pediatric bone marrow transplant patients. Evaluation and management. Arch Otolaryngol Head Neck Surg 1995; 121:1188–1192.
6. Drakos PE, Nagler A, Or R, Naparstek E, Kapelushnik J, Engelhard D, Rahav G, Ne'emean D, Slavin S. Invasive fungal sinusitis in patients undergoing bone marrow transplantation. Bone Marrow Transplant 1993; 12:203–208.
7. Waitzman AA, Birt BD. Fungal sinusitis. J Otolaryngol 1994; 23:244–249.
8. Lueg EA, Ballagh RH, Forte V. Analysis of the recent cluster of invasive fungal sinusitis at the Toronto Hospital for Sick Children. J Otolaryngol 1996; 25: 366–370.
9. Rotstein C, Cummings KM, Tidings J, Killion K, Powell E, Gustafson TL, Higby D. An outbreak of invasive aspergillosis among allergenic bone marrow transplants: a case-control study. Infect Control 1985; 6:347–355.
10. Gillespie MB, O'Malley BW Jr, Francis HW. An approach to fulminant invasive fungal rhinosinusitis in the immunocompromised host. Arch Otolaryngol Head Neck Surg 1998; 124:520–526.
11. Iwen PC, Rupp ME, Hinrichs SH. Invasive mold sinusitis: 17 cases in immunocompromised patients and review of the literature. Clin Infect Dis 1997; 24: 1178–1184.
12. Gillespie MB, O'Malley BW. An algorithmic approach to the diagnosis and management of invasive fungal rhinosinusitis in the immunocompromised patient. Otolaryngol Clin North Am 2000; 33:323–334.
13. Aisner J, Murillo J, Schimpff SC, Steere AC. Invasive aspergillosis in acute leukemia: correlation with nose cultures and antibiotic use. Ann Intern Med 1979; 90:4–9.
14. Cordonnier C, Gilain L, Ricolfi F, Deforges L, Girard-Pipau F, Poron F, Millepied MC, Escudier E. Acquired ciliary abnormalities of nasal mucosa in marrow recipients. Bone Marrow Transplant 1996; 17:611–616.
15. Imamura R, Voegels R, Sperandio F, Sennes LU, Silva R, Butugan O, Miniti A. Microbiology of sinusitis in patients undergoing bone marrow transplantation. Otolaryngol Head Neck Surg 1999; 120:279–282.
16. de Carpentier JP, Ramamurthy L, Denning DW, Taylor PH. An algorithmic approach to aspergillus sinusitis. J Laryngol Otol 1994; 108:314–318.
17. Berlinger NT. Sinusitis in immunodeficient and immunosuppressed patients. Laryngoscope 1985; 95:29–33.

18. Goering P, Berlinger NT, Weisdorf DJ. Aggressive combined modality treatment of progressive sinonasal fungal infections in immunocompromised patients. Am J Med 1988; 85:619–623.
19. Gillespie MB, Huchton DM, O'Malley BW. Role of middle turbinate biopsy in the diagnosis of fulminant invasive fungal rhinosinusitis. Laryngoscope 2000; 110:1832–1836.
20. Talbot GH, Huang A, Provencher M. Invasive aspergillus rhinosinusitis in patients with acute leukemia. Rev Infect Dis 1991; 13:219–232.
21. Washburn RG. Fungal sinusitis. Curr Clin Top Infect Dis 1998; 18:60–74.
22. Rizk SS, Kraus DH, Gerresheim G, Mudan S. Aggressive combination treatment for invasive fungal sinusitis in immunocompromised patients. Ear Nose Throat J 2000; 79:278–280.
23. Samadi DS, Goldberg AN, Orlandi RR. Granulocyte transfusion in the management of fulminant invasive fungal rhinosinusitis. Am J Rhinol 2001; 15: 263–265.
24. Herbrecht R, Denning DW, Patterson TF, Bennett JE, Greene RE, Oestmann JW, Kern WV, Marr KA, Ribaud P, Lortholary O, et al. Voriconazole versus amphotericin B for primary therapy of invasive aspergillosis. N Engl J Med 2002; 347: 408–415.
25. Link H, Bohme A, Cornely OA, Hoffken K, Kellner O, Kern WV, Mahlberg R, Maschmeyer G, Nowrousian MR, Ostermann H, et al. Antimicrobial therapy of unexplained fever in neutropenic patients—guidelines of the Infectious Diseases Working Party (AGIHO) of the German Society of Hematology and Oncology (DGHO), Study Group Interventional Therapy of Unexplained Fever, Arbeitsgemeinschaft Supportivmassnahmen in der Onkologie (ASO) of the Deutsche Krebsgesellschaft (DKG-German Cancer Society). Ann Hematol 2003; 82(suppl 2):S105–117.
26. Peters C, Minkov M, Matthes-Martin S, Potschger U, Witt V, Mann G, Hocker P, Worel N, Stary J, Klingebiel T, Gadner H. Leucocyte transfusions from rhG-CSF or prednisolone stimulated donors for treatment of severe infections in immunocompromised neutropenic patients. Br J Haematol 1999; 106: 689–696.
27. Mirza N, Lanza DC. Diagnosis and management of rhinosinusitis before scheduled immunosuppression: a schematic approach to the prevention of acute fungal rhinosinusitis. Otolaryngol Clin North Am 2000; 33:313–321.
28. Malani PN, Kauffman CA. Invasive and allergic fungal sinusitis. Curr Infect Dis Rep 2002; 4:225–232.
29. Trigg ME, Morgan D, Burns TL, Kook H, Rumelhart SL, Holida MD, Giller RH. Successful program to prevent aspergillus infections in children undergoing marrow transplantation: use of nasal amphotericin. Bone Marrow Transplant 1997; 19:43–47.
30. Malani PN, Kauffman CA. Prevention and prophylaxis of invasive fungal sinusitis in the immunocompromised patient. Otolaryngol Clin North Am 2000; 33:301–312.
31. Rayfield EJ, Ault MJ, Keusch GT, Brothers MJ, Nechemias C, Smith H. Infection and diabetes: the case for glucose control. Am J Med 1982; 72: 439–450.

32. McMahon MM, Bistrian BR. Host defenses and susceptibility to infection in patients with diabetes mellitus. Infect Dis Clin North Am 1995; 9:1–9.

33. Bagdade JD, Nielson KL, Bulger RJ. Reversible abnormalities in phagocytic function in poorly controlled diabetic patients. Am J Med Sci 1972; 263: 451–456.

34. Bagdade JD, Stewart M, Walters E. Impaired granulocyte adherence. A reversible defect in host defense in patients with poorly controlled diabetes. Diabetes 1978; 27:677–681.

35. Mowat AG, Baum J. Chemotaxis of polymorphonuclear leukocytes from patients with rheumatoid arthritis. J Clin Invest 1971; 50:2541–2549.

36. Nolan CM, Beaty HN, Bagdade JD. Further characterization of the impaired bactericidal function of granulocytes in patients with poorly controlled diabetes. Diabetes 1978; 27:889–894.

37. MacRury SM, Gemmell CG, Paterson KR, MacCuish AC. Changes in phagocytic function with glycaemic control in diabetic patients. J Clin Pathol 1989; 42:1143–1147.

38. Jackson RM, Rice DH. Acute bacterial sinusitis and diabetes mellitus. Otolaryngol Head Neck Surg 1987; 97:469–473.

39. Tuazon CU, Perez A, Kishaba T, Sheagren JN. *Staphylococcus aureus* among insulin-injecting diabetic patients. An increased carrier rate. JAMA 1975; 231:1272.

40. Dooley DP, McAllister CK. Candidal sinusitis and diabetic ketoacidosis. A brief report. Arch Intern Med 1989; 149:962–964.

41. Ferguson BJ. Mucormycosis of the nose and paranasal sinuses. Otolaryngol Clin North Am 2000; 33:349–365.

42. Boelaert JR, de Locht M, Van Cutsem J, Kerrels V, Cantinieaux B, Verdonck A, Van Landuyt HW, Schneider YJ. Mucormycosis during deferoxamine therapy is a siderophore-mediated infection. In vitro and in vivo animal studies. J Clin Invest 1993; 91:1979–1986.

43. Yohai RA, Bullock JD, Aziz AA, Markert RJ. Survival factors in rhino-orbital-cerebral mucormycosis. Surv Ophthalmol 1994; 39:3–22.

44. Strasser MD, Kennedy RJ, Adam RD. Rhinocerebral mucormycosis. Therapy with amphotericin B lipid complex. Arch Intern Med 1996; 156:337–339.

45. Parfrey NA. Improved diagnosis and prognosis of mucormycosis. A clinicopathologic study of 33 cases. Medicine (Baltimore) 1986; 65:113–123.

46. Tarp B, Fiirgaard B, Moller J, Hilberg O, Christensen T, Black F. The occurrence of sinusitis in HIV-infected patients with fever. Rhinology 2001; 39: 136–141.

47. Zurlo JJ, Feuerstein IM, Lebovics R, Lane HC. Sinusitis in HIV-1 infection. Am J Med 1992; 93:157–162.

48. Godofsky EW, Zinreich J, Armstrong M, Leslie JM, Weikel CS. Sinusitis in HIV-infected patients: a clinical and radiographic review. Am J Med 1992; 93: 163–170.

49. Rubin JS, Honigberg R. Sinusitis in patients with the acquired immunodeficiency syndrome. Ear Nose Throat J 1990; 69:460–463.

50. Small CB, Kaufman A, Armenaka M, Rosenstreich DL. Sinusitis and atopy in human immunodeficiency virus infection. J Infect Dis 1993; 167:283–290.

51. Lamprecht J, Wiedbrauck C. Sinusitis and other typical ENT diseases within the scope of acquired immunologic deficiency syndrome (AIDS). HNO 1988; 36:489–492.

52. Decker CF. Sinusitis in the immunocompromised host. Curr Infect Dis Rep 1999; 1:27–32.

53. Milgrim LM, Rubin JS, Small CB. Mucociliary clearance abnormalities in the HIV-infected patient: a precursor to acute sinusitis. Laryngoscope 1995; 105: 1202–1208.

54. Barzan L, Tavio M, Tirelli U, Comoretto R. Head and neck manifestations during HIV infection. J Laryngol Otol 1993; 107:133–136.

55. Gurney TA, Murr AH. Otolaryngologic manifestations of human immuno-deficiency virus infection. Otolaryngol Clin North Am 2003; 36:607–624.

56. Lane HC, Masur H, Edgar LC, Whalen G, Rook AH, Fauci AS. Abnormalities of B-cell activation and immunoregulation in patients with the acquired immu-nodeficiency syndrome. N Engl J Med 1983; 309:453–458.

57. Lane HC, Fauci AS. Immunologic abnormalities in the acquired immuno-deficiency syndrome. Annu Rev Immunol 1985; 3:477–500.

58. Currier JS, Williams P, Feinberg J, Becker S, Owens S, Fichtenbaum C, Benson C. Impact of prophylaxis for *Mycobacterium avium* complex on bacterial infections in patients with advanced human immunodeficiency virus disease. Clin Infect Dis 2001; 32:1615–1622.

59. Milgrim LM, Rubin JS, Rosenstreich DL, Small CB. Sinusitis in human immunodeficiency virus infection: typical and atypical organisms. J Otolaryngol 1994; 23:450–453.

60. Upadhyay S, Marks SC, Arden RL, Crane LR, Cohn AM. Bacteriology of sinusitis in human immunodeficiency virus-positive patients: implications for management. Laryngoscope 1995; 105:1058–1060.

61. Meyer RD, Gaultier CR, Yamashita JT, Babapour R, Pitchon HE, Wolfe PR. Fungal sinusitis in patients with AIDS: report of 4 cases and review of the literature. Medicine (Baltimore) 1994; 73:69–78.

62. Teh W, Matti BS, Marisiddaiah H, Minamoto GY. Aspergillus sinusitis in patients with AIDS: report of three cases and review. Clin Infect Dis 1995; 21: 529–535.

63. Marquez-Diaz F, Soto-Ramirez LE, Sifuentes-Osornio J. Nocardiasis in patients with HIV infection. AIDS Patient Care STDS 1998; 12:825–832.

64. Marks SC, Upadhyay S, Crane L. Cytomegalovirus sinusitis. A new manifesta-tion of AIDS. Arch Otolaryngol Head Neck Surg 1996; 122:789–791.

65. Jutte A, Fatkenheuer G, Hell K, Salzberger B. CMV sinusitis as the initial manifestation of AIDS. HIV Med 2000; 1:123–124.

66. Mylonakis E, Rich J, Skolnik PR, De Orchis DF, Flanigan T. Invasive Aspergillus sinusitis in patients with human immunodeficiency virus infection. Report of 2 cases and review. Medicine (Baltimore) 1997; 76:249–255.

67. Dunand VA, Hammer SM, Rossi R, Poulin M, Albrecht MA, Doweiko JP, DeGirolami PC, Coakley E, Piessens E, Wanke CA. Parasitic sinusitis and otitis in patients infected with human immunodeficiency virus: report of five cases and review. Clin Infect Dis 1997; 25:267–272.

68. Rombaux P, Bertrand B, Eloy P. Sinusitis in the immunocompromised host. Acta Otorhinolaryngol Belg 1997; 51:305–313.
69. Rossi RM, Wanke C, Federman M. Microsporidian sinusitis in patients with the acquired immunodeficiency syndrome. Laryngoscope 1996; 106:966–971.
70. Del Borgo C, Del Forno A, Ottaviani F, Fantoni M. Sinusitis in HIV-infected patients. J Chemother 1997; 9:83–88.
71. Belafsky P, Kissinger P, Davidowitz SB, Amedee RG. HIV sinusitis: rationale for a treatment algorithm. J La State Med Soc 1999; 151:11–18.
72. Hern JD, Ghufoor K, Jayaraj SM, Frosh A, Mochloulis G. ENT manifestations of *Pseudomonas aeruginosa* infection in HIV and AIDS. Int J Clin Pract 1998; 52:141–144.
73. Nelson MR, Shanson DC, Barter GJ, Hawkins DA, Gazzard BG. *Pseudomonas septicaemia* associated with HIV. AIDS 1991; 5:761–763.
74. Mendelson MH, Gurtman A, Szabo S, Neibart E, Meyers BR, Policar M, Cheung TW, Lillienfeld D, Hammer G, Reddy S, et al. *Pseudomonas aeruginosa* bacteremia in patients with AIDS. Clin Infect Dis 1994; 18:886–895.
75. Belafsky PC, Amedee R, Moore B, Kissinger PJ. The association between sinusitis and survival among individuals infected with the human immunodeficiency virus. Am J Rhinol 2001; 15:343–345.
76. DiRienzo AG, van Der Horst C, Finkelstein DM, Frame P, Bozzette SA, Tashima KT. Efficacy of trimethoprim–sulfamethoxazole for the prevention of bacterial infections in a randomized prophylaxis trial of patients with advanced HIV infection. AIDS Res Hum Retrovir 2002; 18:89–94.

Index